McDOUGALL'S
MEDICINE
A Challenging Second Opinion

McDOUGALL'S MEDICINE

A Challenging Second Opinion

by

John A. McDougall, M.D.

New Century Publishers, Inc.

CAUTION:

The information provided in this book is for your better health. However, any decision you make involving the treatment of an illness should include the physician of your choice. Particularly, do not change medications without professional advice. Do not change your diet if you are seriously ill or on medication, except while under the care of a medical doctor.

Printing code

11   12   13   14   15   16

Library of Congress Cataloging-in-Publication Data

McDougall, John A.
    McDougall's medicine.

Includes bibliographies and index.
1. Diet therapy. 2. Therapeutics—Popular works. 3. Patient education. I. Title. [DNLM: 1. Diet Therapy—popular works. 2. Preventive Medicine—popular works. WB 400 M478m]
RM217.M37   1985   615.8'54   85-21686
ISBN 0-8329-0407-4

CONTENTS

To Mary and the kids—Heather, Pat, and Craig—
who got me through another one.

ACKNOWLEDGEMENTS

My gratitude and thanks to:

Elaine French, who spent countless hours making my thoughts understandable to the average reader yet not offensive to the well-read health-professional.

Many physicians, who read this material for correctness of context, thinking, and judgment. Each chapter was reviewed by at least three other doctors; their comments were considered and usually acted on positively. Investigators and authors of the original research were contacted, when appropriate, to verify their current feelings on the subject. However, the final editorial decisions were mine. Much appreciation for the valuable time these busy professionals gave me.

Ruth Heidrich, Mary McDougall, and Janice Crowl-Planas who reviewed the book and provided helpful comments.

Gladys Wong, who helped with the word processing and the difficult job of collecting the reference articles from the library shelves. She spent days verifying the references to assure that the curious reader will have little difficulty securing the original source for further study. Dana Proctor, who helped me catch up on the backlog of word processing during one of my many times of panic.

Linda Oszajca who provided the graphic and art works.

Over 4,000 patients, whom I have treated medically according to the philosophy in this book during my past seven years of practice. And many of the thousands more whom I helped care for prior to understanding the importance of diet and lifestyle and more humane and conservative therapy. Each and every one taught me something important about health-care.

The staff of the Hawaii Medical Library, Honolulu, who provided the highest quality reference services for the background on this book.

Last, but not least, my personal IBM computer which provided me with access to the National Library of Medicine and the word processing capabilities to handle the tremendous amount of editing done on this book.

Whenever a new discovery is reported to the Scientific world, they say first, "It is probably not true."

Thereafter, when the truth of the new proposition has been demonstrated beyond question, they say, "Yes, it may be true, but it is not important."

Finally, when sufficient time has elapsed to fully evidence its importance they say, "Yes, surely it is important, but it is no longer new."

Montaigne
1533-1592

FOREWORD

Most consumers of health care, better known as patients, are entirely at the mercy of the doctor they have had the fortune or misfortune to acquire. Medicine is far from an exact science; therefore, the knowledge and biases of the health professional caring for you will result in medical decisions that vary widely. Few patients have the time or money to search out all the various points of view. This book was written to give you other ways of looking at your health-care problems and to help you with making your health- and illness-related decisions. People who are looking for prevention and cure of disease, rather than a patch job once the tragedy strikes, and who are willing to make changes in their diet and lifestyle to obtain better health, will benefit most from the following discussions.

There will be a tendency for many readers to skip to the sections that pertain to themselves. However, I would recommend that you read the entire book to grasp the basic concepts I have expressed. Each chapter, you will find, has something that pertains to your health and well-being. For health problems that personally touch you, specific sections can be explored more thoroughly later. The references to the medical literature are provided for those who wish to read and learn more. Don't be afraid to look at these articles. They are written clearly in most cases, so the average reader will have no trouble comprehending their basic messages. Work with your physician in exploring this information. If something is difficult to understand, then your doctor should feel it is part of his or her service to help you. You want to know more so you can have better health and health-care. Who could object to that?

Hopefully, my opinions will stir controversy, which will bring discussion, which in turn will cause people to think and eventually result in positive changes. I understand that there are other points of view than mine and I certainly do not pretend to have expressed them all in this work. What is expressed is how I feel my patients should be treated and why I believe this way. This book adds support for many of my fellow physicians who have also come to similar conclusions, and care for their patients in a like manner. Many doctors will find this book a helpful tool for patient education.

If you as a reader would like to be treated in this manner, then request such care from your doctor. You may meet some resistance or even a little hostility, but there is much to be gained for everyone by your actions. I wrote this book hoping medical care could be changed more quickly toward providing humane treatments which are sensitive to the patients' total well-being. You can help speed this change by understanding your health needs and requesting care that deals with causes of problems rather than with symptoms.

Factors that lead to disease are rarely flaws in the human design, but rather, are failures in our understanding of proper health care. Believe that your body is the greatest creation ever made and that the true potential for health and healing lies within you. Utilizing these innate strengths will bring you the health you deserve.   John McDougall M.D.

Note:

Throughout the book the nutritive values for foods were taken from one of two sources, unless otherwise indicated:

J. Pennington. *Food Values of Portions Commonly Used.* 14th ed. Harper and Row. New York. 1985.

Nutritive Values of Portions in Common Units. Agriculture Handbook No. 456. Agriculture Research Service. U.S. Department of Agriculture. 1975.

Illustrations are the artist's representations. Exact accuracy has sometimes been sacrificed to better explain a concept.

The people in this book are composites of actual patients. However, any resemblance to actual people from the names, stories, or drawings is purely coincidental and unintentional.

McDOUGALL'S MEDICINE
A Challenging Second Opinion

1

WHY A CHALLENGING SECOND OPINION?

Like most doctors, I entered the profession of health care with many hopes and dreams, and a dedication to the relief of human suffering. During my years of training and as a practicing physician, I have learned that the profession of medicine is more of a profit-oriented business, and less a humanitarian endeavor, achieving far fewer medical miracles than I had once believed it did. Seldom is there a single ideal way to treat the illnesses that people suffer. The modern methods used by health practitioners, calling upon the most technologically advanced drugs, surgical procedures, and radiation techniques, rarely succeed in curing chronic diseases and are never 100% safe because they all have so many side effects. Because these treatments do not fit the ideal of efficacy and safety, there is controversy within the medical profession over how best to care for the diseases that afflict the population in epidemic proportions. The greatest areas of controversy over proper therapy include cancer, osteoporosis, complications of athero-sclerosis (including heart disease), hypertension, diabetes, arthritis, and kidney disease. Almost everyone in the United States is touched personally by one of these conditions or has a close friend or relative who is suffering so. Since there is no ideal form of treatment for these diseases and many justifiable alternatives are available for patients to choose from, you should actively participate in the medical decisions that will affect the quality and length of your life. After all, you will ultimately gain or lose most from the outcome.

To get involved, if you're like most people, you need to know more.

You need to understand as much as possible about the cause and the significance of your illness. Then you need to know the possible solutions to your problems and the advantages and disadvantages of each. Several alternative approaches exist, so you will need help in making these choices. One of the most important roles of your physician is to offer information and expert medical advice about courses of action. You should seek care from a health professional who encourages patient involvement. Develop with your doctor a relationship of mutual respect and participation. Doing so will lead to the best possible resolution of your problem. You should not lose control over your health care by placing your doctor in a position of omnipotence.

As a mortal human being, every physician has personal and professional biases combined with a fund of knowledge that prejudice the decisions made for or with you. Imperfections in judgment occur because of slanted biases and limited knowledge, and they may keep you from getting the care you desire. You can compensate for these limitations by functioning as an informed consumer in the doctor-patient relationship. There are many influences on what your doctor knows and how he or she feels about the treatment of disease. Knowing some of the sources of the influence that mold your personal physician will help you understand why certain treatments are popular.

The molding of a doctor begins with early medical school training and continues throughout the years of practice. We learn to treat with principles and attitudes that are passed on to us by a limited number of authorities first encountered in medical school. Medical textbooks written by many of these same experts provide for an almost cookbook approach to caring for the ills of you and your family. The treatments prescribed vary little from physician to physician across the country. Although several possible approaches to a health problem may exist, at a particular time in a particular place one method of treatment usually becomes more popular than the others. This is not necessarily because it is the best one. The fraternity of physicians practicing in communities and teaching centers is a closely knit group. Once a favorite mode of treatment is established, all other choices are usually unavailable for the patient's consideration. However, even though your personal physician may be disappointed with the treatments prescribed, rarely is there enough time, or sometimes enough interest, to question the knowledge that has been developed with many vested interests and passed on through years of medical tradition. Fortunately, today a few inquisitive professional minds are reevaluating and reshaping the direction medicine is taking. You may have a member of this new breed of physician already working with you.

Consider how the technologically advanced health-care system that has developed in the United States affects your health care. Components of this system have all the characteristics of a business, including the primary goal of maximizing profits. The drug industry is a major part of the health-care system and has been an aggressive business since the days of traveling medicine shows. It spends hundreds of millions of dollars each year on advertising ranging from newsprint to research projects. For many doctors the bulk of continuing medical education has the backing of drug companies. This industry wants to ensure that we know the best way to drug and otherwise treat you and your family. They distribute advertisements in the form of educational handouts for patients, periodicals, academic books, audio cassettes, and video tapes. Hundreds of free publications funded by drug companies are sent to our offices. The medical articles in these publications reflect the interests of the sponsoring companies. Most of us subscribe to medical journals for the purpose of continuing our education, and even the most respected of these journals are filled with colorful ads recommending one drug or another.

Every working day, sales representatives pushing scientific studies and free samples of their products invade your doctor's medical office. These salespeople can be the primary source of any new information many doctors acquire on how to treat your problems. The drug companies often provide free lectures by traveling professors from prestigious universities. These well-educated doctors proceed to hawk a company's wares under the guise of continuing medical education. Week-long conferences are sponsored in part or in full by pharmaceutical companies. Their financial interests are sometimes reflected in the lineup of guest lecturers. A major share of the scientific research carried out is funded directly by drug companies on projects that affect their products. These tactics must be working since the pharmaceutical industry continues to aim the bulk of their advertising dollars directly at the physician. As busy doctors we are certainly eager to hear any news that might help our practice or our patients.

The big-business nature of health care knows no bounds and it encompasses some of our most trusted institutions. You might never have thought of the American Heart Association, the Arthritis Foundation, or the American Cancer Society as businesses. For your own personal well-being, think again. These organizations solicit their income in the form of tax-free contributions from good-hearted people like you. The money thus gained provides for buildings, office furnishings, maintenance, various information-related products and services, and valuable research, just as in many other businesses. The financial livelihood of every employee, from the president to the janitor, depends on the continued successful operation of every part of the organization. And that means they must maintain a good public image to keep those donations coming in.

The public relations department of the American Cancer Society is so well orchestrated that even well-educated doctors are sometimes taken in by their deceptive statistical practices. A brief examination of the claims made by this organization will lead one to suspect that something about their message is misleading. The American Cancer Society brags about winning the war on cancer. It tells the American public that "of all the chronic diseases, cancer is the most curable" and that "nearly half of all cancer patients can be cured by modern treatment methods." Many doctors and lay people who are personally involved with cancer victims soon learn that the wonderful benefits of cancer therapy are hard to see, as we too often watch our patients and loved ones die after suffering from miseries inflicted more by the surgery, the radiation, and the chemotherapy than by the cancer itself. Yet, because of the words of triumph from the Cancer Society, we continue to encourage victims of cancer to participate in human experiments that should still be back in the laboratory instead of unleashed on an entire population of faithful people.

The facts are very different from the Cancer Society's cheerful message. Over 60 percent of all cancer deaths are from cancers of the lung, colon, breast, prostate, pancreas, and ovary. The death rates from these six cancers have either stayed the same or have actually increased during the past fifty-five years. Furthermore, most victims of each of these kinds of cancer sooner or later die of their disease. Similar grim statistics can be described for other cancers, as well. Such indisputable facts attest to the failure of current therapies for most cancers. Only a few of the less common forms of cancer, many of these limited to children, have been cured by cancer therapy. These accomplishments, while important, do not alone warrant the esteem that the Cancer Society gains through its advertisements claiming victory.

One method used by the American Cancer Society to make cancer appear curable is to declare that anyone who survives for five years from the time of diagnosis, free of obvious disease, is cured of cancer. Simply because cancer is a slow-growing disease in most cases, the victims often live over five years even with no treatment at all. When we follow the progress of these people for a few more years, we find that most of them do eventually die from their cancer.

How do the American Cancer Society's public relations experts support their claim that we are winning the war on cancer? They quote statistics saying that "in the early 1900's few cancer patients had any hope of long-term survival." Today they tell us "49% will be alive 5 years after diagnosis." Surgeons operating on cancer in the early 1900's considered a tumor of the breast the size of an orange a small cancer. Many years ago patients sought care for cancer at a much later stage of disease and because of this late diagnosis, the time until death was short. Today a woman usually seeks medical attention for a tumor in her breast when it is only the size of a pea and as a result the time until death from cancer is usually quite long. The Cancer Society fails to tell us that the "improved" survival rate seen over the past eighty years for most cancers is largely the result of earlier detection, not more effective treatment. Finding the cancer earlier does allow more people to live five years from the time of diagnosis. Thus, more people will fit the definition of "cured." However, in most cases early detection does not change the day of death, but only the length of time a person is aware that he or she has cancer. Under this circumstance the real beneficiaries of early detection are the providers of health care, who now have a longer time in which to treat the victims before they die. This means they can charge for more doctors' visits, more procedures, more tests, and longer hospital stays. The American Cancer Society proclaims great success in the treatment of cancer. The best that can be said for this claim is that the Society has put hope up for sale. Unfortunately, to date it has been selling mostly false hope.

The Arthritis Foundation has spent much money and effort spreading the message that diet has nothing to do with the cause or cure of arthritis. This campaign has caused doctors all over the country to squelch any suggestion you might have made that your arthritis was affected by the foods you ate. As painful as such a pronouncement may be for victims of the disease to hear, the truth is much worse; this organization's strong position statement cannot be supported by scientific research. In fact, the relatively small number of investigations done so far clearly show the opposite relationship: an as yet undetermined number of cases of the more serious forms of arthritis, including rheumatoid arthritis and gouty arthritis, are not only caused by improper diet but can be effectively cured by the right choice of foods. This is just one more example of how your charitable contributions are spent in ways that are counterproductive to the health of you and your family.

Knowledge and biases that affect your health care come from some unexpected places. The food industry has become directly involved in the health business by advertising some of its products as being effective for the prevention and treatment of disease. The dairy industry has spent millions of dollars telling women that the secret to preventing osteoporosis is to drink three or more eight-ounce glasses of cow's milk each day and to eat a plentiful supply of other calcium-rich dairy products. This belief in the protective effect of milk products on bone strength is in direct conflict with scientific fact. Worldwide, the countries with the greatest incidence of female osteoporosis, including the United States, Sweden, and Finland also have the highest levels of consumption of dairy products. Therefore, at the very least, dairy products appear to offer little or no protection from this epidemic disease. By way of strong contrast, this bone disease is rare or absent in entire populations of Asian and African women, who consume no milk products.

Even scientific research paid for by the National Dairy Council has shown that the consumption of three eight-ounce glasses of milk daily for a year fails to improve significantly a woman's calcium balance. Bone loss is directly related to calcium balance. The investigators who made this study were honest enough to speculate that the extra protein from the milk had adversely affected calcium balance. High levels of protein in the diet will cause the kidneys to excrete large amounts of calcium, thereby washing this important mineral out of the body. Many other studies confirm the overwhelming effect of excess proteins on the development of osteoporosis. One certain conclusion is that the hazards of consuming a daily diet that includes generous amounts of whole milk and cheese are very serious. A woman eating such a diet may decrease her risk of developing osteoporosis simply by dying earlier from heart disease or cancer—both in part caused by the consumption of more dairy products containing high levels of fats and cholesterol.

McDonald's Corporation entered the health scene with *Good Food, Good Nutrition and McDonald's,* a booklet describing the nutritional benefits of their products. In order to ensure accuracy and gain your trust, this information was reviewed by the Dean of the School of Nutrition of Tufts University Nutrition Institute. According to this colorful booklet, fats and cholesterol are associated with heart disease, and nutritionists recommend that we reduce fats from the current 40 to 45 percent to 25 to 35 percent of total calories consumed each day. You've guessed it. One of McDonald's most popular meals, consisting of a cheeseburger, regular fries, a chocolate shake, and McDonaldland cookies, fits the recommendations for a healthier heart because it provides only 33.5 percent fat. This meal begins with a cheeseburger at 41 percent fat, added to french fries with 47 percent fat, for a total of 44 percent fat. As stated in the booklet, this is much too high in fat and unhealthy for your heart. To accomplish the transformation of greasy fast-food into healthy food, just add sugar and white flour in the form of a chocolate shake (21 percent fat) and cookies (32 percent fat). This dilutes the total fat content down to 33.5 percent and provides over 1200 calories. Are you now convinced of the fast-food industry's interest in safeguarding their customers' health?

The so-called health food industry presents only the selected data that make its products seem desirable and safe. For example, many companies market polyunsaturated vegetable oils to physicians and the general public, advertising that if you eat them they will lower your blood cholesterol level, thus reducing your risk of developing premature atherosclerosis and heart disease. Yet experiments with laboratory animals have indicated that vegetable oils are stronger promoters of cancer than are animal-derived fats. However, the sellers of vegetable oils have said not a word to your medical doctor or the public about the strong possibility of cancer promotion from their products.

It may be hard to believe at first that any health professional would have motives other than interest in the well-being of the patient. In reality, all do. Most of the time these motives remain secondary to the patient's health. However, for some doctors, money, power, ego gratification, tradition, and fear of litigation do take precedence over the health of their patients.

Recently, the good-samaritan images of the community hospital and the personal physician have been somewhat tarnished. At one time, the only public message a hospital wanted to cultivate was that of being a dedicated community servant. Now witness the competitive advertisements for hospitals in your local newspapers, and on television and radio broadcasts: "Guaranteed services, maternity care your way, and meals reminiscent of the finest restaurants." These are only some of the enticements hospitals are using in attempts to improve their business. Ten years ago, advertising by physicians aimed at luring patients was forbidden. The only ethical business promotion permitted to a doctor was lecturing to fellow physicians. Nowadays, eye-catching ads for doctors' services in the newspaper and phone book are hard to distinguish from the ones placed by plumbers, insurance agents, and lawyers.

Competition for your dollar is serious business, but that's not necessarily bad. Well-informed consumers can benefit by receiving more information, more choices, and improved care from health professionals attuned to their needs. Unfortunately, the stiff competition for health dollars can just as well lead to mistreatment of the consumer. Because of the current payment system, competition places pressure on the health professional to provide more goods and services. Doctors and hospitals are paid for their commodities: office visits, hospital visits, physical examinations, laboratory tests, X-rays, EKGs, drugs dispensed, surgical operations, and days of hospital stay. The connection between doing more and receiving more revenue cannot be denied. When confronted with a variety of therapies that have little advantage over one another, some physicians find the more profitable one an easier choice. For you to believe that good moral sense will always win out over good business sense is naive and could be hazardous to your health.

This situation is actually getting worse. Lucrative rewards from the health care business have lured more people into health careers. There is now a glut of hospitals, freestanding emergency centers, and doctors, where only ten years ago there was a serious national shortage of these services. Since no one wants to work for less money, someone must pay more. As a paying patient or a patient with health insurance coverage, you will pay for the rising cost of medical care.

The recent rise in malpractice law suits has had a tremendous impact on the way medicine is practiced. Today doctors expect to be sued a certain number of times during their careers. In an attempt to protect themselves, doctors order many more expensive tests and consultations. These extras rarely benefit the patient and do much to raise the cost of health care. A more harmful effect from frequent malpractice litigation has been the demise of the doctor-patient relationship. Many physicians see themselves working twelve hours a day and trying to provide excellent care for their patients. Even though they're putting out their best effort, a malpractice claim is filed, thus beginning the destruction of the caring nature of such professionals. After a few of these painful experiences, for some physicians the patient simply becomes a potentially hazardous commodity to make as much money from as possible before an early retirement.

The prevailing opinions on the best treatment for each disease are called the community standards of practice. The surest way for a physician to avoid law suits for malpractice is to treat patients according to this community standard. "Just like my colleagues, right or wrong" is a doctor's best defense at all times. This legalized mutual support system stifles free thinking and progress, but it's safe for the fearful doctor. Under this philosophy, outdated and even harmful treatments will take forever to disappear from a physician's repertoire. A more humane and effective procedure is introduced only with difficulty, and its eventual acceptance as a better method becomes next to impossible.

The treatment of breast cancer is an example of sluggish thinking among health professionals that causes unjustifiable suffering in afflicted women today. The death rate from breast cancer has not changed during the past seventy-five years, even with modern advances in surgery, radiotherapy, and chemotherapy. None of the diverse treatments for breast cancer produces any significant advantage in terms of survival time. Nonetheless, doctors continue to prescribe these debilitating treatments.

Treatment choices must be based on the goal of preserving the length of life as well as the quality of life. Since length of life cannot be increased by present day breast cancer surgical therapies, then clearly the most humane approach would be to leave the woman's appearance as normal as possible, thereby preserving the quality of her life at the highest level possible. For almost every case of breast cancer coming before a surgeon today, the best treatment is simple removal of the lump. But each year more than 100,000 women in the United States alone fail to realize this, and their breasts are amputated unnecessarily. To add insult to injury, powerful chemotherapeutic agents make the next year of the patient's life miserable. This physician-induced sickness might be justifiable if it prolonged the woman's life significantly, but it does not.

Of course, a woman with breast cancer should be given a fighting chance for life, and one painless step toward winning this battle is to eliminate the factors that caused the cancer. Even the American Cancer Society now believes that the American diet is one of the major factors involved in causing breast cancer. In addition to having a nondeforming lumpectomy operation, a cancer victim should follow a diet opposite to the one that made her ill. This combined treatment should be standard practice today, but the treatments for disease have always tended to change very slowly. If history repeats itself, at least two more generations of women will have to suffer needlessly before the information now known will be put into practice with breast cancer.

In most cases, the treatments offered by health professionals today certainly are not without short-term beneficial effects. Otherwise they would have been abandoned by both practitioners and consumers long ago. However, along with the benefits there are often serious side effects and drawbacks. Also, with the methods used today the patient is rarely cured of the problem. In almost every case, better methods of treating diseases are available that are backed by scientific study. These alternatives deserve your attention.

For example, women nearing menopause are offered the chance of taking estrogen pills daily to prevent osteoporosis. These hormones do stop bone loss, but they increase the risk of developing uterine cancer by as much as fourteen times. For this reason, uterine biopsies must be done biannually in order to check for possible cancer development. Furthermore, in women taking sequential combinations of hormone that are supposed to reduce the risk of cancer, menstrual periods continue for the rest of their lives. An alternative and far better approach for the prevention of osteoporosis is a low-protein diet and daily exercise. This combination offers the best opportunity to preserve intact the bones of a woman that are meant by nature to last throughout her lifetime, not to begin dissolving away at about age forty-five as they do all too commonly in women who live in our affluent society.

What does a doctor do for those patients who refuse to give up high-protein meals full of beef, fish, chicken, and cottage cheese, and who rebel at going for a daily walk? And what about those unfortunate women who don't even know about the alternatives to hormones or bone loss? Is prescribing estrogen pills an acceptable treatment for them?

Another common treatment that gains no cure and causes some serious side effects is coronary artery bypass surgery. The primary reason why people submit to bypass surgery is the alleviation of chest pain. This surgical intervention does indeed relieve that pain. However, a low-fat diet is also highly effective and much less harmful, not to mention the expense; in patients using such a dietary treatment, chest pain episodes are decreased by 91 percent in only twenty-four days. These good results are obtained without the $25,000 price tag for the operation or the painful foot-long incision across the victim's chest. Furthermore, bypass surgery is associated with an almost certain chance of brain injury, attributed to the heart-lung machine used during the operation. The treatment using a dietary and lifestyle approach enables a person to avoid this injury completely along with the subsequent 15 percent (or greater) risk of persistent brain dysfunction. Still, for those who can't give up their scrambled eggs and roast beef, the only way to stop the chest pains may be painful and expensive surgery.

The existence of the conformist medical opinion, also known as the community standard of practice, might be tolerable if the treatments prescribed were ideal. However, most patients have learned the hard way that this is rarely the case. You went in for a cure, but instead you received a pill to take daily to keep your blood pressure, blood sugar, or uric acid under control or to make the pain tolerable. Removal of your colon was supposed to catch the cancer in time, but it didn't. Look at how much you suffered from the treatments, all for nothing. You are looking for a cure to your illness, not just a patch job to cover up the symptoms.

The standards of community practice by which doctors treat patients today, for the most part are recommended by well-meaning health professionals. It is clear that these people are innocent of purposeful wrongdoing; they believe in these practices enough to subject themselves and their families to the same. Doctors suffering from coronary artery disease undergo bypass operations. They do so even though their medical journals consistently report that lives are not saved by this expensive and painful surgery. As a well-informed consumer, you can do better and make a serious effort to deprive the hospital and the bypass surgeon of their astronomical fees.

Emphasis on financial interests has played a major role in developing the health-care system in America today. Unfortunately, the rewards from the present system are dependent on sickness, not health. Ask your doctor whether he or she would rather have a practice filled with sick patients or one in which everyone was healthy. Our present health-care system might better be labeled an *illness-care system*.

A change in the system of rewarding physicians and hospitals is the most effective way to achieve a change in the way medicine is practiced. The health-care system must reward doctors for keeping their patients healthy. Only then will the measures to prevent disease be stressed, and expensive, ineffective treatments discarded. The federal government and private medical insurance companies have already taken steps to change the ''payment for services rendered'' system in attempts to control escalating medical costs. Health maintenance organizations (HMOs) that cover all costs of health care for a set price are becoming a popular solution to the cost-control problem. If the doctors who are running these organizations can collect your monthly payments and at the same time keep you healthy, then their profits will be high, but so will be your well-being. The judicious use of only the most highly effective treatments, and only when these are necessary, also helps to keep expenses down and profits up.

When money is no longer made by charging for more office visits, tests, and surgeries, then the emphasis on treatment changes. A low-fat diet combined with regular exercise is a lot less expensive form of treatment than a bypass operation for whoever is paying the bill. If the HMO is responsible for the costs, then the doctors profiting from the cost-effective methods of this organization will be more likely to think of the less expensive approach first, at least as an initial try. Besides, after the surgical procedure is done, the patient eventually has to take up the diet and exercise program anyhow, or the new transplanted vessels used for the bypass will likely close up, requiring another expensive surgery. And why take out asymptomatic gallstones if there is no money to be made? Studies show the patient has a greater risk of complications and of dying from the surgery than from leaving the stones alone. Why have a crowd of patients returning every month for refills of pills to control blood pressure and diabetes, especially if the doctor can't charge them for each visit under an HMO plan? A more cost-effective (and also more healing) way is to cure the patient with a low-salt, low-fat, high-fiber, high-carbohydrate diet and a little exercise.

Medicare has introduced a new method of payment to encourage more cost-effective care. Under this new system Medicare no longer reimburses hospitals according to the amount of treatment given to a patient or for the number of days a patient is hospitalized. Instead, they now pay a set amount for a patient's care based on the doctor's diagnosis of the illness. This revised payment system puts pressure on hospitals to have their doctors treat effectively and efficiently in order to keep the costs down and the profits up. Soon private doctors will be under the same payment plan. Will Medicare be bold enough to offer doctors an equal amount of money for treating coronary artery disease with either bypass surgery or with diet and lifestyle training? In that fair exchange, $25,000 wouldn't be bad pay for a doctor who recommends and the hospital that provides a three-week nutrition and exercise course. Perhaps as an alternative solution a payment of $250 will be offered for any treatment for the diagnosis of coronary artery disease with chest pain, be it bypass surgery or education focusing on nutrition and exercise.

When the interests of your doctor do not revolve around surgery, prescribing pills, office visits, and hospital stays, then your chances of being overtreated are decreased. Under this new system, useless treatments, regardless of cost, will be a waste of money. Patients will be grateful to be spared unnecessary treatments and to regain their health. Doctors will receive emotional and financial rewards from helping patients get better, instead of being paid for illness. However, until this state of perfection is a reality, you must be a well-informed consumer with the courage to say no, if you want to obtain humane treatment for yourself and your family.

For your own protection and to get the best possible care, you need to seek opinions that question and, when necessary, challenge the current standards of practice. Your efforts to get such a second opinion and to act on it will have a widespread impact on the health care in your community. Unwillingness to change has its foundations in individuals; therefore, each person who makes a better choice persuades doctors to change and in time helps to improve the entire system by demonstrating the effectiveness of this approach to the people they contact in their daily lives.

A second opinion that challenges the community standards may compel you to stand up to your first physician or dietitian and even concerned friends or relatives. If you are well-informed, you will be able to explain the reasons for your choice of an alternative solution to your health problems, and from that freedom to choose, only benefit can come. Perhaps you will decide after thorough consideration of the facts and opinions available that the standard option is the one you should accept. Even if you do choose that method, at least you have gone through the mental exercise and the psychological preparation of thoroughly evaluating your condition and your choice of therapy. You would do no less if you were buying a new car or a refrigerator; you would certainly compare the advantages and disadvantages of different makes and models. With cars and refrigerators you always have a choice. Unfortunately, until recently the rigid system with a community standard of practice has generally dictated only one way to handle your health problems.

There is one drawback to being actively involved in your own health care: you can no longer lie back and be fixed. Regaining and maintaining your health takes effort on your part, and too many people have to find a reason for expending all this effort. Feeling, looking, and functioning poorly and fear of impending death are all effective motivators for putting effort into recovering one's health. Given these options, most people discover that the effort to improve their health is worthwhile.

You are encouraged to show your physician the arguments in this book that pertain to your individual health problems. You should demand (as tactfully as possible, of course) an explanation of why the approach described here is not the best one for you. Sometimes there are perfectly legitimate reasons why it would not be. Research papers and opinions written by outstanding medical professionals are cited to support the viewpoint presented here. If you or your physician doubt the strength of these arguments, then you are encouraged to read the original articles, as well as other published opinions, and then determine for yourselves the value of the suggestions. You may be surprised to find little resistance, since many doctors have already come to similar conclusions on their own. The opinions I have presented in this book may be new and enlightening to you, but they are not original. Many other doctors share these views. Unfortunately, they are too seldom expressed in a practical way for the patient's consideration.

Some people might argue that the evidence I present does not completely prove that the suggested approach is worthwhile. However, proof is often a matter of willingness to accept supporting evidence. Even in the face of overwhelming data that support a conclusion, personal and financial interests can still work to delay the acceptance of facts affecting certain health information. Consider the representatives of the tobacco industry, who steadfastly deny the overwhelming evidence that supports the dangers of smoking. Their point should be well-taken—there is no proof that smoking tobacco is dangerous to your health—but the incriminating evidence would fill a small library. Nonsmokers have no difficulty believing that smoking is hazardous to health. However, many smokers find emotional comfort in the tobacco industry's efforts, even when their physical discomfort from inhaling smoke constantly reminds them of the health detriments.

This book, *McDougall's Medicine,* provides you with many challenging second opinions for the cause, prevention, and treatment of most of the chronic diseases that affect people in the United States today. These opinions lean toward decisions in the matters of health that will gain the most benefit for a patient with the least suffering, mutilation, and expense. You will quickly learn that as far as treatment is concerned, *less is more.*

The most important question is simple: does the advice offered here work for you? Most of the recommendations presented in *McDougall's Medicine* achieve an immediate effect when followed or ask you for only a few short but faithful weeks to gain success. This book provides you and your doctor with an alternative to the limited choices now available. This is your opportunity to challenge the standard of medical practice in your community. This book and its companions, *The McDougall Plan* and *The McDougall Health-Supporting Cookbooks,* are changing the way people in the United States think about their health. If you, personally or professionally, are looking for a better way, *McDougall's Medicine* will give you the facts and the means to obtain better health and health care beginning today.

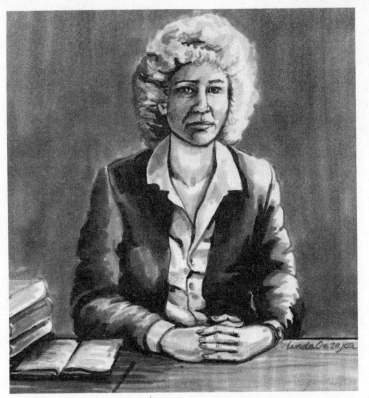

Susan

I am as emotionally sound as any woman nearing forty can be with a tragedy rearranging her life. Just the other day while I was taking a shower I found a small lump. I had minor surgery to remove the tumor. My doctor has told me that I have breast cancer and must have a mastectomy. Now I have so many worries. Maybe last year I could have taken this news better, but I've just been married again and my future was looking so promising. My older daughter will be fine, but can I hope to live long enough to see my ten-year-old graduate from high school?

I've had friends with cancer and they did not do well. The treatments they were given seemed to do more harm to them than the cancer, until their last days. I've read so many things lately about new ways to treat cancer and that there are many controversies among doctors about the best treatments. Certainly I need to know more about what is wrong with me and what I can do to pick up the pieces.

2

CANCER

From what I've told you do you think I should go ahead with a mastectomy?

That depends on what your goals are. If you don't want to defy and offend your doctor or worry your well-meaning friends and relatives, then do what almost everybody does. Have your breast amputated.

If you want to enjoy a healthier life and possibly a longer one, then you need to learn a lot more about your problem and begin making informed decisions. If you don't know much about breast cancer, now is the time to ask questions, not later after you've been through the surgery and the other treatments that will be prescribed "in your best interest."

Why me? How did I get cancer? I can't recall hurting myself.

Yours is a common reaction.[1] But breast cancer does not result from injuring your breast. A sharp or blunt object striking your breast causes no trouble other than the obvious damage from the blow. Scientific evidence is becoming convincing that the actual abuse that led to this cancer was inflicted by way of your knife and fork at the dinner table.

Both men and women eat the same kinds of food. Why does breast cancer affect women most of the time and men only rarely?

Breast tissues are responsive to female hormones, called by the general name of estrogens. The more estrogen a woman produces to stimulate her breast tissues, the more likely it is that cancer will develop. This association of cancer with female hormones is inescapable when you consider that breast cancer is 100 times more common in women than in men.[2] The disease occurs only after puberty, and a longer menstrual life means a greater probability of developing breast cancer. Furthermore, if a woman takes estrogen pills the likelihood of developing breast cancer is increased.[3] In women whose ovaries are removed early in life, the risk of developing breast cancer is greatly reduced. This cancer is almost unknown in women who never develop ovarian function.[2] Also, the amount of estrogen in a women's body will influence the rate of growth of an established breast cancer.[2] Therefore, estrogens appear to be involved closely with the cause and development of breast cancer.

How can something in my diet affect the estrogens in my body and cause breast cancer?

Consider that each day the average woman consumes somewhere between one and four pounds of food. Nutrients and other substances are absorbed through the intestinal wall into the bloodstream and travel to all parts of the body, including the breast tissues. One source of estrogens can be the hormones that are fed to poultry and beef to make them grow faster. In some foreign countries, where the use of food additives is not regulated carefully by the government, significant amounts of estrogen residue can remain in the foods and have dramatic effects on people who eat them. In Puerto Rico and Italy, for example, there are cases where very young boys and girls have developed breasts, and little girls have started their menstrual periods much too early because of hormones in the meats they've been fed.[4,5] Presumably, levels of hormones in poultry and beef raised in the United States are more closely watched. In the American diet, hormone residues in animal products are unlikely sources of increased estrogens.

What is the reason for high estrogens in women in the United States?

In affluent countries like the United States, the biological link between food and diseases of the breast is formed during the metabolism of naturally produced hormones in the human intestine. Estrogens are produced by the ovaries, adrenal glands, and certain other body tissues. After circulating throughout the body, eventually these estrogens are excreted by way of the liver into the intestine. In this process, the estrogens must be combined with another nonabsorbable substance that is produced by the liver and then eliminated in that "complexed" form. If they are not complexed, free estrogens would be reabsorbed into the body through the intestinal wall.[6,7]

Fats in foods encourage certain species of bacteria to grow in the colon. These bacteria have the special ability to split the complex molecule formed by the estrogens and the substance from the liver. As a result, the excreted estrogens are freed and are readily absorbed back into the body. The long-term result is higher levels of these powerful hormones in women who eat foods rich in fats, which, of course, is the typical diet consumed by people in affluent societies.[8]

Another reason for higher estrogen levels is obesity. Being overweight is a common consequence of a high-fat diet centered around dairy and meat products and foods that are processed in oils. The body's fat converts male hormones, generally called *androgens,* and naturally present to some degree in women, into more estrogens.[9] The more body fat a person has, the more estrogen her body will produce. Also, as women grow older their bodies become more efficient at the conversion of androgens into estrogens; because of this conversion, estrogen levels increase from this source with age.[10]

How are estrogens involved in cancer?

Excess amounts of certain kinds of estrogens will overstimulate the growth and activity of hormone-responsive tissues such as those found in the breast. By some mechanism still undetermined, this continuous stimulation contributes to the cancerous changes that eventually give rise to a tumor. The kinds of estrogens that are believed to be involved in the cause of cancer are called *estrone* and *estradiol.* A third kind called *estriol* is believed to be somewhat protective against cancer.[11]

Then most women must be at risk, because we all eat basically the same diet. How common is breast cancer?

Breast cancer is the single most common form of cancer found in women who are middle-aged and older. Approximately one out of ten women living in affluent countries will develop this disease. At the present time in the United States 120,000 new cases are recognized annually, and the numbers are increasing.[12]

What happens in countries where women eat low-fat diets and stay trim? Do they get breast cancer less often?

Bacteria living in the colons of people on low-fat, high-fiber diets centered around starches convert very little excreted estrogen into the absorbable form, and as a result more of this hormone is eliminated from the body.[6] The higher quantity of fiber in a vegetable-based diet may also

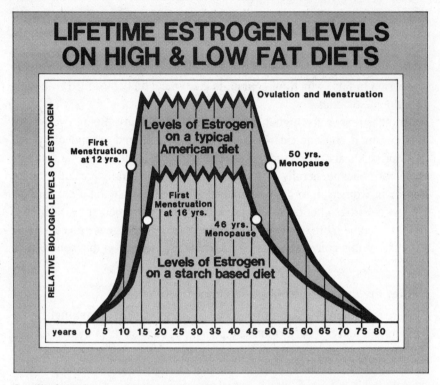

LIFETIME ESTROGEN LEVELS ON HIGH & LOW FAT DIETS

Levels of certain powerful estrogens are 50 percent greater during the reproductive years when women consume a high-fat (typical American) diet compared to women on a low-fat (starch-based) diet.[14] The first menstruation begins four years earlier and menopause starts four years later for women following a high-fat diet.[15,16]

act as a kind of barrier to reabsorption of estrogens.[7] Obesity is rare among women following a starch-based meal plan. As a result, women living in societies where the diet is low in fats and animal products have lower levels of cancer-related estrogens and lower rates of breast cancer.[8,13]

A comparison of vegetarian women with women who eat meat revealed a lower intake of fats in the diets of vegetarians. Vegetarian women excreted two to three times more estrogen in their feces than did nonvegetarians.[14] Also, the level of cancer-related estrogens in the blood of the meat-eating women was 50 percent higher than in vegetarians.[14]

Young girls raised on a high-fat diet start their first menstruation approximately four years earlier than those girls following a low-fat starch-based meal plan—twelve versus sixteen years.[15] A similar effect of lengthening the menstrual life of a woman occurs at the end of her reproductive years.

Menopause begins approximately four years later for those women on a high-fat diet, compared to those on low-fat diets—fifty versus forty-six years.[16] This increase in the years of menstruation are the result of the effects of the additional estrogens in a younger and older woman's body caused by the fat in her diet.[17,18] Early onset of menstruation and late menopause are each associated with approximately twice as high a risk of developing breast cancer as compared to women with a shorter menstrual life.[19,20]

I wish I had known how important fat and estrogens were before I got cancer. Will this information be of any help to me now?

Yes. You must understand the control you can have over your body's estrogen levels because of their importance in your treatment. We will talk about this later.

There is another important reason for you to know about the causal relationship of diet and breast cancer: mother teaches her daughters how to cook and what foods to like. Studies show that because you have developed breast cancer at an early age, your daughters have almost twice the usual risk of developing breast cancer.[21,22] The risk for daughters, and also sisters, of women with breast cancer developing this disease, themselves, can be as great as 50 percent under certain circumstances.[21-23] Some of this increased risk may be from a genetic tendency to be more susceptible to this cancer. More likely, most of this greater risk for breast cancer, as well as many other "family" diseases, is passed along to children through the education they receive in the home while growing up.

Since I'm younger than most women who get breast cancer, is there anything special I should know?

Many investigators believe that younger women with breast cancer have a much worse chance of surviving than older women. However, when all factors are considered, the fact that you are young is not necessarily associated with a worse outcome.[24] Approximately 20 percent of women with breast cancer are diagnosed before menopause and the other 80 percent are postmenopausal when the cancer is discovered.[25]

Some women in the reproductive age group may wonder how a pregnancy might affect their life and their cancer. Hormone levels do change considerably during pregnancy, and therefore a change in the growth of the cancer might be anticipated. Fortunately, all the changes that occur during pregnancy and lactation do not adversely affect the survival of the mother.[26] Termination of pregnancy, although it is recommended by some physicians, does not alter the outcome for the patient.[26] Radiation and chemotherapy, however, can have a serious adverse effect on the unborn baby. A woman with breast cancer must realize that her life expectancy probably will be shortened before she accepts the additional responsibility of bearing more children.

We will discuss some other factors concerning diagnosis and treatment that are related to your age and reproductive status later.

I've had lumps in my breast most of my life that doctors always called fibrocystic disease. Could one of these have turned into cancer?

Fibrocystic disease of the breast is characterized by lumps and bumps and tenderness especially when your estrogen levels are high just prior to your period. At least 50 percent of women in our country have these breast changes during their reproductive years.[27] Fibrocystic disease is believed to be the result of stimulation of the breasts by estrogens along with varying cyclic stimulation with other female hormones.[28] Some studies have indicated that women with fibrocystic disease have about three times the risk of developing breast cancer.[29] This should not be too surprising since estrogen stimulation of the breast seems to be involved in the development of both conditions. A preliminary study has shown that changing to a low-fat diet not only reduced the levels of estrogen, and other breast-stimulating hormones in women with fibrocystic disease, but has also improved the breast pain associated with the condition in all of the women studied.[30]

Other dietary causes of fibrocystic breast disease have been suggested. Caffeine and related chemicals will stimulate the breast tissues and are believed to account for some cases of this disease.[31,32] Reports indicate marked improvement in the painful breast tissues and resolution of lumps after removal of these stimulating chemicals for many women with this disease.[31,32]

Fortunately, of all the biopsies performed on suspicious lumps approximately 75 percent are found to be fibrocystic disease and other noncancerous tumors.[33] The other 25 percent of the time the news is not so good.

It has always been hard for me to tell which lumps I should worry about. However, this one did feel distinctly different. Do you think a yearly mammography would have discovered the cancer early enough to make a difference for me?

Mammography can detect a tumor earlier than self examination can. Studies have found that women over the age of fifty benefit from periodic examinations with mammography; as much as a one-third decrease in death rate is gained in postmenopausal women who undergo screening with mammography.[34-36] However, some questions concerning the usefulness of mammography still need to be answered: are lives actually being prolonged by this screening technique, or are we simply finding the cancers earlier with mammography, and thereby many women only appear to live longer because of an earlier discovery?[37,38] If, on the average, cancer is found a year earlier, and if, on the average, the patients then live a year longer from the time of diagnosis to death, the examination has really not had any beneficial effect. Recent studies have tried to resolve this problem of apparent versus real benefit for women screened with mammography.[34-36] There now appears to be a real improvement in short- to intermediate-term survival for women over fifty years old. Still another unanswered question is related to the advantages suggested by this data. Do the improved survival rates seen in the initial studies of detection by mammography represent permanent cures for these women above the age of fifty, or do they represent only postponement of death from breast cancer?[34,39]

You are in your late thirties; therefore, according to the results of these studies, you would not have benefited from mammography. The reason for the lack of benefit in women under fifty years of age is unknown. One theory proposes that the difference may lie in the possibility that cancers of postmenopausal women may spread more slowly than those found in premenopausal women. Some older women may have their cancers detected and removed before significant spread has occurred.

These findings and the conclusions drawn from them are still preliminary, and changes in recommendations for mammography are likely; they will be based upon the results of ongoing studies.[37-39] At present, most doctors recommend a first mammography for a woman sometime around forty, then yearly examinations after she reaches the age of fifty.[40,41] Certain women who are at higher risk may be recommended for earlier and more frequent examinations. If a tumor is detected by this method, the treatment would be no different from the one for a tumor found, as yours was, by feeling for a lump.

Are mammograms dangerous?

The hazard from radiation is very small, but it is still present, even when proper equipment and technique are used. The human organ most sensitive to the cancer-causing effects of radiation is the female breast.[42] It is even more sensitive than the bone marrow, the lung, and the thyroid gland. Studies done in various X-ray facilities have found that the dosage given for a mammogram can vary as much two hundred-fold with different techniques and equipment.[43] If a woman over fifty decides to have yearly mammographs, she should learn the necessary details about the X-ray department she chooses. She should ask about the age of the X-ray machine, whether or not the equipment was specifically designed for mammography, the number of such studies the department does in a year, and the qualifications of its staff.

One of the biggest concerns about the routine use of mammography is the increased number of biopsies generated solely because of the screening that otherwise would not be done. Between five and ten biopsies turn out to be normal for every one that is cancerous.[37] The emotional and other costs of so many negative biopsies are far from trivial.

I had a mammograph taken just before my biopsy and it was normal. Does this happen often?

Mammographs miss 10 to 30 percent of cancers; therefore, a report that an X-ray is "normal," showing no suspect tumor, does not rule out cancer.[38,44,45] Because of incorrect information from a mammography X-ray, the diagnosis of breast cancer can actually be delayed. For all kinds of cancer, the diagnosis is made only after microscopic examination of surgically removed tissues by a qualified pathologist. Therefore, worrisome lumps, in spite of a negative mammography, must be removed and examined microscopically for the presence of cancer cells.

One more concern is that some tumors found by mammography and classified as cancer never threatened the patients' lives, because actually they were not true cancers. When reviewed by another pathologist at a later date too many of these specimens receive a non-cancerous diagnosis.[37] In one study of 506 small tumors detected by mammography and removed, on later review, 66 were reinterpreted as non-cancerous and 22 others were reinterpreted as "borderline."[46] Extensive surgery when performed on these women was, of course, not justified.

Are better techniques available for finding cancer?

Another early detection method is thermography, which detects differences in the temperatures of the skin and underlying tissues. Cancerous tumors should show up hotter. The technique has no adverse effects. However, the results from screening programs have been very disappointing because so many cancers are missed, and therefore the technique is not considered acceptable for general screening.[47,48] Ultrasound, using high-frequency sound waves, has been limited to the evaluation of breast masses and is not useable for screening.[47,48]

Ninety percent of patients find lumps by themselves. The rest are found by doctors during routine physical examination.[49] Self-examination has been recommended for years as an effective means for early detection. Even though this technique is cheap, safe, and readily available, the evidence to date has not been convincing that routine breast self-examination saves lives through early detection.[38,41]

Deciding which lumps are suspect and in need of further examination is often a difficult problem. A cancer in the breast is rarely painful. Cancers are usually very hard and irregular to the touch and are often attached to surrounding tissues. A lump that is not cancer more likely would be tender and soft and would roll freely under the fingers.[33] An experienced physician can increase the probability of a correct diagnosis and would not order biopsies unless he or she thought they were likely to be confirmed as cancer.

Screening programs also heighten cancerophobia in our society. Some of this fear is justified since a recent autopsy series on women older than 20 years, without a previous history of breast cancer, revealed that nearly 20 percent unknowingly had invasive breast cancer or premalignant lesions.[50] Fortunately, only 10 percent of women in Western societies develop obvious breast cancer in their lifetime.[12]

Do you think it is worthwhile for a woman to have mammography and self-examination?

Yes, routinely for women over fifty who consume the high-fat American diet. With the present general high risk that women in this country have for developing breast cancer, early detection techniques have potential benefits for the individual patient. One unquestionable advantage is that when a breast cancer is found by mammography or frequent self-examination, it is usually very small and therefore easily removed by a nondeforming lumpectomy; mastectomy can be avoided. As mentioned, early studies indicate that for women over fifty life appears to be prolonged when tumors are found by mammography. Women following a low-fat diet have a much lower risk of developing breast cancer, and therefore less potential for benefit from routine mammographs. Yearly mammography in these lower risk women is unlikely to be found justifiable by a cost-risk-benefit comparison.

The most serious problem I see with efforts directed toward early detection is that they divert health dollars away from preventing breast cancer. The cost for screening every woman over the age of fifty in this country with a single examination would be over 2.25 billion dollars each year at 75 dollars per mammogram.[40] The cost for each cancer found by mammography is very expensive: $195,000 per cancer detected.[38]

Currently, efforts are no longer placed on yearly chest X-rays to detect lung cancer early and thereby to reduce the number of deaths from that disease.[40] Instead, people are being taught to stop smoking. I believe that teaching women to follow a low-fat diet is a more sensible approach to preventing breast cancer deaths than annual mammography, and a better way to spend our limited health dollars. Certainly, eating a proper diet would have a far greater impact on the incidence of this disease, since efforts toward early detection can do nothing but increase the number of tumors found. Can you imagine how much valuable information about health and its relationship to diet could be provided to the public with over 2 billion dollars a year? Women would benefit by a decreased incidence of breast cancer among those who followed a more sensible low-fat diet. In addition, most diseases that affect men, women, and children in this affluent society would be reduced in incidence when people accept this effective diet and make other healthful changes in their lifestyles. This all requires a national reeducation program and money to support it.

My other doctor said that because of some law he had to give me a brochure, which listed my options for treatment. His recommendation was a mastectomy. I think he said, "that's the only operation I do, take it or leave it."

Several states now have laws requiring physicians to give breast cancer patients information on options available, and a brochure is usually a part of the packet.

You have many options to choose from and you are the best qualified person to make these important decisions. After all, who has more to gain or lose from the treatments selected? I would like to tell you about the different therapies that are available. You can read more about them in the many articles found in university or medical libraries. Above all, take the time to consider your options and to think things through.

Is very much actually known about this disease?

This kind of tumor is one of the most accessible and easily diagnosed of all major forms of cancers. Breast cancer has been studied for centuries, and it was one of the first kinds of cancers that physicians tried to treat by surgical intervention. In America at the end of the nineteenth century, radical mastectomy was introduced by Dr. William Halsted of Johns Hopkins University Medical School.[51]

Incidentally, Dr. Halsted's operative reports describe breast cancers that measured 8 by 7 centimeters or about the size of an orange, as *small* cancers.[52] Years ago many women delayed seeking medical attention until the tumor was quite large and the disease well advanced. Because of this delay the number of years from surgery until death were fewer than today when the tumors are brought to the doctor's attention much earlier. With more physical self-awareness, frequent breast self-examinations and the use of mammography, tumors found these days by women are often one centimeter or less—the size of a pea. Because the disease is now detected at a much earlier stage, women have many more years from the time of surgery until they die of their breast cancer.

What are my choices?

Since the introduction of radical surgery by Dr. Halsted more than ninety years ago, a number of surgical approaches have been devised to remove the tumor. In addition, radiation has been tried at different stages of therapy in hopes of improving the length and quality of life for women affected by this disease. The effectiveness of each method of treatment has been tested by many practitioners, and the results of their observations are available to doctors and patients who make the effort to study them.

This list presents a brief summary of several surgical procedures that have been used.

Biopsy: removal of a small piece of the suspected tumor for laboratory analysis.

Lumpectomy: removal of the entire tumor only, not adjoining tissues.

Partial or segmental mastectomy: removal of a large section of breast with tumor and surrounding tissues.

Simple mastectomy: removal of entire breast.

Modified radical mastectomy: removal of entire breast as well as adjacent lymph nodes in the axilla (armpit).

Radical mastectomy: removal of entire breast, lymph nodes in axilla and underlying chest muscles.

Extended radical mastectomy: removal of entire breast, lymph nodes in axilla, underlying chest muscle, and lymph nodes next to the sternum (breastbone).

I heard that many doctors consider the radical mastectomy as the best treatment.

The radical mastectomy has been used as the standard with which to compare other procedures. However, to date no significant advantage of one surgical approach over another has been found, as far as survival of the patient is concerned.[38,53-71] A disappointing but well-researched conclusion for you to know is that, despite improved surgical techniques, advanced methods of radiotherapy, and the widespread use of chemotherapy, the death rate from breast cancer has not changed during the last seventy-five years.[53]

I'm sorry to present you with such dismal facts, but you must be informed enough to make the decisions that will have profound effects on your life.

Do other doctors really understand that all these treatments are not prolonging lives?

Most of them do. Unfortunately, a few share with their patients a world of hopes and dreams. Actually, the lack of appreciable differences in the results from various methods has led to a fatalistic attitude in the medical profession regarding the effectiveness of surgery in treating breast cancer. C. Barber Mueller, head of the Department of Surgery of McMaster University in Ontario, analyzed data collected over nineteen years on 3558 women with breast cancer from the Cancer Registry at Syracuse, New York. He concluded that "age, stage, or type of growth, operative therapy, or time at risk do not determine the time of death or alter the 90 percent certainty that death will be due to cancer of the breast."[63] Long-term studies of patients, treated by the best therapies medical science had to offer, confirm that at least 75 percent of the women who are diagnosed as having breast cancer will die with evidence of active disease in their bodies.[54,57,67,71] In other words, it is beyond denying that the treatments given have failed to cure these women. One startling finding is that twenty years after diagnosis, 80 percent of the women diagnosed as having breast cancer will be dead; 88 percent of these deaths will be due to breast cancer.[71]

Why don't surgery and radiation succeed in curing this cancer?

The use of extensive local therapies, such as mastectomies and radiation is based on the belief that breast cancer is a disease confined to the breast at the time of diagnosis and that removing the tumor in the breast will halt the disease.[72] Failure to improve survival rates by treatments directed at the tumor in the breast indicates that this theory is wrong.

A review of the natural history of the disease will help you to understand why cancer of the breast is rarely curable, if ever, with present treatments.[73] Studies have shown that breast cancer begins with the change of a healthy cell into a malignant one.[73] This transformed cell then grows at a steady rate. The time one cell requires to divide into two cells is called the doubling time. The average doubling time for breast cancer cells is approximately 100 days. In other words, 100 days after the beginning of the cancer in one cell, two malignant cells are present in the breast; at 200 days, four such cells are lurking there; and after one year, twelve cells have formed. At this rate of *doubling,* in six years the cancer mass contains one million cells and is the size of the point of a pencil. A mass of this size is less than one millimeter in diameter and is undetectable by palpation or mammography.[73] In ten years, the mass is finally detectable, having grown to a size comparable to the eraser of a common pencil. At that stage it consists of about one billion cells and is one centimeter in diameter.[73]

It sounds like I don't have to rush back to the operating room, since I probably have had this cancer for ten years by now.

This information may sound very discouraging, but you must know these facts in order to avoid unnecessary treatments that can disfigure and otherwise harm you.

When the full course of the disease is followed from the start of the cancer to the death of the woman, 75 percent of the time during which the woman has been a victim of cancer neither she nor her physician has known that it exists.[73,74] This fact, combined with the rarity of cure, leads to the conclusion that by the time the diagnosis is made, cells have already spread from the original tumor to other parts of the body.[38,53-71] This is true in most, if not all, cases of breast cancer.

Studies show that before the tumor is discovered in the breast, when the cancer is still virtually microscopic in size, cancer cells are entering the bloodstream. At the time of a diagnostic lumpectomy, these cancer cells can be found in the circulating blood of women with breast cancer.[75] These cancer cells, distributed by the blood, eventually settle in healthy tissues, and there many develop new tumors.[76] The cancer cells from the original tumor in the breast that lodge and grow in other parts of the body are called *metastases*. These metastatic cancers also have the same average doubling time of 100 days.[73] They eventually grow in the victim's critical organs, replacing tissue in the brain, liver, and lung. Rarely, if ever, does a woman die as a direct result of the tumor growing in her breast.

Doctors have understood the natural history of breast cancer for more than thirty years.[74] Yet, little of this understanding is reflected in the surgical treatments that have been prescribed for women over the past three decades.

I never realized before that lumpectomy and mastectomy are equally effective because both treatments are usually too late to stop the spread of the cancer. After the lump was removed from my breast I had a chest X-ray, bone scan, and blood tests. My doctor told me the cancer hadn't spread. Can that be true?

These tests are not sensitive enough to detect small tumors.[77] A lump developing from a metastasis must be almost a centimeter in diameter for a bone scan or an X-ray to detect it. Such areas of metastatic cancer would have been growing for an average of ten years in order to reach that size.[73] When these metastatic cancers finally reach detectable sizes, they seem to have spread like wildfire, overnight. Actually, many small tumors have

This diagram will illustrate the growth of breast cancer:

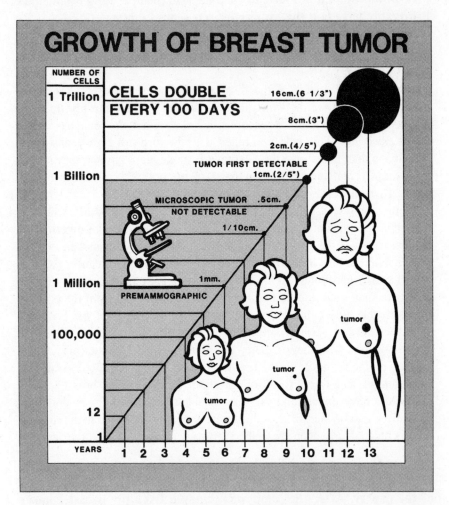

Three-fourths of the time a woman has been a victim of breast cancer has been without her knowledge.[73,74] Only during the final stages of this disease is the tumor detectable by any method. Unfortunately, by this time spread to other parts of the body has occurred in almost every case and the disease is incurable.[71] Because most of the years of cancer growth are hidden at microscopic levels, efforts toward early detection are unlikely to ever yield much success in saving lives. Our precious health-care dollars would be better spent on efforts toward prevention, such as teaching a low-fat (starch-based) diet.

been busily doubling in size for years until they become detectable to the touch or to X-rays and bone scans. When metastatic lesions appear two years or so after a small breast tumor was found, the spread through the bloodstream probably occurred about two years after the original cell in the breast became cancerous, or eight years before diagnosis!

The most effective and least expensive tests to determine if metastases have occurred are a physical examination, chest X-ray and simple blood tests.[78] These should be routinely performed just after diagnosis of cancer, because this may influence the choice of therapy, especially if the cancer has spread extensively. Bone and liver scans, X-rays of the full skeleton, and examinations of the bone marrow for cancer should be reserved for specific indications.[77,78] The value of any of these tests performed at routine intervals for follow up is questionable, since there is little effective therapy available for women when the tumor has been found to have spread. Therefore, in most cases, there is no reason for breast cancer victims to undergo routine testing to detect spread of cancer.[79] When symptoms appear, then appropriate examinations should be performed. There is value in contacting a physician regularly in order to detect any recurrence of the tumor in the affected breast or chest area and in the opposite breast. Frequent breast self-examination is valuable for detecting recurrences.

My previous doctor told me I must have my whole breast removed because other places in the same breast may also be cancerous.

He is right about the likelihood that other parts of your breast will be involved. The dietary factors, as well as other factors, that are involved in the cause of breast cancer affect all the breast tissues. Breast cancer, therefore, develops not just as a disease of the one detected site but as a disease that affects all breast tissues. The lump you found, the growth from one original cancer cell, is just more advanced than the other sites in your breast that are developing from a later starting time but at about the same rate of growth. After a mastectomy, when breast tissues outside the site of the actual tumor that was removed are examined microscopically, in most instances, these tissues too show evidence of cancer.[80] This is why surgeons often recommend a mastectomy, complete removal of the breast. Fortunately, these other and newer cancers grow to a size where they become detectable in only about 10 percent of women who, for one reason or another, do not have mastectomies or radiation to the breast.

Remember that breast cancer is a disease of all breast tissues. When the opposite breast is examined in women diagnosed as having breast cancer, in almost 100 percent of the cases various stages from precancerous changes to actual cancerous lumps are found there too.[50,81] Therefore, the same rationale your doctor gave you for a mastectomy, the probability of "satellite" tumors in the same breast, should also demand that all mastectomies be bilateral in order to remove all breast tissues that are involved with this disease. But a surgeon who suggested such madness would find few women paying for his or her skills. Fortunately, such new precancerous and cancerous sites in the opposite breast grow to problem sizes in only 10 percent of the cases.[82]

There doesn't seem to be much hope for cure. How long can I expect to live?

Now we can start talking about information that is a little more encouraging. Although this may seem contrary to some of the pessimistic messages I have been giving you, most likely you will live a long time.

Studies of cases of breast cancer demonstrate that most women who have this disease live for many years after initial diagnosis. For example, half the women in your age group twenty-one to fifty are alive thirteen years after learning they had cancer.[71] Many women live 30 years and longer after diagnosis.[65-69] This should be your goal.

But I've heard that if you live for five years without recurrence you're cured.

Because the metastatic cancer cells are slow-growing and hidden in vital areas of the body, some people are fooled into believing that cure has been achieved by the initial surgery. Usually these microscopic tumors produce no symptoms until near the time of death. The largely silent nature of the disease, combined with the fact that in up to 90 percent of cases the ultimate cause of death will be cancer of the breast, shows why five-year survival rates don't represent anything close to a cure.[63,71]

Medical professionals and representatives of cancer organizations who use such short-term survival statistics to support the success of present-day therapy are seriously misrepresenting to the public the actual course and outcome of breast cancer.[38,83]

What is the minimum treatment? How little surgery is actually required for control of the cancer in the breast?

Many patients have been treated by a lumpectomy, a simple nondeforming procedure that removes all of the tumor with little disfigurement of the surrounding breast tissue. Survival rates are as good as those of more radical therapies used for removal of the tumor, such as mastectomy.[60,61,84] One drawback to such limited surgery is that there is a greater risk of a recurrence of the cancer in the remaining breast tissues following a lumpectomy. The risk of this local recurrence is related more to the stage of development of the tumor at the time of diagnosis than to the skill of the surgeon. The later the stage at the time of diagnosis, the more likely will be a local recurrence.[85,86]

These recurrences in the breast that originally held the tumor are usually the result of metastatic cancer cells that have spread through the blood vessels and lymphatics to the skin and other breast tissues long before the discovery of the original lump.[85] Sometimes recurrence is because the surgeon performed an inadequate resection of the original tumor and left parts behind.[61] When the pathologist examines the specimen, the margins are checked and the pathologist's report tells if they are free of cancer cells. If the surgery was incomplete the surgeon can easily perform a slightly wider excision to include all of the cancer, and this must be done before the treatment is considered adequate.

These recurrences, if they do happen because of tumor cell spread or inadequate resection, are easily treated with further surgery or radiation.[87,88] Conservative surgery avoids treating everyone with extensive methods when, in reality, only a few will need a mastectomy or supplementary radiation therapy. Just remember, you will not sacrifice survival time later by choosing minimal surgery now.[38,60,61,84]

If all the cancerous tumor is removed by any procedure, in the case where spread has not already occurred, than even the simplest treatment of a lumpectomy has "cured" the patient. On the other hand, no amount of aggressive treatment to the affected breast will change the course of breast cancer that has already spread. All of the alternative surgeries offered today by surgeons, from simple lumpectomy to extended radical mastectomy, do one thing only: remove the tumor from the chest! Radiation therapy can do no more.

Doctors have been questioning the need for extensive surgery for breast cancer for many years. In 1951, a thorough review article on breast cancer treatment was written in a widely read medical journal. The authors concluded that the evidence strongly suggests that treatment is quite ineffectual in reducing the incidence of death from metastatic breast cancer.[89] They further suggested that minimal surgery was as effective as the more extensive procedures for treatment of localized breast cancer. Over the last three decades there has been too little change in the direction recommended by these pioneers in breast cancer surgery.

Removal of the cancerous mass in the breast is certainly necessary. Otherwise, the tumor may grow into an unsightly mess, eventually breaking through the skin, developing into a draining, ulcerated condition, which is difficult to care for.

I understand now that regardless of the kind of surgery I choose to remove the lump, it will not prolong my life. There must be other things I should consider?

Because no procedure has been convincingly shown to offer an advantage over others as far as survival, secondary considerations should guide you. Your physical appearance, as well as the mental, emotional, and physical suffering associated with the therapy, not to mention its cost, should help you to choose the best course of therapy for you.

Loss of function and swelling of the arm on the affected side are complications that occasionally follow the more extensive forms of surgery. The dangers from general anesthesia and postoperative complications are risks inherent in any kind of major surgery. With extensive surgery the cost is measured in the thousands of dollars, compared with a few hundred dollars for a minor lumpectomy performed on you as an outpatient with only local anesthesia. However, the most important issue is this: For most women, removal of the breast is an unnecessary form of mutilation that can destroy self-esteem and sexual identity and often results in severe psychological depression.[90] Every day physicians and patients are recognizing that the less surgery a woman receives in order to remove the obvious tumor, the better off she will be in every respect.[38,86,91]

Is a lumpectomy with radiation a good treatment to choose for me?

Just at the time in medical history when the use of X-ray treatment after a mastectomy has been almost discarded, the use of X-ray in the treatment of breast cancer has found a new role. More popular every day is combined therapy using a nondeforming lumpectomy and radiation. Radiation is given over a six-week period beginning soon after surgery. This combined approach achieves survival rates and risks of local recurrence that are comparable to those obtained with mastectomy.[92] The use of combined radiation and lumpectomy was recommended as adequate treatment of breast cancer in 1954.[93] More than thirty years have passed since this recommendation, yet today only a small minority of women are offered this therapy, which is much less deforming than any form of mastectomy. Occasionally, radiation is used as the only form of therapy after a small portion of the tumor is removed for diagnosis.

Radiation is a treatment not to be taken lightly. Radiation therapy to the breast can have significant adverse side effects and possible disastrous complications that reduce immunity and maybe even chance of survival. Early complications include radiation sickness, depression, and loss of appetite. Later on, breast deformity, rib fractures, and inflammation of the lung can be real problems.[92,94] In most cases, the breast keeps a reasonably normal appearance, although often the deeper tissues are more firm to the touch, and the skin will be discolored and leathery.

Radiation has definite harmful effects on the immune system. Most studies done today show comparable survival rates between women treated with lumpectomy and radiation and those treated by mastectomy. However, the safety of radiation therapy must continue to be questioned because of earlier studies that demonstrate harmful effects of radiation on women who had mastectomies. Women receiving radiation after mastectomy have been shown to die sooner than those for whom this additional therapy was not prescribed.[95-97] One review of the results of radiation therapy reports that in six controlled clinical trials, including more than 3400 patients, the decrease in survival ranged from 1 to 10 percent in irradiated patients, compared to those treated with mastectomy alone.[95] Women treated with lumpectomy and radiation have not had major surgery or blood transfusions, which also depress the immune system.[98-100] This may be one reason that the harmful affects of radiation have not shown up in recent comparisons of lumpectomy and radiation with mastectomy which does include these two insults to the immune system function.

Certain kinds of white blood cells known as *lymphocytes* are important in the body's defense against cancer. Both the numbers and the activities of these cells are depressed after radiation to the chest in the treatment of breast cancer.[101,102] There is evidence that this decreased immunity increases the risk of metastatic disease and thereby worsens survival rate.[95-97]

The routine use of postoperative irradiation in early breast cancer must seriously be questioned, even though there is an advantage of decreased local recurrences in the affected breast. Why subject every woman with breast cancer to the effects of radiation when only a few will benefit from it?

Is there ever a reason to do a mastectomy or radiation?

From what I said, you might think there is little reason to choose any therapy besides a lumpectomy. For some women, the thought of the tumor recurring after initial treatment of whatever kind is psychologically devastating. These women may choose more extensive treatment hoping to reduce the risk of recurrence in the breast or the muscles of the chest wall. After lumpectomy, local recurrences occur in about 15 to 25 percent of the cases; with mastectomies and lumpectomy with radiation therapy, the recurrence risk is about 10 percent.[61,86,103] Remember, these recurrences are effectively treated at the time they occur with additional surgery or radiation.[87,88]

In a very few cases the tumor is so large by the time the patient comes in for medical care that extensive procedures, such as a mastectomy and/

or extensive radiation, are the only way to remove all of the obvious cancer. Such a case is encountered in only a very small percentage of patients today. Sadly, many of these women have delayed seeking care only because of their very real fear of losing a breast, since most of them believe that mastectomy is the only therapy available.

I was also told that I must have surgery on the lymph nodes under my arm. I'm an artist and need full use of my right arm. Is that surgery really necessary?

Today women are subjected routinely to removal of a sample or all of the lymph nodes that drain a cancerous breast. Only by microscopic examination can physicians determine if those specimens are involved in the early stage of cancer. In about 50 percent of the cases so examined, enlarged nodes are found not to be cancerous. On the other hand, 25 percent of the time in cases in which no nodes can be felt, cancer is present when the nodes are examined microscopically.[104] Most of the surgeries performed on the lymph nodes today are only samplings rather than removal of all of the nodes, which was once done routinely when radical mastectomies were popular. This sampling method has been considered unreliable in predicting actual node involvement.[102]

Some doctors have questioned the wisdom of removing the armpit, or axillary, lymph nodes from the affected side either by surgery or by destroying them with radiation.[97,106-111] During the years when the Cleveland Clinic performed the more limited treatments of lumpectomy or simple mastectomy without radiation or removal of the axillary lymph nodes, the survival rates for women with breast cancer were better and the risk of local recurrence was suprisingly lower than they had been during the years when the clinic employed the more extensive treatments that destroyed the lymph nodes.[97]

Animal experiments have shown that lymph nodes that drain the area of a cancerous breast play important roles in the body's defenses against spread of the cancer.[97] Further investigations have shown that in laboratory experiments the lymph nodes in breast cancer patients exhibit a definite activity against cancer cells taken from the breast tumor.[111] The hypothesis suggests that the lymph nodes that drain the affected breast produce white blood cells, lymphocytes, that circulate through out the body and are able to destroy cancer cells that have metastasized.

Current evidence does question the wisdom of removing or otherwise destroying the lymph nodes, even though a definite detrimental effect has not been established. It is certain, however, that removing lymph nodes already showing the presence of cancer cells does not benefit the patient by decreasing the chances that the cancer will spread or by increasing the length of survival for a cancer victim.[38,62]

There must be reasons why so many doctors are recommending this additional surgery. What would I gain from having the lymph nodes under my arm removed?

The primary reason why doctors remove the axillary nodes is to determine whether or not a women would receive any benefit from chemotherapy.[54] The number of nodes that have become cancerous by the time of surgery has been used to predict the likelihood of a favorable response from the use of "cancer-killing" drugs, or *chemotherapy*, which are administered for a period of time following surgery.

If you decide that you will not take chemotherapy after surgery because of the ineffectiveness and toxicity of this therapy, then there is very little need to know if your nodes are involved.

Another reason for performing surgical removal of the lymph nodes is to determine the stage that the disease has reached and the patient's chance of surviving a certain number of years. When no nodes are involved, the five-year survival rate is about 80 percent; with involvement of axillary nodes the survival rate drops to about 50 percent.[54] Ten years after the diagnosis the survival rate in patients without initial node involvement drops to 65 percent and in women with involvement of nodes it drops to about 25 percent.[54] Approximately 50 percent of women operated on for breast cancer are in the early stages of disease where the lymph nodes are free of cancer. The other 50 percent at the time of initial surgery, have "positive nodes" or even more advanced distribution of obvious cancer cells spread throughout the rest of the body.[34]

Even though involvement of the lymph nodes generally indicates that the disease is in an advanced stage, many women who have reached this stage at the time of diagnosis live for twenty years or longer after their cancer is discovered. In one study of women who lived for more than twenty years, the lymph nodes of 35 percent were cancerous at the time of initial diagnosis.[112] Therefore, prediction for the probability of survival in cases with lymph node involvement cannot be relied upon in individual cases. Predictions, I should emphasize, are based upon statistics; therefore, women who are aware of lymph node involvement may worry unnecessarily, and for them pessimism may be unwarranted.

The issue of whether or not to remove axillary nodes is easily resolved by recognizing that few women will find that the knowledge of the stage their disease has reached is worth the risk and the cost of surgery. The possibility of side effects of continual pain and the cosmetic deformity of swelling and scarring of the arm, not to mention possible adverse effects on the immune system's fight against cancer cells, are additional reasons to refuse to submit to this surgery.

I'm wondering, what does a person do if the lymph nodes can be felt at the time the breast cancer is found?

Enlarged lymph nodes suspected of containing cancer cells have been reported to regress in size within three months after the removal of the cancer in the breast in 75 percent of patients with breast cancer and enlarged lymph nodes.[113] Some of these nodes probably contained cancer, however most of the nodes were enlarged only as the result of a reaction from the tumor in the breast. This observation of node regression eliminates another reason some doctors give for radiation or removal of the affected axillary nodes. If the lymph nodes should grow and become uncomfortable or unsightly, then they can be treated by radiation or surgery without sacrificing survival time.[38,62,87,88]

Please tell me more about chemotherapy. Shouldn't I take these drugs to kill the cells that have already spread?

The obvious failure of locally directed therapies such as surgery and radiation to improve survival by ''catching'' the cancer before it has spread has led to the practice of administering chemotherapeutic agents during surgery and for variable periods of time afterward. This approach, called *adjuvant* chemotherapy, is regarded as an enhancer of surgical and radiation therapies. The chemical agents administered to the patients are supposed to inhibit or kill cancer cells that have already spread throughout the body. The drugs chosen for these purposes are toxic to cancer cells that are grown in tissue cultures or in animal models. A second criterion for these agents is they must affect the cancer before they kill the patient.

In the United States, adjuvant chemotherapy was accepted with enthusiasm by most physicians at first, in part out of the desperation surrounding the failure of previous therapies to prolong the lives of breast cancer victims. The initial enthusiasm, induced by early findings of improved survival rates in all women for the first two years after surgery, was quickly tempered by results three to five years after therapy. In one widely publicized long-term study performed by proponents of chemotherapy, the advantage to survival dwindled after five years to 4 percent over those patients who did not receive chemotherapy.[114] When separated into groups, premenopausal women had a 12 percent survival advantage, and women who were past menopause had a 5 percent decrease in chances of survival compared with those who did not take the therapy.[115]

A recent study in England concerning the effectiveness of adjuvant chemotherapy failed to show any advantage in survival rates, even for the premenopausal group.[116] The authors of this study have asked the medical community to weigh more carefully the benefits of chemical agents against their toxicity before recommending widespread use of postoperative chemotherapy. Effects of psychological and physical toxicity are considerable, as more than half the patients reported feeling anxious or depressed, and virtually all were found to suffer from physical illness, and interference with blood cell production from the bone marrow was common.[116]

I've heard that chemotherapy has terrible side effects. What can I expect?

The side effects of adjuvant chemotherapy are unpleasant, to put it mildly. In fact, they are so severe that 79 percent of the women treated reported that they were disturbing enough to interfere with their lifestyle and 29 percent declared that never again would they submit to the experience.[117] Many women, if not most, stop taking chemotherapy before the course of injections and pills is finished, because of the drugs' serious adverse effects.[115] These include hair loss, nausea, loss of nerve function, depressed blood cell counts causing anemia and allowing infections, diarrhea, cystitis, vomiting, and oral ulcers. The drugs used in chemotherapy depress the immune system and decrease the body's ability to fight off microbial infection and to defend itself against cancer.[118] Progressive growth of the breast cancer, and the formation of new cancers, are real possibilities because of this experimental therapy.[118,119] Viral infections are twice as common in women while taking adjuvant chemotherapy for breast cancer.[120]

Giving chemotherapy to women routinely after surgery subjects all women to the powerful toxic effects of these drugs. Evidence indicates that even the small improvement in survival rates that is seen in selected women who receive adjuvant chemotherapy can be obtained as effectively when chemotherapy is reserved until the time when the cancer recurs.[121] If chemotherapy has any significant advantage for survival, withholding these powerful drugs for use only in the late stage of the disease will spare many women needless suffering.

Since the benefit of adjuvant chemotherapy is seriously questioned and its toxicity to the body is definite, this kind of experimentation should be reserved for clinical investigative studies, sparing women until an effective therapy can be developed.[116,118,121-126]

You are really saying that I'm better off doing as little as possible in the way of surgery, radiation, and chemotherapy. I just want to live as long as possible.

The burden of proving the benefits of a procedure rests on those physicians who recommend these mutilating and dangerous treatments. Considering our present state of knowledge, we should reserve extensive surgery, radiation, and chemotherapy for women who develop recurrences, instead of subjecting all women with breast cancer to the mutilations, risks, and complications associated with these therapies. Every one of them, along with blood transfusions and the high-fat hospital diet, has been convincingly demonstrated or strongly suspected to decrease immunity and thereby may give the cancer an added advantage.[95,97-100,110,118,127,128]

Here is a list of experiences that can happen to cancer patients while they're hospitalized, and may adversely affect their recovery from cancer:

FACTORS THAT DEPRESS THE IMMUNE SYSTEM AND HAVE BEEN SUSPECTED OF DECREASING SURVIVAL BY LOWERING THE BODY'S DEFENSE AGAINST CANCER:

Major surgery

Blood transfusions

Radiation

Chemotherapy

Lymph node irradiation

Lymph node removal

High-fat diet

Why add insult to injury? Because of the evidence obtained during the last ninety years of scientific observations on the treatment of breast cancer, every health practitioner and cancer patient must ask what advantage can really be gained by any or all of the alternative surgeries, radiation therapies, and chemotherapies that are being prescribed for breast cancer victims.

Would cutting down on my body's estrogen production by removing my ovaries be of any help?

Removing the ovaries, which produce estrogen, or the pituitary gland, which controls the ovaries, by surgery or radiation is popular therapy for breast cancer in premenopausal women. With the subsequent decrease in estrogen production, tumor growth is slowed and some regression in size is seen. Stopping estrogen function can give dramatic relief of symptoms to some breast cancer victims. However, advantage to survival is small at best.[129] It is important to know that the same benefits are obtained when surgery is either done shortly after diagnosis of cancer or reserved for later stages of the disease.[130] Waiting until later to remove ovarian function shortens the time a woman would have to suffer with menopausal symptoms and spares many women the need for major surgery or extensive radiation to remove the ovaries or pituitary gland altogether.

One interesting theory holds that the benefits from chemotherapy come solely from destruction of the ovarian function, specifically of estrogen production, by the chemotherapy agents. Most women cease menstruation soon after beginning chemotherapy. According to these investigators, the slight benefits in survival rates and slowed tumor growth that are seen following chemotherapy can be obtained by surgical or radiation therapies designed to reduce estrogen production.[131] These direct approaches to lowering estrogen production avoid the long lasting and debilitating side effects of chemotherapy.

Can I take a drug that will lower the stimulating effects of estrogen in my body?

An antiestrogen drug called *tamoxifen* has shown a beneficial effect on breast cancer. Tumors will decrease in size in patients taking this drug, and the survival time of women with metastatic disease may be lengthened somewhat.[132-134] Recent studies even suggest that prolonged survival and delayed recurrence of disease may be achieved when tamoxifen is given for a couple of years after initial surgery, before any sign of spread.[135-137] In other words, tamoxifen appears to be of value as an adjuvant therapy in a few studies.

The real advantage to this hormone approach is that the results are as good as those obtained with any of the more toxic adjuvant chemotherapy programs, and the adverse side effects are much less.[135] Only 2 percent of women stop taking the drug because of side effects; most of these are due to the decreased effects of the estrogens and are similar to the symptoms of menopause.[135] The most recent trial using tamoxifen as adjuvant therapy has demonstrated a 34 percent decrease in death rate after six years of study.[136] This most likely represents a prolongation of life and not a cure. You must understand that when disease has spread to other parts of the body, no hormone therapy or chemotherapy will cure the patient.[138]

My other doctor told me my tumor was estrogen-receptor-positive. Does this mean that tamoxifen will work any better?

There are sites on the inside of breast cancer cells to which the estrogen attaches. These sites are called receptors. Molecules of tamoxifen will also attach to these same sites and block the activity of the estrogens. These sites have been found to have some prognostic value; the more receptor sites the tumor has, the better the prognosis and the more effective any antihormone therapy, like tamoxifen, is likely to be.[139] Breast cancer cells in premenopausal women usually have fewer estrogen receptors than cancer cells in postmenopausal women. In general, postmenopausal women and those with slow growing tumors respond better to all forms of hormone therapy, whether it is designed to diminish estrogen levels or even to add to them. Premenopausal women with fast growing cancers do not respond as well.[54] Contrary to what is expected, some encouraging results have been seen with adjuvant tamoxifen therapy even in women with low levels of estrogen receptors on the inside of their cancer cells.[136]

The biggest question on my mind is still this: How can I live longer?

The clinical course of breast cancer is highly variable. Some women will die soon after the lump in their breast is discovered, while others will survive twenty years or more in apparent good health, only to die eventually from their original cancer.[65-70] Your goal is to be one of those women who live for many years. The course of breast cancer and, ultimately, the time of death are determined by the patient's ability to resist the aggressiveness of the tumor. This contest is commonly referred to as the *host versus tumor relationship*.[63]

Present modes of treatment, including surgery, radiation, and chemotherapy, try to change this relationship with techniques aimed at removing or weakening the tumor. However, as we have discussed, many years of experience with these treatments have been generally disappointing and have left investigators wondering if any real progress has been made in the war against breast cancer.[38,53-71]

Are you suggesting I try treatments that are designed to improve my defense system?

Many researchers are looking for ways to improve the cancer patient's natural immunity.[54] Agents that stimulate the immune system, such as *levamisole* and *BCG vaccine*, have produced mixed results. *Interferons* are proteins secreted by certain body cells which can be taken up by other cells rendering them resistant to infection with viruses. These proteins are synthesized in a laboratory and then given to patients with a variety of diseases. Interferon has been used experimentally in cancer patients and regression of breast cancer nodules has been seen with interferon.[140] To date, however, the overall results have shown only limited promise. Another possibly useful, but still experimental, approach to fighting the cancer is to induce an *artificial fever*, either by administering bacterial toxins that cause a rise in body temperature or by employing techniques, called *hyperthermia*, that heat the body internally or externally.[141]

So what else can I do to increase my strength to fight the tumor?

Compared to the efforts that physicians have made in attempting to destroy the cancer, very little attention has been given to the possibility of strengthening the host defenses. However, nutritional factors have long been recognized as important in affecting our ability to resist disease and to recover from illness.[142]

Dietary advice about preventing cancer was proposed by the Senate Select Committee on Nutrition and Human Needs in 1977, the National Cancer Institute in 1979, the National Academy of Sciences in 1982, and the American Cancer Society in 1984.[143-146] These organizations agree that we should cut down our intake of meat, dairy products, and fats from all sources and that we should increase grains, fresh fruits and vegetables in our diets.

I'm afraid it's a little late for me to worry about prevention. Do you really believe that by adopting a certain diet I can make a difference even after the disease has started?

Many knowledgeable people believe that our rich American diet is involved as an important factor in the cause of breast cancer. Logically, then, we should stop adding fuel to the fire and apply the dietary advice for preventing breast cancer to those unfortunate women who already have become victims of this disease. By changing from the rich diet that promotes breast cancer to a diet that best supports good health, further growth of cancer could be slowed and the woman's life would be prolonged.

I certainly could use a fresh approach to my cancer. If I do change my diet now, how can I know if I'm getting any better?

Several observations have been made on factors related to the rate of progress of breast cancer. Four of these factors, obesity, cholesterol, estrogen and prolactin, are associated with a poorer prognosis.[147-150]. Overweight women with high levels of cholesterol live for less than half the five-year survival rates compared with slimmer women who have low levels of cholesterol.[147] Reducing the levels of the hormones estrogen and prolactin by means of drugs or surgery can retard the growth of established breast cancer and cause regression of tumors.[151] Of particular importance to you is the recognition that these four prognostic factors are a direct consequence of your nutrient intake; therefore, they may be altered by a conscious and consistent change in diet.

In affluent Western societies where the incidence of breast cancer is high, diets are typically rich in fat and cholesterol, and low in fiber content, and obesity is a common consequence.[146] People eating such diets have levels of cholesterol, estrogen and prolactin that are higher than the levels produced by the diets of underdeveloped countries, where breast cancer is much less common.[8,152,153] Investigators have found that when starch-centered diets, low in fat and cholesterol and high in fiber, are fed to volunteers, weight reduction occurs and the levels of cholesterol, estrogen, and prolactin in the blood are reduced.[18,153-156] When postmenopausal women with breast cancer were fed a starch-centered meal plan, similar favorable reductions were observed.[157]

You can easily and inexpensively check on your weight and cholesterol level to determine if you are making progress toward better health. Tests for estrogen and prolactin levels are expensive and more difficult to obtain; with a lower-fat diet, these will likely decrease. I would recommend that you not depend on these tests and only check your weight and cholesterol periodically.

If I do change my diet do you think the cancer will actually grow slower?

Factors that cause cancer are also believed to encourage its growth. For example, patients with a form of lung cancer caused by cigarettes live longer if they quit smoking than those who continue the habit.[158] Animal studies show that fats and oils promote the growth of tumors and that animals receiving a diet with higher cholesterol show more frequent occurrence of tumors and metastases.[159-161] Several investigators have observed that women with breast cancer who live in countries where low-fat diets are followed survive longer, with less progression of their disease, than do women on higher fat diets.[162-164] For example, the five-year survival rate for breast cancer patients in Japan is 74.9 percent as compared with 57.3 percent for breast cancer patients in Boston.[162] Japanese women have a considerably lower fat intake in their diets.[165]

How strict do I need to be with my diet?

How strictly you follow my recommendations is something you must decide. I will tell you what I believe is best. Victims of breast cancer, as well as women wanting to prevent that kind of cancer, should adopt the best diet designed for maintaining the body's health and healing processes. This health-supporting diet is low in fats of all kinds, is high in fiber, and contains no cholesterol. Like the diet eaten in societies where breast cancer is rare, this diet is centered around a variety of delicious starches, such as rice, potatoes, sweet potatoes, corn, breads and pasta, along with all the fresh or frozen vegetables and fruits you may want to eat.[166]

Do you have any proof this will help me?

Proof is a very difficult thing to provide, but the evidence is very convincing that a diet change will help you. I regard the benefits from changes in diet and lifestyle not from the point of view of cure but as improvements in the quality and possibly length of life for the cancer victim. Could five years expected survival time be lengthened to seven, ten or even fifteen by improving the health of the host? Studies still to be done will tell us how valuable a dietary change will actually be for women with breast cancer. The National Cancer Institutes have ten year studies in progress that will provide evidence on the effects of a lower-fat diet on women with a diagnosis of breast cancer.[167] At the present time no harm can come from trying. Even though much further study in this subject is needed, the probable advantages to be gained from this approach should persuade women with breast cancer to adopt a healthier diet immediately. These recommendations are free of adverse effects and of the expenses that are common to most other forms of medical therapy. In addition, a starch-centered diet has been found to improve health in many ways, from loss of weight and relief of constipation to lowering blood pressure and blood sugar levels.[166] Without question, women with breast cancer have every reason to maintain the best level of health they can possibly achieve.

Has anyone ever been cured once cancer has spread throughout her body?

A woman with breast cancer must never give up hope. We know about very rare but documented cases of women with metastatic breast cancer spreading throughout their bodies who have experienced spontaneous regression, or disappearance of the cancer for reasons unknown.[168,169] These cures in the face of almost hopeless odds demonstrate that the body has the potential to win its battles, and possibly the war, with cancer. Common sense would declare that a body in good health will have a better chance than one that is ill. Therefore, a victim of breast cancer should make every effort to eat correctly and to support her general health in every possible way.

Are any other cancers similar to breast cancer in the way they get started and their resistance to treatment?

Most cancers that are found as a solid mass have similar characteristics. These include cancer of the prostate, ovary, lung, kidney, pancreas, liver, gallbladder, esophagus, stomach, and colon. Although they may have different environmental causes, they are all advanced by the time of diagnosis and survival is affected little, if at all, by various forms of therapy.[170]

Colon cancer, which affects between twenty and thirty percent of the families in the United States, for example, is thought to be caused by the foods we eat; in particular the high-fat, high-cholesterol, low-fiber diet consumed by most Americans.[143-146,171] Efforts to prolong survival by detecting colon cancer earlier through finding minute quantities of blood in the stool have been largely disappointing.[172,173] In almost all cases the disease is far advanced by the time of discovery.[174] Cancer cells can be found in the blood of the veins draining from the tumor even in stages of colon cancer that are considered early.[175] As with most other cancers, cells that spread long before the cancer is discovered cause the metastases that kill their victim.

Long-term survival rates are very poor and actually worse than those for breast cancer at five and ten years, possibly because the detection is more difficult and tumors are found at a more advanced stage of growth.[174,176-179] Treatment appears to have little effect on the ultimate survival.[176-180] Because of lack of appreciable improvement in survival from extensive surgery, more conservative therapy is being used. For example, cancer of the very last part of the large intestine, the rectum, has been traditionally treated with an extensive surgery called an *abdominoperineal resection* which often employs two surgical teams, one working above and the other below, to remove the cancer. Recently, treatment by simply burning off the cancer with an electrocautery has been found to be as effective with even better survival rates than from extensive surgery.[181]

Polyps of the colon are found more commonly in populations with a high incidence of colon cancer, and both diseases are suspected of sharing the same dietary cause.[182] Polyps often precede the development of colon cancer and the polyp may actually become the site of the cancer with time.[183] The interval between the appearance of a polyp and progression to cancer has been reported to be as long as fifteen years, which suggests a slow rate of change to cancer.[183] Early detection and removal of polyps is believed to decrease the risk of colon cancer.[184] Operations that divert the flow of stool away from the segment of colon with polyps have resulted in regression of the polyps.[185,186] This would suggest there is a stage in the transition toward the development of cancer of the colon that is reversible. Investigations should be done to determine if a low-fat, high-fiber diet— the diet opposite to the one believed to be the cause of colon polyps and cancer—would result in similar regression.

Colon cancer patients should seriously consider that a change in diet may be beneficial for them for the same reasons that a change in diet may help women with breast cancer. Furthermore, since the change does no harm and has many known benefits, there is no reason not to switch to a low-fat, no-cholesterol, high fiber diet, even after developing colon cancer. Animal studies have demonstrated that the removal of cholesterol from the diet of rats with established colon cancer reduces the incidence of metastases and improves survival rates over animals fed the standard food with cholesterol.[187] Survival varies between ethnic groups in the United States, and this may be the result of differences in diets they follow.[188] Like breast cancer, there have been a few cases of spontaneous regression of advanced colon cancer.[189,190]

You may think this is an unusual question, but I'd like to hear your answer: is it possible that another reason why women are treated so aggressively, and with so little concern for their personal feelings, is that most doctors are men?

Certainly the dominant role of men over women is an ancient issue, and today it is under direct challenge in every aspect of our lives, including medicine. One observation leading me to believe that this has something to do with the slowness of change is the way a similar cancer in men is treated. Prostate cancer in men is very much like breast cancer in women.[191] Here too, high-fat diets are involved in the cause and this is also a hormone-dependent cancer.[18] Like breast cancer, prostate cancer is about ten years old before it is diagnosed, and it has spread in almost every case by the time diagnosis is made.[191] Treatment by radical prostate surgery is as ineffective as mastectomy is in breast cancer surgery.[191] However, several years ago radical prostate surgery became unpopular. These days, the treatment of choice for prostate cancer is radiation after a diagnostic biopsy.[192] You could surmise from this that the male-dominated medical profession is more sympathetic to men with prostate cancer and more responsive to men's problems.

Why is all of this information on breast cancer so little known among women and their doctors?

People are slow to change and accept new ways, even when the evidence is convincing. Several years ago after a hospital conference, I asked a well known surgeon: "Doctor, I have just listened to you talk for the past hour on the failure of surgery, including the time-honored mastectomy, to cure breast cancer or prolong life. Why do you still perform mastectomies when you fully realize the ineffectiveness of this approach in saving lives?" His answer was simply, "That is the way I was trained." I pursued the matter by asking what would change this common surgical practice in our health care system. He replied, "A whole new generation of surgeons trained differently."

What about other women who are being treated for breast cancer by their doctors? What can be done to make doctors change their methods faster?

Inertia within the medical system is the main factor that has delayed progress in the treatment of breast cancer. The time has come for people outside the medical system to demand appropriate changes in all aspects of medical care. During the past few years, three states, Massachusetts, California, and Hawaii, have enacted informed consent laws that require a physician to explain to women with breast cancer the alternative methods of treatment that are available. Information about the importance of nutrition is also given to women in Hawaii. Similar legislation designed to involve the patient in her care and to help cut back on excessive and unnecessary surgical procedures is being introduced in Michigan, Minnesota, Pennsylvania, Virginia, and Wisconsin. As women who have breast cancer become fully informed about the disease, they will cause their doctors to give up old thoughts and outmoded techniques, and they will demand more humane treatments for themselves.

℞
BEFORE BREAST CANCER DEVELOPS
- Prevention with a low-fat, high-carbohydrate, high-fiber diet is the ideal approach to breast cancer.
- Self-examination should be performed by all women
- Women over fifty following high-fat diets should have mammography, however, how often such examinations should be performed has not been determined. For now, consider every other year reasonable.

AFTER BREAST CANCER DEVELOPS
- Initial evaluation for spread of the disease should include a physical examination, chest X-ray, and blood tests.
- Select the minimal surgery that will remove all of the obvious cancer from the affected breast. A lumpectomy will suffice for most women.
- Do not choose axillary node sampling surgery unless special circumstances warrant it (such as need to remove uncomfortable nodes).
- Do not choose postoperative radiation unless special circumstances warrant it (such as need to control recurrent disease in the breast, axilla or on the chest wall.)
- Do not choose adjuvant chemotherapy with highly toxic drugs unless special circumstances warrant it (I can't think of any special circumstances that warrant adjuvant chemotherapy with highly toxic chemical agents. However, future experimentation may find a worthwhile therapy).
- Adjuvant chemotherapy with tamoxifen may be a reasonable choice for many women, especially those who are estrogen-receptor-positive.
- Reserve mastectomy and other extensive surgery for removal of a tumor that cannot be controlled by more limited surgery.
- Recurrences after a lumpectomy should be treated by more surgery unless breast deformity will be severe. In this case radiation should be the next choice for most women interested in maintaining a "normal" appearance.
- Chemotherapy with toxic agents and operations to decrease the estrogen production—ovary and pituitary surgery—should be reserved for late stages of the disease to control symptoms and gain whatever limited survival advantage is possible with these therapies.
- Regardless of the stage of disease, a low-fat diet is a sensible change for all women.
- Routine follow-up for most women should be limited to checking for recurrences in the remaining breast tissues and chest wall. No routine tests, X-rays, or scans are advisable.

REFERENCES

[1]Breast CA- What every woman knows. *Hospital Practice,* February 1981, p 29-37.

[2]Kirschner M. The role of hormones in the etiology of human breast cancer. *Cancer* 39:2716, 1977.

[3]Judd H. Estrogen replacement therapy: Indications and complications. *Ann Intern Med* 98:195, 1983.

[4]Fara G. Epidemic of breast enlargement in an Italian school. *Lancet* 2:295, 1979.

[5]Saenz de Rodriguez C. Environmental hormone contamination in Puerto Rico. *N Engl J Med* 310:1741, 1984.

[6]Gorbach S. Estrogens, breast cancer, and intestinal flora. *Rev Infect Dis* 6 (Suppl I):S85, 1984.

[7]Goldin B. Estrogen excretion patterns and plasma levels in vegetarian and omnivorous women. *N Engl J Med* 307:1542, 1982.

[8]MacMahon B. Urine oestrogen profiles of Asian and North American women. *Int J Cancer* 14:161, 1974.

[9]MacDonald P. Effect of obesity on conversion of plasma androstenedione to estrone in postmenopausal women with and without endometrial cancer. *Am J Obstet Gynecol* 130:448, 1978.

[10]Hemsell D. Plasma precursors of estrogen. II. Correlation of the extent of conversion of plasma androstenedione to estrone with age. *J Clin Endocrinol Metab* 38:476, 1974.

[11]Zumoff B. Hormone profiles in hormone-dependent cancers. *Cancer Res* 35:3365, 1975.

[12]Cancer Statistics, 1985. The National Cancer Institute's Surveillance, Epidemiology and End Results Program (Seer) (1977-1981). *CA* 35:19, 1985.

[13]Lea A. Dietary factors associated with death-rates from certain neoplasms in man. *Lancet* 2:332, 1966.

[14]Goldin B. Effect of diet on excretion of estrogens in pre- and postmenopausal women. *Cancer Res* 41:3771, 1981.

[15]Kagawa Y. Impact of Westernization on the nutrition of Japanese: Changes in physique, cancer, longevity and centenarians. *Prev Med* 7:205, 1978.

[16]Frommer D. Changing age of the menopause. *Br Med J* 2:349, 1964.

[17]Armstrong B. Diet and reproductive hormones: a study of vegetarian and nonvegetarian postmenopausal women. *JNCI* 67:761, 1981.

[18]Hill P. Environmental factors and breast and prostatic cancer. *Cancer Res* 41:3817, 1981.

[19]Staszewski J. Age at menarche and breast cancer. *J Natl Cancer Inst* 47:935, 1971.

[20]Trichopoulos D. Menopause and breast cancer risk. *J Natl Cancer Inst* 48:605, 1972.

[21]Anderson D. A genetic study of human breast cancer. *J Natl Cancer Inst* 48:1029, 1972.

[22]Ottman R. Practical guide for estimating risk for familial breast cancer. *Lancet* 2:556, 1983.

[23]Lynch H. Management of familial breast cancer. II. Case reports, pedigrees, genetic counseling, and team concept. *Arch Surg* 113:1061,1978.

[24]Rosen P. Breast carcinoma in women 35 years of age or younger. *Ann Surg* 199:133, 1984.

[25]Leis H. Epidemiology of breast cancer: identification of the high-risk woman. In: Gallager H.S. (ed) *The Breast.* St Louis. C. V. Mosby, 1978,pp 37-48.

[26]Max M. Pregnancy and breast cancer. *S Med J* 76:1088, 1983.

[27]Devitt J. Clinical benign disorders of the breast and carcinoma of the breast. *Surg Gynecol Obstet* 152:437, 1981.

[28]Greenblatt R. The role of estrogens in mastopathy and mammary cancer in perimenopausal women. *J Am Geriatr Soc* 30:165, 1982.

[29]Coombs L. A prospective study of the relationship between benign breast diseases and breast carcinoma. *Prev Med* 8:40, 1979.

[30]Rose D. Low fat diet in fibrocystic disease of the breast with cyclical mastalgia: a feasibility study. *Am J Clin Nutr* 41:856, 1985.

[31]Minton J. Caffeine, cyclic nucleotides, and breast disease. *Surgery* 86:105, 1979.

[32]Brooks P. Measuring the effect of caffeine restriction on fibrocystic breast disease. The role of graphic stress telethermometry as an objective monitor of disease. *J Reprod Med* 26:279, 1981.

[33]Pilnik S. Clinical diagnosis of benign breast diseases. *J Reprod Med* 22:277, 1979.

[34]Shapiro S. Ten- to fourteen-year effect of screening on breast cancer mortality. *JNCI* 69:349, 1982.

[35]Collette H. Evaluation of screening for breast cancer in a non-randomised study (the DOM project) by means of a case-control study. *Lancet* 1:1224, 1984.

[36]Tabar L. Reduction in mortality from breast cancer after mass screening with mammography. *Lancet* 1:829, 1985.

[37]Bailar J. Mammographic screening: a reappraisal of benefits and risks. *Clin Obstetr Gynecol* 21:1, 1978.

[38]Skrabanek P. False premises and false promises of breast cancer screening. *Lancet* 2:316, 1985.

[39]Editorial: Breast screening: New evidence. *Lancet* 1:1217, 1984.

[40]ACS report on the cancer-related health checkup. *CA* 30:194, 1980.

[41]Health and Public Policy Committee, American College of Physicians; Philadelphia Pennsylvania. The use of diagnostic tests for screening and evaluating breast lesions. Position Papers. *Ann Intern Med* 103:143, 1985.

[42]Gregg E. Radiation risks with diagnostic x-rays. *Radiology* 123:447, 1977.

[43]Bicehouse H. *Survey of mammographic exposure levels and techniques used in eastern Pennsylvania.* Presented at the Seventh Annual National Conference on Radiation Control, April 27-May 2, 1975, Hyannis, Mass. DHEW Publication 76-8026.

[44]Martin J. Breast cancer missed by mammography. *AJR* 132:737, 1979.

[45]Hicks M. Sensitivity of mammography and physical examination of the breast for detecting breast cancer. *JAMA* 242:2080, 1979.

[46]Thier S. Editorial: Breast-cancer screening: a view from outside the controversy. *N Engl J Med* 297:1063, 1977.

[47]Mushlin A. Diagnostic tests in breast cancer. Clinical strategies based on diagnostic probabilities. *Ann Intern Med* 103:79, 1985.

[48]Kopans D. Breast imaging. *N Engl J Med* 310:960, 1984.

[49]Greenwald P. Estimated effect of breast self-examination and routine physician examinations on breast-cancer mortality. *N Engl J Med* 299:271, 1978.

[50]Nielsen M. Precancerous and cancerous breast lesions during lifetime and at autopsy. A study of 83 women. *Cancer* 54:612, 1984.

[51]Editorial: Treatment of early carcinoma of breast. *Br Med J* 1:417, 1972.

[52]Lewison E., Montague A. (eds) *Diagnosis And Treatment Of Breast Cancer.* International Clinical Forum. Williams & Wilkins Baltimore/London 1981. p. 5-7.

[53]Greenberg D. "Progress" in cancer research-Don't say it isn't so. *N Engl J Med* 292:707, 1975.

[54]Henderson I. Cancer of the breast. The past decade. Part 1 and 2. *N Engl J Med* 302:17 & 78, 1980.

[55]Baum M. The curability of breast cancer. *Br Med J* 1:439, 1976.

[56]Stehlin J. Treatment of carcinoma of the breast. *Surg Gynecol Obstet* 149:911, 1979.

[57]Brinkley D. The curability of breast cancer. *Lancet* 2:95, 1975.

[58]Meyer A. Carcinoma of the breast. A clinical study. *Arch Surg* 113:364, 1978.

[59]Fisher B. Comparison of radical mastectomy with alternative treatments for primary breast cancer. *Cancer* 39:2827, 1977.

[60]Crile G. Results of partial mastectomy in 173 patients followed for from five to ten years. *Surg Gynecol Obstet* 150:563, 1980.

[61]Fisher B. Five-year results of a randomized clinical trial comparing total mastectomy and segmental mastectomy with or without radiation in the treatment of breast cancer. *N Engl J Med* 312:665, 1985.

[62]Fisher B. Ten-year results of a randomized clinical trial comparing radical mastectomy and total mastectomy with or without radiation. *N Engl J Med* 312:674, 1985.

[63]Mueller C. Bilateral carcinoma of the breast: frequency and mortality. *Can J Surg 21:459,* 1978.

[64]Langlands A. Long-term survival of patients with breast cancer: a study of the curability of the disease. *Br Med J* 2:1247, 1979.

[65]Mueller C. Cancer of the breast: Its outcome as measured by the rate of dying and causes of death. *Ann Surg* 182:334, 1975.

[66]Brinkley D. Long-term survival of women with breast cancer. *Lancet* 1:1118, 1984.

[67]Adair F. Long-term follow-up of breast cancer patients: the 30-year report. *Cancer* 33:1145, 1974.

[68]Hibberd A. Long term prognosis of women with breast cancer in New Zealand: study of survival to 30 years. *Br Med J* 286:1777, 1983.

[69]Le M. Long-term survival of women with breast cancer. *Lancet* 2:922, 1984.

[70]Rutqvist L. Is breast cancer a curable disease? A study of 14,731 women with breast cancer from the cancer registry of Norway. *Cancer* 53:1793, 1984.

[71]Mueller C. Breast cancer in 3,558 women: age as a significant determinant in the rate of dying and the causes of death. *Surgery* 83:123, 1978.

[72]Fisher B. The contribution of recent NSABP clinical trials of primary breast cancer therapy to an understanding of tumor biology—an overview of findings. *Cancer* 46:1009, 1980.

[73]Gullino P. Natural history of breast cancer. Progression from hyperplasia to neoplasia as predicted by angiogenesis. *Cancer* 39:2697, 1977.

[74]MacDonald I. The natural history of mammary carcinoma. *Am J Surg* 3:435, 1966.

[75]Webster D. The prognostic significance of circulating tumour cells: A five-year follow-up study of patients with cancer of the breast. *Can Med Assoc J* 96:129, 1967.

[76]Fidler I. Recent concepts of cancer metastasis and their implications for therapy. *Cancer Treat Rep* 68:193, 1984.

[77]Brewin T. Point of view: The cancer patient-too many scans and x-rays? *Lancet* 2:1098, 1981.

[78]Coombes R. Assessment of biochemical tests to screen for metastases in patients with breast cancer. *Lancet* 1:296, 1980.

[79]Editorial: Follow up of patients with breast cancer. *Br Med J* 290:1229, 1985.

[80]Qualheim R. Breast carcinoma with multiple sites of origin. *Cancer* 10:460, 1957.

[81]Gallager H. Early phases in the developement of breast cancer. *Cancer* 24:1170, 1969.

[82]Leis H. Managing the remaining breast. *Cancer* 46:1026, 1980.

[83]Inquiry: fighting cancer. Interview with Vincent T. Devita Jr. by Richard Pyatt. *USA Today* Dec. 3, 1984.

[84]Hermann R. Results of conservative operations for breast cancer. *Arch Surg* 120:746, 1985.

[85]Doa T. The clinical significance of skin recurrence after radical mastectomy in women with cancer of the breast. *Surg Gynecol Obstet* 117:447, 1963.

[86]Mueller C. Editorial: Surgery for breast cancer: less may be as good as more. *N Engl J Med* 312:712, 1985.

[87]Chu F. Locally recurrent carcinoma of the breast. Results of radiation therapy. *Cancer* 37:2677, 1976.

[88]Madoc-Jones H. Evaluation of the effectiveness of radiotherapy in the management of early nodal recurrences from adenocarcinoma of the breast. *Breast* 2:31, 1976.

[89]Park W. The absolute curability of cancer of the breast. *Surg Gynecol Obstet* 93:129, 1951.

[90]Maguire G. Psychiatric problems in the first year after mastectomy. *Br Med J* 1:963, 1978.

[91]Editorial: Treatment of breast cancer—is conservative safe? *Lancet* 1:964, 1985.

[92]Danoff B. Conservative surgery and irradiation in the treatment of early breast cancer. *Ann Intern Med* 102:634, 1985.

[93]Mustakallio S. Treatment of breast cancer by tumour extirpation and roentgen treatment instead of radical operation. *J Fac Radiol* 6:23, 1954.

[94]Ferguson D. Late effects of adjuvant radiotherapy for breast cancer. *Cancer* 54:2319, 1984.

[95]Stjernsward J. Decreased survival related to irradiation postoperatively in early operable breast cancer. *Lancet* 2:1285, 1974.

[96]Bond W. The prognostic implication of treatment. *Proc Roy Soc Med* 63:111, 1970.

[97]Crile G. Rationale of simple mastectomy without radiation for clinical stage 1 cancer of the breast. *Surg Gynecol Obstet* 120:975, 1965.

[98]Park S. Immunosuppressive effect of surgery. *Lancet* 1:53, 1971.

[99]Han T. Postoperative immunosuppression in patients with breast cancer. *Lancet* 1:742, 1972.

[100]Blumberg N. Relation between recurrence of cancer of the colon and blood transfusions. *Br Med J* 290:1037, 1985.

[101]Meyer K. Radiation-induced lymphocyte-immune deficiency. A factor in the increased visceral metastases and decreased hormonal responsiveness of breast cancer. *Arch Surg* 101:114, 1970.

[102]Stjernsward J. Lymphopenia and change in distribution of human B and T lymphocytes in peripheral blood induced by irradiation for mammary carcinoma. *Lancet* 1:1352, 1972.

[103]Crile G. Results of conservative treatment of breast cancer at ten and 15 years. *Ann Surg* 181:26, 1975.

[104]Wallace I. Axillary nodes in breast cancer. *Lancet* 1:217, 1972.

[105]Kissin M. The inadequacy of axillary sampling in breast cancer. *Lancet* 1:1210,1982.

[106]Crile G. Possible role of uninvolved regional nodes in preventing metastasis from breast cancer. *Cancer* 24:1283, 1969.

[107]Fisher B. Studies concerning the regional lymph node in cancer. III. Response of regional lymph node cells from breast and colon cancer patients to PHA stimulation. *Cancer* 30:1202, 1972.

[108]Fisher B. Studies concerning the regional lymph node in cancer. IV. Tumor inhibition by regional lymph node cells. *Cancer* 33:631, 1974

[109]Fisher B. Studies concerning the regional lymph node in cancer. II. Maintenance of immunity. *Cancer* 29:1496, 1972

[110]Krajcovic D. Routine axillary node removal in the treatment of breast cancer—an illogical approach. *In Controversy In Surgery.* (eds) Varco R. Delaney J. W.B. Saunders Co. Philadelphia, 1976, p 75-80.

[111]Gewant W. Lymph node-breast carcinoma interrelations in tissue culture. *Surg Gynecol Obstet* 133:959, 1971.

[112]Fentiman I. Which patients are cured of breast cancer? *Br Med J* 289:1108, 1984.

[113]Edwards M. Regression of axillary lymph-nodes in cancer of the breast. *Br J Surg* 59:776, 1972.

[114]Vorherr H. Adjuvant chemotherapy of breast cancer: reality, hope, hazard? *Lancet* 2:1413, 1981.

[115]Vorherr H: Adjuvant chemotherapy of breast cancer : tumour kinetics and survival. *Lancet* 2:690, 1981.

[116]Howell A. Controlled trial of adjuvant chemotherapy with cyclophosphamide, methotrexate, and fluorouracil for breast cancer. *Lancet* 2:307, 1984.

[117]Palmer B. Adjuvant chemotherapy for breast cancer: side effects and quality of life. *Br Med J* 281:1594, 1980.

[118]Costanza M. Adjuvant chemotherapy: eight years later. *JAMA* 252:2611, 1984.

[119]Kerbel R. Facilitation of tumour progression by cancer therapy. *Lancet* 2:977, 1982.

[120]Lenders J. Viral infections during chemotherapy for breast cancer. *Br Med J* 290:1626, 1985.

[121]Blamey R. Trials of adjuvant chemotherapy in breast cancer. *Lancet* 1:920, 1979.

[122]Kushner R. Is aggressive adjuvant chemotherapy the Halsted radical of the '80s? *CA* 34:345, 1984.

[123]Smith I. Regular review: Adjuvant chemotherapy for early breast cancer. *Br Med J* 287:379, 1983.

[124]Henderson I. Adjuvant chemotherapy of breast cancer: a promising experiment or standard practice? *J Clin Oncol* 3:140, 1985.

[125]Rubens R. Controlled trial of adjuvant chemotherapy with melphalan for breast cancer. *Lancet* 1:839, 1983.

[126]Editorial: Breast cancer: adjuvant chemotherapy. *Lancet* 1:761, 1981.

[127]Santiago-Delpin E. Prolonged survival of skin and tumor allografts in mice on high fat diets. Brief communication. *J Natl Cancer Inst* 59:459, 1977.

[128]Meade C. The mechanism of immunoinhibition by arachidonic and linoleic acid: Effects on the lymphoid and reticulo- endothelial systems. *Int Arch Allergy Appl Immunol* 51:2, 1976.

[129]Ravdin R. Results of a clinical trial concerning the worth of prophylactic oopherectomy for breast carcinoma. *Surg Gynecol Obstet* 131:1055, 1970.

[130]Kennedy B. Therapeutic castration versus prophylactic castration in breast cancer. *Surg Gynecol Obstet* 118:524,1964.

[131]Pourquier H. Adjuvant chemotherapy of breast cancer: is it a direct cytotoxic or has it an indirect hormone effect? *Int J Radiat Oncol Biol Phys* 4:917, 1978.

[132]Rose C. Treatment of advanced breast cancer with tamoxifen. *Rec Results Cancer Res* 91:230, 1984.

[133]Campbell F. Quantitative oestradiol receptor values in primary breast cancer and response of metastases to endocrine therapy. *Lancet* 2:1317, 1981.

[134]Editorial: Tamoxifen. *Lancet* 1:1199, 1983.

[135]Controlled trial of tamoxifen as adjuvant agent in management of early breast cancer. Interim analysis at four years by Nolvadex Adjuvant Trial Organisation. *Lancet* 1:257, 1983.

[136]Controlled trial of tamoxifen as single adjuvant agent in management of early breast cancer. Analysis at six years by Nolvadex Adjuvant Trial Organisation. *Lancet* 1:836, 1985.

[137]Senanayake F. Adjuvant hormonal chemotherapy in early breast cancer: Early results from a controlled trial. *Lancet* 2:1148, 1984.

[138]Henderson I. Chemotherapy of breast cancer. A general overview. *Cancer* 51:2553, 1983.

[139]Rose C. Beneficial effect of adjuvant tamoxifen therapy in primary breast cancer patients with high oestrogen receptor values. *Lancet* 1:16, 1985.

[140]Editorial: Can interferons cure cancers? *Lancet* 1:1171, 1979.

[141]Dickson J. Hyperthermia in the treatment of cancer. *Lancet* 1:202, 1979.

[142]Mann G: Food intake and resistance to disease. *Lancet* 1:1238, 1980.

[143]Statement by Arthur C. Upton, M.D. Director, National Cancer Institute: Status of the diet, nutrition and cancer program before the Subcommittee on Nutrition. State Committee of Agriculture, Nutrition and Forestry Oct. 2, 1972.

[144]Committee on Diet, Nutrition, and Cancer: Assembly of Life Sciences, National Research Council. *Diet, Nutrition, and Cancer.* National Academy Press, Washington D.C. 1982.

[145]Nutrition and Cancer: Cause and Prevention. An American Cancer Society Special Report. *CA* 34:121, 1984.

[146]U.S. Senate Report: Dietary Goals for the United States. Government Printing Office, Washington, DC, 1977.

[147]Tartter P. Cholesterol and obesity as prognostic factors in breast cancer. *Cancer* 47:2222, 1981.

[148]Donegan W. The association of body weight with recurrent cancer of the breast. *Cancer* 41:1590, 1978.

[149]Smithline F. Prolactin and breast carcinoma. *N Engl J Med* 292:784, 1975.

[150]Vihko R. Estrogen and progesterone receptors in breast cancer. *Acta Obstet Gynecol Scand Suppl* 101:29, 1981.

[151]Legha S. Hormonal therapy of breast cancer: New approaches and concepts. *Ann Intern Med* 88:69, 1978.

[152]Stamler J. Lifestyles, major risk factors, proof and public policy. *Circulation* 58:3, 1978.

[153]Hill P. Diet and prolactin release. *Lancet* 2:806, 1976.

[154]Duncan K. The effects of high and low energy density diets on satiety, energy intake and eating time of obese and nonobese subjects. *Am J Clin Nutr* 37: 763, 1983.

[155]Fraser G. The effect of various vegetable supplements on serum cholesterol. *Am J Clin Nutr* 34:1272, 1981.

[156]Hill P. Effect of diet on plasma and urinary hormones in South African black men with prostatic cancer. *Cancer Res* 42:3864, 1982.

[157]McDougall J. Preliminary study of diet as an adjunct therapy for breast cancer. *Breast* 10:18, 1984.

[158]Johnston-Early A. Smoking abstinence and small cell lung cancer survival. An association. *JAMA* 244:2175, 1980.

[159]Hill P. Diet and endocrine-related cancer. *Cancer* 39:1820, 1977.

[160]Cruse P. Dietary cholesterol is co-carcinogenic for human colon cancer. *Lancet* 1:752, 1979.

[161]Littman M. Effect of cholesterol-free, fat-free diet and hypocholesteremic agents on growth of transplantable animal tumors. *Cancer Chemother Rep:* 50:25, 1966.

[162]Morrison A. Some international differences in treatment and survival in breast cancer. *Int J Cancer* 18:269, 1976.

[163]Wynder E. A comparison of survival rates between American and Japanese patients with breast cancer. *Surg Gynecol Obstet* 117:196, 1963.

[164]Nemoto T. Differences in breast cancer between Japan and the United States. *J Natl Cancer Inst* 58:193, 1977.

[165]Armstrong B. Environmental factors and cancer incidence and mortality in different countries, with special reference to dietary practices. *Int J Cancer* 15:617, 1975.

[166]McDougall J. *The McDougall Plan*, New Century Publ. Piscataway, 1983.

[167]NCI to study effect of low-fat diet on breast cancer, recurrence. *Intern Med News* 18:21, 1985.

[168]Lewison E. Spontaneous regression of breast cancer. *Natl Cancer Inst Monogr* 44:23, 1976.

[169]Cole W. Spontaneous regression of cancer: The metabolic triumph of the host? *Ann N Y Acad Sci* 230:111, 1974.

[170]Cancer Surveillance, Epidemiology, and End Results (SEER) Program, *Cancer Patient Survival—report no. 5*, DHEW publ no. (NIH) 77-992, 1976.

[171]McConnell R. Genetic aspects of gastrointestinal cancer. *Clin Gastro* 5:483, 1976.

[172]Ribet A. Occult blood tests and colorectal tumours. *Lancet* 1:417, 1980.

[173]Editorial: Screening for colorectal cancer. *Lancet* 2:1222, 1979.

[174]Evans J. Management and survival of carcinoma of the colon: results of a national survey by the American College of Surgeons. *Ann Surg* 188:716, 1978.

[175]Fisher E. The cytologic demonstration and significance of tumor cells in the mesenteric venous blood in patients with colorectal carcinoma. *Surg Gynecol Obstet* 100:102, 1955.

[176]Polk H. Surgical mortality and survival from colonic carcinoma. *Arch Surg* 89:16, 1964.

[177]Ederer F. Survival of patients with cancer of the large intestine and rectum, Connecticut, 1935-54. *J Natl Cancer Inst* 26:489, 1961.

[178]Holliday H. Delay in diagnosis and treatment of symptomatic colorectal cancer. *Lancet* 1:309, 1979.

[179]Stefanini P. Surgical treatment of cancer of the colon. *Int Surg* 66:125, 1981.

[180]Kies M. Editorial: Fluorouracil for colorectal cancer: A sobering look. *JAMA* 247:2826, 1982.

[181]Madden J. Electrocoagulation as a primary curative method in the treatment of carcinoma of the rectum. *Surg Gynecol* Obstet 157:164, 1983.

[182]Bremner C. Polyps and carcinoma of the large bowel in the South African Bantu. Cancer 26:991, 1970.

[183]Winawer S. Screening for colon cancer. *Gastroenterology* 70:783, 1976.

[184]Gilbertsen V. The prevention of invasive cancer of the rectum. *Cancer* 41:1137, 1978.

[185]Dunphy J. Etiologic factors in polyposis and carcinoma of the colon. *Ann Surg* 150:488, 1959.

[186]Williams R. Multiple polyposis, polyp regression, and carcinoma of the colon. *Am J Surg* 112:846, 1966.

[187]Cruse P. Dietary cholesterol deprivation improves survival and reduces incidence of metastatic colon cancer in dimethylhydrazine-pretreated rats. *Gut* 23:594, 1982.

[188]Hirohata T. Survival patterns from large bowel cancer in Hawaii. *Hawaii Med J* 36:343, 1977.

[189]Fergeson J. Disappearance, probably spontaneous, of locally inoperable carcinoma of the descending colon: report of a case. *Proc Mayo Clin* 29:407, 1954.

[190]Shapiro C. Remission of metastatic adenocarcinoma of the colon: case reports. *JAMA* 250:2503, 1983.

[191]Stamey T. Cancer of the prostate: An analysis of some important contributions and dilemmas. *Monographs in Urology,* 1982.

[192]Conant J. Survival with localized carcinoma: radical prostatectomy vs radiation therapy. *Urology* 25:347, 1985.

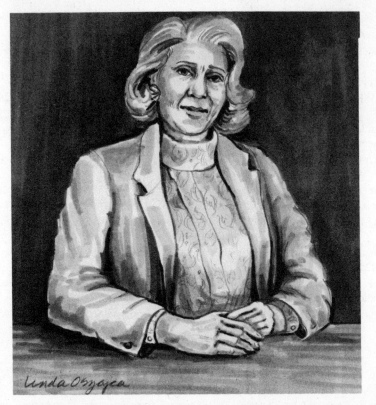

I've just turned fifty, my menstrual periods are stopping, and I'm worried sick that one of these days I'm going to break a hip and end up in the hospital. This happened to my mother without any warning when she was sixty-five. She didn't trip over something and fall. She was just walking across the kitchen floor when all of a sudden her leg gave way under her.

I've heard how important calcium is for strong bones, yet I can't drink milk because it gives me a stomachache and diarrhea. I'm afraid to take hormones; I think that's how mother got cancer. Besides, I don't believe in pills, whether they are prescribed by doctors or sold in health food stores. What a dirty deal! This is one of those times when I wish I was born a man.

3

OSTEOPOROSIS

What is osteoporosis? Everybody is talking about it these days.

Osteoporosis is a disorder related to aging, which is characterized by loss of enough bone minerals so that, even with little force, one or more bones can be broken.[1] The more bone material that is lost, the greater is the risk of breaking your bones.[2] Such a break is known as a *fracture*. Fractures due to osteoporosis are most common in the wrists, the backbone, and the hips, but they can occur in almost any bone in the body. Victims of this disease are not aware that anything is wrong because in the beginning osteoporosis is subtle and painless until a bone breaks. In some women, but certainly not all, the bones become so weak that they cannot withstand even minor physical forces encountered in daily living. Thus, a cough can break a rib, riding over a bumpy road can fracture a backbone, or nothing more than the weight of a woman's own body can cause her hip bones to crumble.

Osteoporosis sounds very serious. How common is it?

Osteoporosis is one of the most common bone diseases affecting women in affluent Western societies. It also occurs, but to a lesser extent, in aging men in those same societies. In fact, with all of the media coverage it has received during recent years, osteoporosis has become a household word. Even so, few people know very much about this condition.

Let me give you some facts about the disease as it occurs in the United States:[1,2-5]

• As many as 15 to 20 million persons are affected by osteoporosis in this country alone. It has reached epidemic proportions.

• In women over age sixty-five, 35 to 40 percent have suffered from one or more osteoporosis-related fractures.

• About 1.3 million fractures attributed to osteoporosis occur annually in people forty-five years and older.

• Approximately 100,000 wrist fractures occur annually from osteoporosis.

• Hip fractures are especially serious, with 190,000 occurring each year at a cost in excess of 1 billion dollars, and 80 percent of these fractures are in postmenopausal women.

• For people who reach the age of ninety, 32 percent of women and 17 percent of men will suffer from an osteoporosis-related hip fracture.

• At least 15,000 women die each year as a direct result of hip fractures. Of those who recover, only 25 percent regain full mobility.

• The diagnosis and care of people suffering from this disease has become a 4-billion-dollar-a-year health business in the United States.

Women should rightly fear this epidemic disease that can shorten not only their stature, but also their lives.

Does everyone eventually get osteoporosis if he or she lives long enough?

Loss of bone material with increasing age does not occur uniformly, and some people actually gain bone in their later years.[6] Furthermore, people in other societies of the world who observe different dietary practices and lifestyles suffer very rarely, if at all, from this bone disease.[7] Therefore, osteoporosis should not be accepted as part of getting older.

How do I find out if I have osteoporosis? Will an X-ray tell me?

The strength of a bone is estimated from the compactness or density of the bone material as measured by a variety of methods. With most standard X-ray techniques, it is difficult to estimate bone density accurately. By the time the earliest signs of osteoporosis appear in an X-ray film, about one-third of the bone has already disappeared.[3] Even then the diagnosis is based most often on the types of fractures that are seen in the X-ray film, rather than by how "thin" the bones appear to be in the picture.

Some doctors use a new method called a *photon absorptiometry bone scanner* to estimate bone thickness. Very small electromagnetic particles called *photons* are shot through the bone. The density of the bone is determined by the amount of photons it absorbs. Compact bone, being denser, absorbs more photons. As a result of public concern about this disease, screening clinics are being established all over the country. The cost for annual screening is about 40 to 100 dollars per examination.

How do the bones become so weak?

Osteoporosis is an actual decrease in the amount of bone material. The loss includes minerals such as calcium and phosphorus, as well as the protein-rich structural material that forms the bed in which the minerals are deposited.

This generalized loss of bone material can occur under several different circumstances. Osteoporosis is found most often in women after menopause. However, immobilization of a person due to an illness or an accident, as well as certain metabolic conditions such as diabetes or kidney and thyroid diseases, and some medications, such as corticosteroids, can also cause significant bone loss that may lead to early and severe osteoporosis.

You mentioned that most fractures occur in women past the menopause. How is this condition related to menopause?

At the time of menopause, the ovaries' production of the female hormones, *estrogens,* gradually ceases. As a result the menstrual periods become irregular at first and later stop altogether. Estrogens play an important role in bone metabolism.[1,2] Bone material everywhere in the body is constantly being formed and broken down throughout life. Estrogens slow the rate of bone breakdown. But hormones do little to increase the rate of formation of new bone tissue. Because of this, giving estrogen pills to postmenopausal women suffering from osteoporosis will not cause bone tissues to regenerate to premenopausal levels; it will only slow the rate of loss from the remaining bone.

Maximum bone thickness is reached at around age thirty-five. After the age of forty a woman who is destined to suffer from osteoporosis loses about 0.5 percent of her skeleton per year. After menopause the rate of loss accelerates to 1 to 2 percent or more per year.[8,9] The rate of bone loss is most rapid right after menopause, and then it slows down approximately ten years later. By the age of sixty-five 40 percent of the initial adult skeleton is gone.[10]

When a women loses the function of her ovaries earlier than the normal age of menopause in most women, the loss of bone material is even more rapid and her condition is more severe.[3] Usually this premature loss of ovary function is the result of surgery, radiation, or chemotherapy that has been used to treat some other illness.

Tell me more about osteoporosis in men.

The condition does occur in men, but in them it is less severe and rarely begins to appear before age seventy-five, whereas most women begin to show signs of the disease in their fifties and sixties.[9] Men do not naturally pass through a period of rapid decrease in production of reproductive hormones that is comparable to menopause in women. The sustained levels of male androgen hormones and, to some extent, the greater physical activity of men help to maintain their bone strength longer than is likely with women.[11]

I don't understand how something as natural as menopause could be the cause of such a serious disease as osteoporosis. What really causes it?

The cause of osteoporosis involves many factors, but a flaw in the design for females is not one of them. What's the sense in designing a body intended to last eighty-five years and then equipping it with a set of bones that holds up for only sixty years? We must conclude that osteoporosis is a disease, not an expected, natural condition in life. And, as with other diseases, a cause or causes must exist.

Racial background is considered by many investigators to be important because of the high incidence of the disease in American Caucasian women and its low incidence in Asians and African blacks.[7] However, the protective effects of heredity are difficult to separate from diet and lifestyle. Rarity of osteoporosis in certain populations probably has little to do with their genetic strength. More likely it is a benefit passed on to successive generations through safeguards in diet and custom.

What kind of cultural differences would have an effect on osteoporosis?

Several factors in lifestyle and nutrition have been found to cause bone loss. Smoking tobacco, drinking alcohol and caffeine, and lack of exercise have been associated with greater than usual loss of calcium and other bone matter from the body.[12-15] These factors, unlike age and gender, can be controlled and changed; therefore, they can be used as measures in the prevention and treatment of osteoporosis.

Most investigators have considered that the foods we eat exert the strongest influence on the strength of the bones we make.[16] This should not be surprising. Each day we take in from one to five pounds of foods which provide the raw materials that our bodies use to function and grow. The building blocks for our bones also come from the foods we eat each day. Because the incidence of osteoporosis varies among different populations that are following a variety of diets, researchers have looked to the kinds of foods that people eat for clues to the causes of weakness or strength of their bones.

What nutrients have an effect on my bones?

The important components of the diet that have been thought to affect the bones are vitamin D, phosphorus, fluorides, calcium, and proteins.

A deficiency in vitamin D has been suspected for a long time because of the important role this vitamin plays in bone metabolism. However, several reasons have been found to explain why osteoporosis is not a disease caused by vitamin D deficiency. In the first place, vitamin D is actually a hormone synthesized in our bodies by the action of sunlight on the skin. The vitamin D levels in a person's body are a direct result of the amount of sunlight received and are not dependent upon dietary sources of this hormone, which is synthesized in the body.[17] Only under very unusual circumstances would someone fail to receive the small amount of sunlight that is required to produce adequate levels of vitamin D.[17] Elderly people who are confined indoors would be most susceptible to vitamin D deficiency. However, even then the lack of vitamin D is not likely to contribute in any way to the development of osteoporosis.[18]

Much research has been done on the treatment of osteoporosis with vitamin D. This approach has not met with success in reducing the numbers of fractures in patients with osteoporosis.[9,19-21] Furthermore, vitamin D taken in excess is toxic and can cause serious illness. When used alone to treat osteoporosis, this vitamin can have a harmful effect because it is actually a potent hormone that stimulates reabsorption of bone material.[22]

I don't know much about fluorides and phosphorus. How do they affect bones?

Fluorides and phosphorus are simple chemicals that are incorporated in the bone structure along with calcium. The amount of each in the diet has an effect on bone metabolism.[16] *Fluoride* salts are present in all natural foods and in some places they are present naturally in higher concentrations in drinking water, while elsewhere they are added intentionally to foods and water supplies. The fluoride element is one of the most effective stimulators of new bone growth, and people living in areas supplied with fluoridated water have greater bone densities than those who are not exposed to higher concentrations of this mineral.[16] However, treatment of osteoporosis with fluoride supplements alone or in combination with calcium and vitamin D has been disappointing.[20,21,23] Bone tissue formed under the influence of large doses of fluoride appears to have less strength, as shown by the unfortunate fact that this treatment fails to reduce the rate of fractures.[20,23] A further disadvantage to the deliberate use of this mineral is that almost 40 percent of the patients who are treated with fluoride develop significant side effects, including vomiting, bleeding stomach ulcers, and joint pains.[24]

Dietary *phosphorus,* present in all foods, is found in high amounts in meats, dairy products, additives, and soft drinks. Problems of bone metabolism develop when the intake of phosphorus is much greater than that of calcium, and this imbalance has been suspected as a cause of bone loss related to age.[10] However, several studies have failed to show any deleterious effects from high-phosphorus diets.[10] Treatment of osteoporosis by changing the calcium-phosphorus balance has been without benefit.[10]

What about calcium? I see advertisements wherever I look, telling me to drink milk to keep my bones strong. Should I just force it down, even if it makes me sick?

The latest recommendation from the National Institutes of Health to help women prevent early bone loss advises them to consume 1000 to 1500 milligrams of calcium a day.[1] This message has the solid backing of the National Dairy Council and has also made millionaires out of manufacturers and distributors of calcium supplement pills.

However, these recommendations for additional calcium intake are based on conflicting data from studies on natural populations and experimental groups of humans.[3] In most published studies about calcium, the correlation between dietary calcium intake and bone density has been weak or non-existent.[25,26] In other words, people who consume more calcium in their diets have not been found to develop stronger bones than people who have low-calcium diets. Studies actually have shown that an intake of 150 to 200 milligrams of calcium daily is adequate to meet the needs of most normal people, even during pregnancy and lactation.[27] The controversy over recommendations of increased calcium intake will continue for a long time because of one undeniable fact: most of the world's population ingests 300 to 500 milligrams of calcium daily, which is much less than the recommended daily amount of 800 milligrams now being promoted in the United States. Nevertheless, those people receiving the smaller amounts are able to grow and maintain normal adult skeletons.[25]

Let's look at some of these values for comparison.

SOURCE	Milligrams (mg)
Minimum calcium need, determined by experiment	150-200 mg
Worldwide calcium intake in most populations	300-500 mg
World Health Organization recommendation for minimum intake for adults	400-500 mg
Food and Nutrition Board recommendation for the USA	800 mg
Recent proposal for USA by the National Institutes of Health	1000-1500 mg

It must be very confusing for you to see such a wide discrepancy in figures for our daily calcium needs. As we talk further, I shall explain why so much confusion has arisen over this basic dietary component.

All my life I have believed that added calcium, especially from dairy products, is necessary for my health. I thought that people living in third-world countries were deprived of good nutrition because they couldn't drink three or four glasses of milk every day.

Throughout history, in every part of the world, people have had no trouble making bones that lasted a lifetime, without the need to include any dairy products or calcium pills in their daily diet until recently. Actually, the inclusion of dairy products in the diet had been limited to only a few people because of the lack of refrigeration or the cost of owning a dairy cow. But during the last century technology has advanced to the point where milk can be produced, preserved, and distributed to millions of people in Western nations. Now dairy products are available to most people living in developed countries; and, paradoxically, now too we have this outburst of osteoporosis.

If we examine the worldwide distribution of cases of osteoporosis today, we are struck by the fact that this disease is most common in countries where dairy products and calcium supplements are consumed in the largest quantities: the United States, Sweden, Finland, and United Kingdom.[28-31] The occurrence of osteoporosis is rare in Asian and African countries, where milk is not consumed because it is not available or because of a very high incidence of *lactose intolerance*.[7,28-31] As many as 90 percent of Asians and blacks have this inability to digest lactose, or milk sugar.[32] People with lactose intolerance learn to avoid most milk products because they often develop diarrhea, stomach cramps, and intestinal gas from milk sugar. On the evidence of the distribution of osteoporosis in the many countries of the world, we can conclude that eating dairy products does not appear to have a significant protective effect against whatever agent is causing this disease.

Location	Hip fractures rate /100,000	Dairy intake grams/day/person	Protein intake grams/day/person total	animal
United States	98	462	106	72
Sweden	70	502	89	59
Israel	59	315	105	57
Finland	44	711	93	61
United Kingdom	43	455	90	54
Hong Kong	32	95	82	50
Singapore	20	113	82	39
South Africa/ Black townships	6	10	55	11

OSTEOPOROSIS AND SELECTED NUTRIENTS[29-31]

Worldwide, the incidence of osteoporosis has a direct correlation to the total protein, and especially, the animal protein intake of a population of people; the more animal protein consumed by the people, the more the osteoporosis in the population. Furthermore, a high consumption of dairy products offers little protection for the bones, since countries with the highest intakes of these products— United States, Sweden, Israel, Finland, and the United Kingdom— also have the highest rates of osteoporosis-related hip fractures. Likewise, a low intake of dairy products appears to in no way harm the bones since the countries with the lowest intakes of dairy products— Hong Kong, Singapore, and rural Africa—have the lowest rates of osteoporosis.[28-31] (All numbers have been rounded off to whole numbers. Figures for hip fractures from some countries may actually be from the population of a large city in that country).

If calcium intake has no relation to bone strength, then why are so many people being told to take calcium pills and eat lots of dairy products?

Some studies have shown that bone loss is reduced when postmenopausal women are treated with daily calcium supplements.[33-37] These are the studies that are emphasized whenever recommendations for increasing calcium intake are made. However, many other studies disagree with those findings and report no benefit to bone density from daily calcium supplements.[20,38-40] Large doses of calcium have been given intravenously to women with osteoporosis, and even this aggressive therapy has not shown consistent benefit for the bones.[41,42] The many studies showing no positive effects of calcium supplementation have apparently had little influence on advice we have received recently from health experts. Although undoubtedly one's diet should be adequate in its content of minerals and vitamins, the present evidence is far from convincing that osteoporosis is effectively treated, much less prevented, with supplements of calcium in the form of tablets or milk products.[3]

A recent study observed the effect of calcium supplements on the bones of 103 postmenopausal women.[40] The calcium intakes these women received from the foods they ate were supplemented with 500 milligrams of calcium tablets per day. After two years, women who consumed less then 550 milligrams of calcium daily showed bone loss similar to that in those who took as much as 2000 milligrams per day. The investigators concluded that calcium intakes of 1000 to 2000 milligrams a day were ineffective in preventing bone loss in early menopause.

If I don't get my calcium from dairy products or calcium pills, from what other sources can I get this essential nutrient?

Calcium is found in all foods, and the amounts are sufficient to easily supply enough of this essential nutrient to meet the requirements for growing children and adults. Many green and yellow vegetables and fruits give plentiful amounts of calcium. Meats, poultry, and fish are low in calcium unless you eat their bones. Dairy products, as we have all learned, are concentrated sources of calcium.

The primary source of calcium, as for other minerals, is the soil. Plants absorb minerals from watery solutions in the soil and incorporate them in their tissue cells to serve varying needs. Animals consume the plant parts and absorb the calcium from them. Humans have a highly efficient intestinal tract that, under almost every circumstance, will absorb the correct amount of calcium to meet the body's needs. The intestinal cells act as regulators of the amount of calcium that enters the body. The amount absorbed is relatively independent of the amount of calcium that is present in the foods eaten. When the calcium content of the diet is low, then a relatively higher percentage of this mineral is absorbed from the foods.[43] If the diet is high in calcium, then a smaller percentage of the calcium is absorbed.[43] But the body's need is always the controlling factor regulating the entry of calcium into the cells of the intestinal wall.

I've heard that the fiber in plant foods prevents the calcium from being absorbed. Can too many vegetables can lead to calcium deficiency and osteoporosis?

Not only fiber, but also oxylates and phytates, which are found in high concentrations in plants, will combine with calcium and other minerals and prevent them from being absorbed. Experimental studies have shown that this combining action decreases the amounts of those minerals that the body can absorb.[44] This concern is largely experimental and theoretical because actual cases of mineral deficiency caused by these components in vegetable foods are, however, almost nonexistent. While there is a suggestion that in actual living situations, increased consumption of cereals and vegetables will reduce the amounts of minerals that can be absorbed, the added cereals and vegetables themselves will increase the intake of calcium and other minerals, and thereby limit any deleterious effects on mineral status that might be caused by fibers or phytates in vegetable foods.[45] A recent study found no evidence of mineral deficiencies in people maintained on long-term, high-fiber, vegetarian diets.[46] The case for the adverse effects of fiber, oxylates, and phytates has been exaggerated way out of true perspective and unfortunately has become one excuse for many people who protest against adding more vegetables to their diet.

I couldn't become a strict vegetarian. I'm still worried that I would get a disease from calcium deficiency if I relied only on starches, vegetables, and fruits for my calcium.

An important fact to remember is that all natural diets, including purely vegetarian diets without a hint of dairy products, contain amounts of calcium that are above the threshold for meeting your nutritional needs. In fact, the scientific literature states clearly that a "calcium deficiency disease" due to a low calcium intake from natural diets simply does not exist.[27,28,47,48] In other words, all diets provide adequate calcium to meet our health needs, and for most people in the world today milk is not a part of their diet. The same is true for all adult animals. The guilty agent that causes osteoporosis is not a deficiency in calcium.

Since every one of us takes in as much as or more calcium than he or she needs, the excess that is not needed is either passed out of the body with the feces or by way of the kidneys into the urine.

Do you know of any specific examples of people who live on a starch-centered diet and still have healthy bones?

Because of widespread famine in many parts of Africa, many of us have difficulty in thinking of those people as examples of good health. Nonetheless, in times of plenty most Africans eat a diet that gives them ample amounts of grains, vegetables, and fruits. The health of these people does offer an excellent contrast to that of people living in our society, who eat a diet centered on meats and dairy products. A specific example of people with strong bones who after weaning are raised on milk-free diets is the Bantu women of Africa.[49] These women consume 240 to 450 milligrams of calcium a day which is present in grains, fruits, and vegetables. Those amounts are one-half to one-third the amounts of calcium that are consumed each day by American women. Not uncommonly, Bantu women bear as many as ten babies during a lifetime. And they nurse each child for ten months, which places a further demand upon their calcium needs. Yet even with this requirement for large amounts of calcium; and so low an intake by our standards, osteoporosis is almost unknown among these hardy women, and many live to an old age.[7,28,49] An estimated 10 percent of the population is more than sixty years old; therefore, these Bantu women reach an age when osteoporosis would certainly appear if it were going to do so.[50]

Couldn't the low incidence of osteoporosis in blacks be due to their genetic makeup?

Heredity is not likely to be very important, because when African blacks move to affluent countries and change their diets and lifestyles, osteoporosis becomes common among them.[51] Like almost everyone else living in the United States, black women choose a diet centered around meat and dairy products. Through generations of living in this country they have learned the general American way of eating that increases their calcium intake considerably, as well as their protein intake. The incidence of osteoporosis in black women approaches that of Caucasian women eating a high-protein diet.[51]

What does increasing the intake of proteins have to do with bone loss?

An important point about the Bantu women is that their diet provides only about 50 grams of proteins a day. That is less than half the protein intake of most American women.

The first clue implicating proteins in the diet as an important cause of osteoporosis came from studies of different populations, such as Africans and Americans. The more proteins, especially those from animal sources, that are consumed by a group of people in a society, the greater is the incidence of osteoporosis in that population.[7,29,31] This strongly positive relationship between protein consumption and osteoporosis is very different from the evidence that little or no correlation exists between strong bones and consumption of dairy products for their content of calcium.[25,26,28-30,52] See chart page 68.

How does eating proteins damage the bones?

Proteins in excess cause the body to lose large amounts of calcium and other minerals, which are excreted through the kidneys into the urine. This loss is not compensated for by a sufficient increase in absorption of calcium from the intestines. The net result is that more calcium leaves the interior of the body than is absorbed into it. This creates a condition that is called *a negative calcium balance*. The measurement of calcium balance is useful because a reasonable correspondence exists between this value and bone loss in postmenopausal women.[53] Therefore, studies of calcium balance in groups of patients can be used as one measurement of the influence of different nutrients on bone metabolism and to judge the effectiveness of various therapies in altering the rate of bone loss.

One common method of determining the calcium balance begins with measuring the total amount of calcium in the foods the subjects are to eat during the test period. Then, during the test, all urine and fecal material from each subject is collected and analyzed for calcium content. Calcium balance is calculated as the total intake minus the sum in the urine and fecal discharges. If this value is positive—that is, if the amount of calcium introduced is greater than the amount lost—the difference represents the amount of calcium that is added to the body and presumed to be stored in the bones. If the value is negative, this indicates that more calcium is lost from the body than is absorbed and that the bones are likely to be sources of this extra calcium that is lost.

I thought I needed lots of proteins in order to grow and be strong. Now you tell me that proteins can damage my bones. I need a whole reeducation about what to eat.

The idea that if a little protein is good then more is better is a common fallacy. The beef industry recently launched a big advertising promotion to tell us that "beef gives strength", taking advantage of the widely accepted myth that high-protein beef is a body-building food. Considering that the giants in the food industry, those marketing meats, dairy products and eggs, sell foods that are high in proteins, we can see why people continue to misunderstand the true place of proteins in their diets.

At most, an adult needs no more than 20 grams of proteins a day, or about two-thirds of an ounce. These proteins are needed to grow hair, replace skin, produce hormones, form tissue cells, and for many other uses.[54] Most Americans consume 105 to 120 grams and more of proteins each day (different studies give a range of estimates). What happens to the excess 100 grams of proteins?

Excess calories from fats and carbohydrates are stored in the form of body fats, but there is no such storage system for proteins.[55] If we did store proteins they would pile up in our muscles, and, after years of gorging on high-protein diets, most of us would resemble body builders, like Arnold Schwarzenegger and the Hulk.

What happens to those excess proteins if they are not stored?

Most of the proteins we eat are broken down into their component amino acids, which are the ingredients that pass through the intestinal wall into the bloodstream. Once they enter the blood, some of the amino acids are used for the body's various needs and some of the excess is metabolized in the liver into urea, a powerful diuretic. Many people who have tried high-protein diets in order to lose weight have experienced the diuretic effect of urea: they lose almost eight pounds of water weight during the first week.

When urea and amino acids enter the kidneys on the way to elimination in urine, they cause not only the loss of excess water but also the excretion of large amounts of minerals.[56] One of the most important minerals lost in that way is calcium. The more proteins that are consumed, the greater is the loss of calcium. Researchers estimate that doubling the amount of proteins in the diet will increase by 50 percent the amount of calcium lost in the urine.[57] Many experimental studies have shown that when healthy adults consume amounts of proteins representative of the amounts many Americans eat every day, a negative mineral balance develops.[57-61] I'd like to show you the results of some typical calcium-balance studies of people on low- and high-protein intakes.

EFFECTS OF LOW AND
HIGH-PROTEIN DIETS ON CALCIUM BALANCE

Principal Investigator (initials)	Calcium Intake (milligrams)	Balance with a low-protein intake	Balance with a high-protein intake
C.A.	500	+31	−120
M.H.	500	+24	−116
R.W.	800	+12	−85
N.J.	1400	+10	−84
H.L.	1400	+20	−65
Average	**920**	**+19**	**−94**

Low-protein diets contained 47 to 50 grams of proteins, and the high-protein diets offered 141 to 150 grams of proteins.[57-61] Calcium balance figures are calculated for twenty-four hours. These studies used supplementary mixtures of proteins added to the normal diet in order to raise the protein content to higher levels.

In these experiments, the net loss of calcium for subjects eating the high-protein diet averaged a negative 94 milligrams per day. In order for a woman to develop osteoporosis, she'd need to maintain a negative balance of calcium of only 30 to 40 milligrams each day.[62] Considering that the average protein intake in America is around 120 grams each day, and many estimates are higher, we can believe that most Americans are living each day in negative calcium balance and are losing more calcium from their bodies each day than they are absorbing from the quantities of food they devour.

Please note also from these studies that reducing the intake of proteins consistently leads to an average positive calcium balance; this positive balance means that loss of calcium from the bones has stopped. A further reasonable assumption would be that the positive mineral balances mean remineralization of the bones is occurring and thereby the reversal of bone loss.

These examples may start you thinking for the first time that stuffing yourself with more portions of all those favorite foods should no longer be your primary goal at the table. Only a very few ounces of chicken added to the other protein foods in your daily menus could easily swamp your system with enough proteins to cause a negative calcium balance. You can fill yourself up on rice and potatoes and still stay in a safe range of protein intake without the pangs of hunger. In terms of familiar foods, 50 grams of proteins could mean portions like any one of the following: 6 ounces of chicken without skin, 7 ounces of broiled cod, or 1 2/3 cups of low-fat cottage cheese. In contrast, from vegetable sources fifty grams of proteins would be the equivalent of 25 medium boiled potatoes or 11 cups of cooked rice.

Will adding more calcium to my daily intake compensate for the loss of calcium caused by the proteins in my diet?

Increasing calcium intake may improve the balance, especially when a person is on a high-protein diet.[26] However, the studies described here and others consistently show that even large increases in the calcium intake fail to compensate for the calcium losing effects of the proteins.[57-61,63] Note in particular that a calcium intake in two of the studies of 1400 milligrams daily, which is consistent with the most recent recommendations by the National Institutes of Health, did little to resolve the negative balance caused by such a high protein level, as is consumed by many people in affluent countries. Investigators have shown that the body does not adapt over long periods of time to the calcium-losing effects of protein.[63] And the losses go on day after day until the bones are so weak an affectionate hug fractures several ribs and a backbone.

On very high protein intakes of 225 grams a day it has been estimated that adults will lose 4 percent of their skeleton per year, even while taking 1400 milligrams of calcium a day.[63] Although a diet providing 225 grams of protein per day offers more than most people would eat, even in affluent countries, many individuals do exceed this level. People on high-protein weight-reducing diets, body builders taking protein powders, and those who indulge a passion for eating chicken, beef, fish, and cottage cheese to the exclusion of vegetable foods are most likely to develop this alarming degree of calcium loss and consequent osteoporosis.

When a low-protein diet is consumed the amount of calcium given has little or no effect on calcium absorption through the intestine into the body.[61] As these studies show, when the diet provides around 50 grams of proteins, an amount closer to our actual needs, all levels of calcium create a positive balance, and raising the intake of calcium makes no improvement in the balance.[57-61]

I would like to emphasize that the calcium-losing effect of protein on the human body is not an area of controversy in scientific circles. The many studies performed during the past fifty-five years consistently show that the most important dietary change that we can make if we want to create a positive calcium balance that will keep our bones solid is to decrease the amounts of proteins we eat each day.[64] The important change is not to increase the amount of calcium we take in.

Is it simply the diuretic effect of proteins that washes the calcium out of the body, or do proteins have other effects?

Other properties of proteins also affect calcium metabolism in the kidneys and in the bones. Proteins are made up of different combinations of approximately twenty assorted building blocks called *amino acids*. Some of these amino acids have a direct effect upon the tubules of the kidneys, preventing the reabsorption into the body of calcium that enters the tubules from the bloodstream. As a result, that soluble calcium is lost in the urine.

Proteins and amino acids are weak acids. These acids act by still another mechanism that prevents the reabsorption of calcium by the kidney.[56] Also, as these weakly acidic proteins and amino acids enter the bloodstream, they must be neutralized to prevent them from causing harm to the body. To accomplish this, bone material must be dissolved to provide calcium and phosphates. The alkaline phosphate from this combination neutralizes the amino acids, and the freed calcium ions are available to be excreted by the kidneys and lost to the body.[65,66]

Another adverse effect on calcium balance is caused by those amino acids which contain sulfur. All twenty of the common amino acids are made of different arrangements of the elements carbon, hydrogen, oxygen, and nitrogen. Three of these twenty amino acids also incorporate the element sulfur in their structures, and they have a very powerful calcium-losing effect on the kidneys.[67] Animal proteins have an especially high content of sulfur-containing amino acids. Methionine is a typical sulfur-containing amino acid. Roughly twice as much of this amino acid is present in meats as in grains, and five times as much methionine is found in meats as in beans.[68] In 1930, the first study was published that showed that in humans a diet with a high meat content caused the loss of large amounts of calcium and a negative calcium balance.[69] And yet, fifty-five years later, our learned medical authorities are still pondering the cause of osteoporosis!

So you're saying that too much protein is the most important cause of osteoporosis, and that animal protein is the worst of all. Are there any examples of people who eat lots of animal protein and have very "thin" bones?

One well-studied example is the Eskimos. The Eskimos' traditional diet consists almost entirely of meats from fishes, walruses, seals, and whales, and it provides 200 to 400 grams of protein daily.[70] Eskimos also eat plenty of calcium in fish bones; their intake is estimated to be as much as 2500 milligrams of calcium per day, which is a very large amount indeed. Both men and women, as they age, show early and large loss of bone material. Eskimos over the age of forty have an average of 10 to 15 percent less bone than do comparable Caucasians in the United States. Eskimo women lose 10 to 12 percent of their skeleton per decade, compared with a 9.5 percent loss estimated for American white females.[70] In general, Eskimo bones appear to be ten years older than those of American women. This condemns even more a high-protein diet when we consider that Eskimos have the protective advantage of being very active physically.

If all this information is this well supported by research, then why do so many health professionals ignore the effects of proteins and simply say that adding more calcium to our diet will prevent osteoporosis?

That is a simple question to ask and a difficult one to answer, when we consider what the scientific studies that have been performed to date show about the effects of proteins and calcium on our calcium balance. Consider these factors as possible influences upon present recommendations. To prevent bone loss by lowering the protein content in the diet is a therapy that the food industry, not to mention most consumers, just will not accept. Lowering the protein intake in our national diet would cause meat, egg, and dairy industries to suffer great economic hardship. Approaching the problem by ignoring the role that proteins play and recommending instead that we gulp down more calcium each day offends no established industrial interest. In fact, recommending more calcium boosts the business of the dairy industry and the companies that produce calcium supplements. Then, too, from the consumers' viewpoint, if high-protein foods are blamed for causing osteoporosis, we might have to give up all those tasty delicacies we've learned to love, like steaks, chicken, fish, and cottage cheese. Instead we'd have to like lower-protein grains and fresh fruits and vegetables. Some very big changes will be required from everyone if and when this issue ever comes to public and scientific attention, where it belongs.

Once I heard a dietitian say that even though the meats we eat are high in proteins, they contain lots of phosphorus that prevents calcium loss. Is this true?

Phosphorus will decrease the loss of calcium caused by the high protein content of a diet, but in most studies the improvement seen is not sufficient to correct the negative calcium balance and prevent the devastating effects on bones. Meat is high in both proteins and phosphorus. In most experiments, eating meat caused a negative calcium balance in subjects fed such a diet.[57] Two recent studies have shown an increase of 23 percent or more in calcium excretion when tuna fish and other meats are added to the diet.[71,72] Another experiment specifically designed to demonstrate the effects of phosphorus on calcium metabolism in human subjects, showed a 28 percent increase in calcium loss when a low-protein intake was raised to a high-protein intake, even when a high phosphorus level was provided by the diet.[57] Again, the adverse effects of meat in a population are demonstrated by the exaggerated bone loss seen in Eskimos who eat little else besides meats.[70]

Controversy over the effect of meats on calcium balance continues today because of the opinions expressed by one group of investigators whose work is supported by research grants from the National Livestock and Meat Board and the National Dairy Council.[73,74] They claim that meats do not adversely effect calcium balance, presumably because of the high phosphorus content of the meats.[73,74] The discrepancy in results between this group's work and that of others has yet to be explained. However, the selection of the human subjects studied by these investigators has been criticized.[10] Because of existing health problems with some of the subjects used in their experiments, a negative calcium balance may not have been observed as expected when meats were added to the diet.

Perhaps milk is a better source of calcium than pills. All my life I have heard that milk will build strong bones and teeth. Won't drinking milk cause the calcium balance to become positive?

Although the effect of milk consumption on calcium balance seems like an obvious issue to investigate, almost no research has been done on this important subject. Actually, the first study done to determine the effects of milk consumption on the calcium metabolism of healthy postmenopausal women was reported in February 1985.[75] This study, funded by the National Dairy Council, attempted to show the benefits of drinking milk for women susceptible to osteoporosis. However, the study's results failed to show a significant increase in calcium balance when the diets of these women were supplemented with three 8-ounce glasses of low-fat milk daily for one year. According to these investigators, "...this may have been due to the average 30 percent increase in protein intake during milk supplementation." In their scientific wisdom, they concluded by recommending a reduction in protein intake in the diet from other sources than milk (such as chicken and fish) in order to improve calcium balance. The women drinking the milk supplement were still in negative calcium balance after one year of taking nearly 1500 milligrams of calcium daily![75]

All my life I've believed that milk was nearly a perfect food. It's hard for me to adjust to what you're telling me now.

Let's suppose you actually do need 1000 to 1500 milligrams of calcium a day and that this need is satisfied by drinking three or four 8-ounce glass of milk a day in addition to calcium in other foods you eat. Even if it is recommended, so much milk could mean that as much as one-third of the calories in the diets of many older women would be derived from milk alone.

Taking dairy products in order to obtain the additional calcium invites some serious risks to health. Three classes of components in cow's milk provide calories: fats, proteins, and carbohydrates. Each of these is associated with known health hazards. The fats are believed to be involved in the cause of heart attacks, cancer, and obesity; the proteins can cause food allergies, mineral imbalance, and possibly kidney damage; and lactose, the major carbohydrate in milk can cause a number of digestive problems in many people.[76] Dairy products are deficient for human needs in iron, fiber, as well as essential fatty acids, vitamin B1 and vitamin C. Also, dairy products all too often are highly contaminated with chemicals from the environment, bacteria and viruses.[76] In the United States more than 20 percent of the dairy cows are infected with leukemia viruses.[77] When these viruses are fed to chimpanzees, the experimental animals have developed leukemia.[77]

How can a food having so much potential to cause so many different illnesses in people be the source of a nutrient necessary for human health? Nature was never so unkind; only people prevent nature's intentions. By observing the way in which milk is used by animals, we see that after the weaning period, no animals depend on milk for calcium, and no other animal living in a natural setting drinks the milk of another species.

Another concern with the multi-million dollar advertising campaign laid on us by the dairy industry is based on the fact that the increased consumption of fats from all those dairy products may decrease the incidence of osteoporosis in women in our country by a means no one in the dairy industry will point out: simply by increasing the number of women dying early in life from heart disease or cancer, long before they reach an age when they would be at risk for osteoporosis. Women who think they are sensible by choosing to eat the low-fat forms of dairy products are still contributing to their risks for food allergies, kidney and bone damage from excess proteins, and problems of lactose intolerance.[76]

I can certainly agree with you that my nutritional needs are not the same as those of a baby calf. So from now on I won't drink milk. Will calcium pills hurt me also?

The human intestinal tract has built-in safety mechanisms that protect us from much of our dietary foolishness. When we drink cow's milk or swallow pills loaded with potentially toxic minerals such as calcium, the active intestinal lining blocks the entry into our bloodstream of high doses of this mineral that otherwise could kill us.[43] Without this protection our blood calcium levels would rise, and soft tissues, such as those in muscles and kidneys, would develop calcium deposits. Calcification of the kidneys can result in kidney failure and early death.

"Calcium overdose" can actually be caused by a once-popular form of therapy for duodenal "stomach" ulcers called the Sippy Diet.[78] This regimen consisted of antacids and milk products taken at alternate hours. The diet's purpose was to lower the acid content of the stomach to speed healing of the ulcer. But, unfortunately the Sippy Diet led to a high level of calcium in the blood, an alkaline system, and calcification of the soft tissues.[78] Apparently the antacids hindered the body's ability to protect itself from the high calcium content of the dairy products.

Another recent finding with a few popular calcium supplements should discourage you from using certain products. This is the additional hazard of contamination with dangerous chemicals. Some brands of bone meal and dolomite contain harmful amounts of lead, arsenic, mercury, and other toxic metals.[79]

Could taking an uncontaminated calcium supplement without antacids offer a little added benefit without causing any harm?

As I've mentioned, some studies have shown that benefits can be gained from calcium supplements taken daily, but only when people are on a high-protein calcium-losing diet. Because of the virtual absence of toxic reactions to calcium pills, you will not harm yourself by taking daily an additional 500 to 1000 milligrams of calcium in tablet or capsule form. Furthermore, the extra calcium is not likely to increase your risk of developing kidney stones.[25] Also, as mentioned, if you have already learned the benefits of a diet sensible in protein content, then the additional calcium will simply pass on through the intestine.[61]

The concern I have about calcium supplements is that people who take them will focus their attention on the wrong issues. Instead of concentrating on eating the right foods and being physically active, they may believe that a single pill swallowed each day will compensate for the choices of an incorrect diet and a disinclination to exercise. Also, as a minor point, for most of us the money spent on these calcium pills could be better used for other things.

Certainly I can see that we were never naturally intended to take calcium pills in order to keep our bones intact. And I find it just as hard to believe that taking estrogen pills daily is reasonable. Most of my friends are on these pills. Do you think I should be too?

Estrogen supplements definitely prevent bone loss in postmenopausal women. However, some studies have shown that once a woman stops taking the supplements her bones rapidly decrease in density, meaning that they lose calcium.[80] Therefore, estrogen therapy to prevent osteoporosis appears to be a commitment for a woman to take this hormone for the rest of her life.

Once osteoporosis has begun, estrogen replacement therapy will do little or nothing to replace the lost bone material. The estrogens work by slowing down the rate of bone loss, not by increasing bone production. If estrogen therapy is not started within the first few years after the beginning of menopause, before a significant amount of bone is lost, then estrogens given after that will come too late to have beneficial effects for most women.

Are you trying to tell me that all postmenopausal women should be taking this hormone?

No! The present trend among physicians to prescribe estrogens is causing millions of women numerous health problems.[81] The addition of daily estrogens stimulates, beyond the intended period for a "normal life," the uterus, breasts, and ovaries, and thereby increases the risk of developing cancer in these estrogen-responsive organs.[81,82] The risk depends on the duration of treatment and the dosage of estrogens. The evidence for the relationship between estrogens and the development of uterine cancer is very well established: risk levels are estimated to be as much as 5 to 14 times greater for women receiving estrogens than they are for women not receiving the hormones.[83-85] This means that an additional forty to fifty cases of cancer of the uterus can be expected in every 1000 women who take estrogen pills for fifteen years. Compare that figure with the five to ten cases of uterine cancer that occur in untreated women.[86] Once the estrogens are stopped the risk of cancer decreases over the next two years to non-user levels.[87]

Furthermore, gallbladder disease occurs two to three times as frequently in women receiving estrogen therapy as in those not taking it.[88] Some evidence also suggests that the risk of cardiovascular complications, such as strokes and heart attacks, is increased with this form of therapy. However, other evidence does not support these predictions.[81]

Estrogen supplements have been found to cause or worsen diabetes and high blood pressure in some women.[89,90] These hormones are also found to increase the likelihood of a woman developing inflammation and blood clots in the veins which can lead to pulmonary embolism, where blood clots travel to the lungs, and can cause death.[81]

Estrogen therapy to prevent osteoporosis also has a few other important drawbacks. Because of the increased risk of endometrial cancer, women being treated will need biannual uterine biopsies to check for any evidence of such cancer. A uterine biopsy is a painful procedure and few women will permit its repetition for screening purposes. Most women will suffer also from the nuisance and discomfort of a lifetime of monthly menstrual periods while they are taking the popular program of estrogen therapy that includes a combination of female hormones. Frequent visits to the doctor's office for refills of prescriptions can also be expected.

Because of all these adverse consequences, many doctors feel that the widespread use of estrogen replacement therapy in postmenopausal women is not really achieving the purposes for which it is designed. These doctors encourage diet and exercise as the first line of defense against osteoporosis.[91]

I've heard that I can take another pill in place of estrogen for one week in the month in order to prevent cancer of the uterus. Is this right?

The female hormone *progesterone* is commonly prescribed along with estrogen because of preliminary evidence that this combination will reduce the high risk of cancer of the body of the uterus.[92] However, not enough studies have been done to assure physicians that the cancer-causing effects of estrogens are eliminated with the addition of progesterone.[86] Sequential birth control pills which contain progesterone have not prevented the development of uterine cancer in young women.[93]

The recent popularity of prescribing progesterone along with estrogens may lead to more blood vessel disease, because progesterone raises the levels of harmful cholesterol in the blood.[94] Furthermore, taking a pill every day leaves many women with the feeling that they are incurably ill. All considered, estrogens, even in combination with progesterone, are far from an ideal answer to the problem of premature bone loss in postmenopausal women.

How about younger women who have had their ovaries removed. Should they take estrogens?

When, as a result of surgery, radiation, or chemotherapy, a woman's production of estrogens from her ovaries is interrupted before the normal time of natural menopause, then estrogen therapy may be indicated in addition to a healthy diet and regular exercise.[95] However, for some women, especially those with cancer, the use of estrogens may be contraindicated. The estrogen pills will improve menopausal symptoms, known as hot flashes. These symptoms occur more intensely with the sudden ending to the production of estrogens after surgical removal of the ovaries. Estrogens also prevent thinning and dryness of vaginal linings which make sexual intercourse painful.

Vaginal problems caused by the lack of natural estrogens may be treated with estrogen creams. The hormones in these creams are absorbed into the body, but in amounts much smaller than those from pills taken by mouth. Women who wish to continue an active sexual life after menopause may choose to use these vaginal creams. No association between vaginal estrogen creams and cancer of the uterus has been observed as yet.[96] Benefits still must be weighed against the slight risks because of the internal absorption.

When a woman who has lost the function of her ovaries early in life reaches the age of natural menopause, at about the age of forty-six, then a decision should be made to stop taking the estrogen pills. Of course, the healthier low-protein diet and program of regular exercise must be maintained.

How do I prepare a diet low in proteins that will still provide all the proteins I need for body repair and functions?

According to the calcium balance studies mentioned earlier, this would mean lowering the intake to about 50 grams of proteins per day for most people. This level agrees with the recommendations for minimum daily requirements set by the Food and Nutrition Board of the United States, which are 47 grams for women and 56 grams for men. The World Health Organization suggests a lower minimum level of proteins per day: 29 grams for women and 37 grams for men. Both of these recommendations include safety margins to satisfy the protein needs of all people and actually are requirements set two to three times higher than the need for most healthy adults.[54] Therefore, a level of protein intake that is healthy for your bones is also healthy for the rest of your body and easily satisfies all your protein needs.

The high-protein diet that causes experimental subjects to be in a negative calcium balance is realized when subjects are fed a synthesized protein mixture in addition to regular food. The natural proteins in food have less calcium-losing effect than these synthetic mixtures because of the phosphorus content in the natural foods and a decreased availability of the proteins in natural foods. Also, vegetable sources of proteins have less of an adverse effect on calcium balance because these foods are less acidic and lower in their content of sulfur-containing amino acids than animal sources of proteins. Actually, considerably more than 50 grams of proteins from vegetable sources can be eaten daily while still keeping most people in a positive calcium balance.

You won't need a nutrition handbook to figure out the number of grams of proteins you'll want in your daily menu. The margins for safety and effectiveness are really quite large when you plan a diet that is based on plant sources of food. First of all, it is virtually impossible to design a diet too low in proteins when you use unprocessed starches and vegetables, as long as you eat enough to satisfy your caloric needs.[54] Second, basing your meal plan on starches, vegetables, and fruits and limiting the high-protein vegetable foods such as beans, peas and lentils will provide a low enough level of proteins to assure a positive calcium balance. Pick your favorite starch for the main part of your meal, such as sweet potatoes, white potatoes, rice, or whole wheat pasta. Add to that plenty of fresh fruits and vegetables. Red meats, poultry, fish, shellfish, eggs, and dairy products are quite high in protein and therefore should be kept to a rare feast in your diet.

A trend today is to select foods lower in fats in order to avoid obesity, heart disease, and cancer. Chicken, shrimp, tuna canned in water, low-fat cottage cheese, and skim milk have become "healthier" food choices for many Americans. However, animal foods promoted as being low in fat are just the very ones that are highest in proteins. In following the trend, many people are only trading the problems of artery disease for those of bone disease.

Look at these examples:

FOOD	% CALORIES OF PROTEINS	% CALORIES OF FAT
Whole milk	21	49
Skim milk	41	2
Cottage cheese (regular)	51	36
Cottage cheese (low-fat)	79	3
Pork	23	75
Beef	30	70
Chicken	76	18
Cod fish	89	5

Starchy foods, most vegetables, and almost all fruits have protein contents that are the most sensible for humans to eat. Important exceptions to this general rule are beans, peas, and lentils, which are starchy foods high in proteins. They should be restricted to one cup per day or less, on the average, for people without bone disease, and should be eliminated entirely from the diet of someone with osteoporosis who is attempting to make large improvements in their calcium balance. On the other hand, most fruits are lower in proteins and can be eaten more liberally.

Let's take a look at the protein and fat contents of some fresh fruits and vegetables.

FOOD	% CALORIES OF PROTEIN	% CALORIES OF FAT
Pears	5	6
Sweet potatoes	6	3
Oranges	8	4
Rice	8	5
Potatoes	11	1
Corn	12	8
Spaghetti	14	3
Kidney beans	26	4
Lentils	26	3
Peas	30	4

One effective way to decrease protein intake is to use sweet "empty-calorie" foods containing little protein, such as sugar, honey, maple syrup, molasses, and fruit juices. However, some people will not be able to tolerate these simple sugars because of medical problems such as elevated triglyceride levels, hypoglycemia, or obesity. Tooth decay and the development of a nutritional imbalance can occur if these "empty-calorie" foods are used in too large amounts.

Will exercise help prevent osteoporosis?

Exercise is another very important factor in keeping your bones strong. People who are confined for a long time to bed because of illness or injury lose substantial amounts of bone.[13,97,98] This loss is estimated to range from 200 to 300 milligrams per day. Astronauts in space, even for short periods of time, show a measurable loss of bone.[25] Fortunately, bone lost as a result of immobilization is rebuilt when weight-bearing activities are resumed.[13,25] Experimental studies show that postmenopausal women with "thin bones" can increase the density of their bones with a regular daily exercise program.[99,100]

You must realize that once the factors that cause bone loss are corrected, the body has the ability to rebuild the bones as is clearly seen in cases of osteoporosis caused by lack of physical activity. However, lack of activity is not a major problem for most women. The excess protein content of their diets is the real villain. Therefore, correcting the negative calcium balance is most effectively accomplished by lowering the protein content of the diet. Daily exercise and proper nutrition provide the circumstances that will most effectively strengthen bones weakened by years of poor diet and physical inactivity.

You're saying that even after my bones have been weakened through years of wrong eating and laziness, they will get stronger if I change my diet and exercise regularly?

Correcting the negative calcium balance is one of the major goals of all therapies for osteoporosis, including diet therapy. Many studies have shown that a positive calcium balance is easily achieved when the dietary protein level is decreased to around 50 grams a day, even on lowest calcium intakes.[57-61,64] The effect of diet on people with severe osteoporosis was recently demonstrated in a hospital study.[101] A high-protein diet and a low-protein diet were fed at different times to five patients with severe osteoporosis who had received no kind of treatment. A negative calcium balance of 64 milligrams a day was observed on the high-protein diet. On the low-protein diet the calcium balance was a positive 40 milligrams a day in favor of bone remineralization. The protein levels in this study and the results obtained are consistent with the many other studies that have been done on healthy young men and women. Then these investigators added estrogen and calcium supplements to the diets and found that the effects of these therapies on calcium balance were inconsistent.

I've heard that some doctors are giving another kind of hormone that comes from fish to treat osteoporosis. Does this work?

The hormone you're referring to is called calcitonin. The calcitonin concentrations are surprisingly higher than normal in postmenopausal women with untreated osteoporosis.[102] Although this hormone is formed naturally in our bodies, the commercial product available in pharmacies today is derived from salmon and inhibits bone loss without the serious adverse effects of estrogens. However, calcitonin must be given daily as an injection, and local and generalized allergic reactions have been reported. This approach is experimental, and results from the studies performed so far are somewhat conflicting.[103] The claim that calcitonin can prevent bone loss in patients with postmenopausal osteoporosis appears to be based on a single controlled study.[104] This drugs acts by slowing down breakdown, similar to the effect of estrogens, and therefore can not be expected to rebuild lost bone.

The cost of the drug is 10 dollars a day, to which the cost of the injections must be added. And the therapy is given over a period of two years or longer, making it impractical for most people even if future evidence should show a definite benefit for those who suffer with osteoporosis.

I have read that exercise can stop a woman's menstrual periods and cause her to develop osteoporosis, and also that fat women have less chance of developing osteoporosis. How can this be?

These issues make sensational news stories, and there is a bit of truth in both. Very strenuous exercise, not just moderate daily exercise, reduces the ovaries' production of estrogens in some athletic women. This is often seen with long-distance runners.[105] A decrease in menstrual function is especially common when the calorie intake of the diet is also inadequate. Menstrual periods stop or become irregular. And there is some evidence that these women are more likely to develop exercise-related fractures.[105]

Estrogens are also part of the explanation of fewer cases of osteoporosis in overweight women. Body fat converts male hormones, called *androgens*, into estrogens.[106] The more fat that is available, the more estrogens are produced. As we have discussed, estrogens decrease bone loss, and as a result these obese women have fewer osteoporosis-related fractures.[107] Because of their extra pounds, they must carry around more weight each day, and that in itself may help to strengthen their bones.

Thus, one common factor for both of these apparently paradoxical situations is the estrogen levels in a woman's body. These issues should not lead anyone to making incorrect conclusions. Obesity is never a sign of good health. And remember, moderate exercise is always beneficial to health.

How can someone know if they are getting better from eating a low-protein diet and taking more exercise?

Determining success from these approaches is difficult. Tests for calcium balance are complicated and expensive. Sensitive measurements of bone density by the photon absorption test will show the benefit over a period of time, but equipment for this test is not readily available to most physicians even though the cost is quite reasonable. If available and affordable, then photon absorptiometry bone scanner tests every six months may give you valuable information on your progress. However, the most important information you can look for is fewer new fractures. Since treatment using a healthier diet and a little exercise is without cost or danger, there is no reason to delay.

I certainly don't feel like a helpless victim of osteoporosis now that we've had this talk. I really don't foresee any difficulty in changing my diet and lifestyle. I can clearly understand the value of this alternative approach.

You have learned enough about the ideal state of health and your nutritional needs to avoid being conned by the commercial messages and advertising approaches that will do you little good, if any, and might do much harm. I'm sure you will no longer believe the self-proclaimed guardians of your health, who recommend quantities of milk and handfuls of calcium pills without considering the probable damaging impact on your health that these products can cause. You also understand that the risks from estrogen therapy may not be worth the potential benefits. However, as with all therapies, the patient has the most to lose or gain, whatever he or she does. Therefore, ultimately you will have to make the choice yourself.

Most people—and, sad to say, our health and dietary professionals are included among them—are focusing their attention on the minor dietary influences affecting bone metabolism. Although calcium, phosphorus, and fiber in the diet do have a small effect on calcium balance, the overriding determinant of calcium and bone metabolism in osteoporosis is the excessive amount of protein, and especially animal protein, in the foods most people eat.

Osteoporosis is not an inevitable part of growing older, but is rather a degenerative disease resulting from improper care of your body during your younger and middle years. Now that you know a better set of rules to live by, your efforts can be directed towards preventing osteoporosis by eating a proper diet and choosing to follow a healthful lifestyle.

Osteoporosis cannot be reasonably considered to be a disease from cow's milk deficiency, a calcium pill deficiency, nor an estrogen pill deficiency. That it is a disease from too much meat and other high-protein foods and inadequate physical activity is a lot easier for us to believe. Until the dangers from eating excess amounts of animal proteins is recognized, when we plan our personal diets ourselves, and when national health policies are established by our guardian authorities, osteoporosis will continue to be a major disease of epidemic proportions for postmenopausal women in affluent societies.

℞

- A low-protein diet is essential in preventing and treating osteoporosis.
- A low-protein diet is centered around a variety of starchy foods, with the addition of fresh or frozen fruits and vegetables:

Limit or avoid entirely high-protein starchy foods such as beans, peas, and lentils.

Unless contraindicated for other reasons, you may use "empty calorie" simple sugars in limited amounts. Contraindications would be sensitivity to sugar with resulting high triglyceride levels or hypoglycemia.

All animal products should be excluded initially. With improvement of osteoporosis or in healthy individuals about 1 cup on the average of beans, peas, and lentils can be used daily and high-protein animal products can be consumed on festive occasions, like turkey for Thanksgiving.

- Moderate daily physical activity is very important in maintaining or regaining bone density and strength.
- Avoid caffeinated beverages, alcoholic beverages, and smoking tobacco.
- Estrogens should not be taken routinely by women as they pass through menopause. However, women who are unable to adopt a low-protein diet and daily physical activity must weigh the risks of taking estrogens with the probable benefits.
- Estrogens should be taken by women who lose their ovarian function prematurely if there are no other contraindications.
- Estrogen vaginal creams may be a small compromise acceptable to women wanting to remain sexually active after menopause.
- The addition of 500 to 1000 milligrams of an uncontaminated calcium supplement to the above will do no harm, but probably no good, for anyone able to lower their dietary protein intake to a sensible level. Those unable to give up the high-protein foods will gain a slight benefit from the addition of calcium in the form of a daily supplement to their diet. Also, people with a diagnosis of osteoporosis may wish to include a supplement in hopes of gaining a slight additional benefit from the added calcium.
- Dairy products should never be considered as the calcium supplement because of associated health hazards.

REFERENCES

[1]Consensus Conference: Osteoporosis. *JAMA* 252:799, 1984.

[2]Smith D. The loss of bone mineral with aging and its relationship to risk of fracture. *J Clin Invest* 56:311, 1975.

[3]Stevenson J. Postmenopausal osteoporosis-regular review. *Br Med J* 285:585, 1982.

[4]Nordin B. Osteoporosis and osteomalacia. *Clin Endo Metab* 9:177, 1980

[5]Marx J. Osteoporosis: new help for thinning bones. *Science* 207:628, 1980.

[6]Milne J. A five-year follow-up study of bone mass in older people. *Ann Hum Biol* 4:243, 1977.

[7]Solomon L. Osteoporosis and fracture of the femoral neck in the South African Bantu. *J Bone Joint Surg* 50B:2, 1968.

[8]Smith D. Age and activity effects on rate of bone mineral loss. *J Clin Invest* 58:716, 1976.

[9]Raisz L. Osteoporosis. *J Am Geriatr Soc* 30:127, 1982.

[10]Marcus R. The relationship of dietary calcium to the maintenance of skeletal integrity in man-an interface of endocrinology and nutrition. *Metabolism* 31:93, 1982.

[11]Foresta C. Osteoporosis and decline of gonadal function in the elderly male. *Hormone Res* 19:18, 1984.

[12]Daniell H. Osteoporosis of the slender smoker: vertebral compression fractures and loss of metacarpal cortex in relation to postmenopausal cigarette smoking and lack of obesity. *Arch Intern Med* 136:298, 1976.

[13]Donaldson C. Effect of prolonged bed rest on bone mineral. *Metabolism* 19:1071, 1970.

[14]Bikle D. Bone disease in alcohol abuse. *Ann Intern Med* 103:42, 1985.

[15]Heaney R. Effects of nitrogen, phosphorus, and caffeine on calcium balance in women. *J Lab Clin Med* 99:46, 1982.

[16]Parfitt A. Dietary risk factors for age-related bone loss and fractures. *Lancet* 2:1181, 1983.

[17]Fraser D. The physiological economy of vitamin D. *Lancet* 1:969, 1983.

[18]Stevenson J. Calcitonin and the calcium-regulating hormones in postmenopausal women: effect of oestrogens. *Lancet* 1:693, 1981.

[19]Jensen G. Treatment of postmenopausal osteoporosis. A controlled therapeutic trial comparing oestrogen/gestagen, 1,25- dihydroxy-vitamin D3 and calcium. *Clin Endo* 16:515, 1982.

[20]Christiansen C. Prevention of early postmenopausal bone loss: controlled 2-year study in 315 normal females. *Eur J Clin Invest* 10:273, 1980.

[21]Christiansen C. Effect of 1,25-dihydroxy-vitamin D3 in itself or combined with hormone treatment in preventing postmenopausal osteoporosis. *Eur J Clin Invest* 11:305, 1981.

[22]Raisz L. Hormonal regulation of bone formation. *Recent Prog Horm Res* 34:335, 1978.

[23]Editorial: Fluoride and the treatment of osteoporosis. *Lancet* 1:547, 1984.

[24]Riggs B. Effect of the fluoride/calcium regimen on vertebral fracture occurrence in postmenopausal osteoporosis. Comparison with conventional therapy. *N Engl J Med* 306:446,1982.

[25]Heaney R. Calcium nutrition and bone health in the elderly. *Am J Clin Nutr* 36:986, 1982.

[26]Draper H. Calcium, phosphorus, and osteoporosis. *Fed Proc* 40:2434, 1981.

[27]Paterson C. Calcium requirements in man: a critical review. *Postgrad Med J* 54:244, 1978.

[28]Walker A. The human requirement of calcium: should low intakes be supplemented? *Am J Clin Nutr* 25:518, 1972.

[29]Lewinnek G. The significance and a comparative analysis of the epidemiology of hip fractures. *Clin Ortho Related Res* 152:35, 1980.

[30]*Food balance sheets. 1979-1981 average.* Food and Agriculture Organization of the United Nations. Rome. 1984.

[31]*FAO production yearbook.* 37:263,1984.

[32]Gilat T. Lactase deficiency: the world pattern today. *Israel J Med Sci* 15:369, 1979.

[33]Heaney R. Menopausal changes in calcium balance performance. *J Lab Clin Med* 92:953, 1978.

[34]Recker R. Effect of estrogens and calcium carbonate on bone loss in postmenopausal women. *Ann Intern Med* 87:649, 1977.

[35]Schwartz E. Radioactive calcium kinetics during high calcium intake in osteoporosis. *J Clin Invest* 44:1547, 1965.

[36]Riggs B. Effects of oral therapy with calcium and vitamin D in primary osteoporosis. *J Clin Endocrinol Metab* 42:1139, 1976.

[37]Horsman A. Prospective trial of oestrogen and calcium in postmenopausal women. *Br Med J.* 2:789, 1977.

[38]Moore W. The evaluation of bone density findings in normal populations and osteoporosis. *Trans Am Clin Climatol Assoc* 86:128, 1974.

[39]Shapiro J. Osteoporosis: evaluation of diagnosis and therapy. *Arch Intern Med* 135:563, 1975.

[40]Nilas L. Calcium supplementation and postmenopausal bone loss. *Br Med J* 289:1103, 1984.

[41]Dudl R. Evaluation of intravenous calcium as therapy for osteoporosis. *Am J Med* 55:631, 1973.

[42]Jensen H. Treatment of osteoporosis with calcium infusions: an osteodensitometric study. *Scand J Clin Lab Invest* 32:93,1973

[43]Spencer H. Influence of dietary calcium intake on Ca47 absorption in man. *Am J Med* 46:197, 1969.

[44]Cummings J. Nutritional implications of dietary fiber. *Am J Clin Nutr* 31:S21,1978.

[45]Nutrition: the changing scene. Proposals for nutritional guidelines for health education in Britain. *Lancet* 2:835, 1983.

[46]Anderson B. The iron and zinc status of long-term vegetarian women. *Am J Clin Nutr* 34:1042, 1981.

[47]Symposium on human calcium requirements: Council on Foods and Nutrition. *JAMA* 185:588, 1963.

[48]Goodhart and Shils, *Modern Nutrition in Health and Disease (Dietotherapy)*, 5th ed. Lea and Febiger, Philadelphia, 1973, p274.

[49]Walker A. The influence of numerous pregnancies and lactations on bone dimensions in South African Bantu and Caucasian mothers. *Clin Sci* 42:189, 1972.

[50]Solomon L. Rheumatic disorders in the South African Negro. Part 1. Rheumatoid arthritis and ankylosing spondylitis. *S A Med J* 49:1292, 1975.

[51]Smith R. Epidemiologic studies of osteoporosis in women of Puerto Rico and Southeastern Michigan with special reference to age, race, national origin and to other related or associated findings. *Clin Orthop* 45:31, 1966.

[52]Smith R. Concurrent axial and appendicular osteoporosis. Its relation to calcium consumption. *N Engl J Med* 273:73, 1965.

[53]Horsman A. The relation between bone loss and calcium balance in women. *Clin Sci* 59:137, 1980.

[54]McDougall J. *The McDougall Plan,* New Century Publ. Piscataway, 1983, p. 95-109

[55]McLaren D. Stores, sumps, and sinks. *Lancet* 1:242, 1980.

[56]Schuette S. Studies on the mechanism of protein-induced hypercalciuria in older men and women. *J Nutr* 110:305, 1980.

[57]Hegsted M. Urinary calcium and calcium balance in young men as affected by level of protein and phosphorus intake. *J Nutr* 111:553, 1981.

[58]Anand C. Effect of protein intake on calcium balance of young men given 500 mg calcium daily. *J Nutr* 104:695, 1974.

[59]Walker R. Calcium retention in the adult human male as affected by protein intake. *J Nutr* 102:1297, 1972.

[60]Johnson N. Effect of level of protein intake on urinary and fecal calcium and calcium retention of young adult males. *J Nutr* 100:1425, 1970.

[61]Linkswiler H. Calcium retention of young adult males as affected by level of protein and of calcium intake. *Trans NY Acad Sci* 36:333, 1974.

[62]Whedon G. Editorial: Osteoporosis. *N Engl J Med* 305:397, 1981.

[63]Allen L. Protein-induced hypercalciuria: a longer term study. *Am J Clin Nutr* 32:741, 1979,

[64]Altchuler S. Dietary protein and calcium loss: a review. *Nutr Res* 2:193, 1982.

[65]Wachman A. Diet and osteoporosis. *Lancet* 1:958, 1968.

[66]Barzel U. The effect of excessive acid feeding on bone. *Calc Tiss Res* 4:94, 1969.

[67]Zemel M. Role of the sulfur-containing amino acids in protein-induced hypercalciuria in men. *J Nutr* 111:545, 1981.

[68]Brockis J. The effects of vegetable and animal protein diets on calcium, urate and oxalate excretion. *Br J Urology* 54:590, 1982.

[69]McClellan W. Prolonged meat diets with a study of the metabolism of nitrogen, calcium, and phosphorus. *J Biol Chem* 87:669, 1930.

[70]Mazess R. Bone mineral content of North Alaskan Eskimos. *Am J Clin Nutr* 27: 916, 1974.

[71]Robertson W. The effect of high animal protein intake on the risk of calcium stone-formation in the urinary tract. *Clin Sci* 57: 285, 1979.

[72]Cummings J. The effect of meat protein and dietary fiber on colonic function and metabolism; 1. Changes in bowel habit, bile acid excretion, and calcium absorption. *Am J Clin Nutr* 32:2086, 1979.

[73]Spencer H. Effect of a high protein (meat) intake on calcium metabolism in man. *Am J Clin Nutr* 31:2167, 1978.

[74]Spencer H. Further studies of the effect of a high protein diet as meat on calcium metabolism. *Am J Clin Nutr* 37:924,1983.

[75]Recker R. The effect of milk supplements on calcium metabolism, bone metabolism and calcium balance. *Am J Clin Nutr* 41:254, 1985.

[76]McDougall J. *The McDougall Plan,* New Century Publ, Piscataway, 1983 p. 49-62.

[77]Ferrer J. Milk of dairy cows frequently contains a leukemogenic virus. *Science* 213:1014, 1981.

[78]Orwoll E. The milk-alkali syndrome: current concepts: review. *Ann Intern Med* 97:242, 1982.

[79]Roberts H. Potential toxicity due to dolomite and bonemeal. *S Med J* 76:556, 1983.

[80]Lindsay R. Bone response to termination of oestrogen treatment. *Lancet* 1:1325, 1978.

[81]Judd H. Estrogen replacement therapy: indications and complications. *Ann Intern Med* 98:195, 1983.

[82]Hoover R. Stilboestrol (diethylstilbestrol) and the risk of ovarian cancer. *Lancet* 2:533, 1977.

[83]Zeil H. Increased risk of endometrial carcinoma among users of conjugated estrogens. *N Engl J Med* 293:1167, 1975.

[84]Smith D. Association of exogenous estrogen and endometrial carcinoma. *N Engl J Med* 293:ll64, 1975.

[85]Mack T. Estrogens and endometrial cancer in a retirement community. *N Engl J Med* 294:1262, 1976.

[86]Ljunghall S. Postmenopausal osteoporosis. *Br Med J* 285:1504, 1982.

[87]Hulka B. Estrogen and endometrial cancer: cases and two control groups from North Carolina. *Am J Obstet Gynecol* 137:92, 1980.

[88]Boston Collaborative Drug Surveillance Program. Surgically confirmed gallbladder disease, venous thromboembolism, and breast tumors in relation to postmenopausal estrogen therapy. *N Engl J Med* 290:15, 1974.

[89]Ajabor L. Effect of exogenous estrogen on carbohydrate metabolism in postmenopausal women. *Am J Obstet Gynecol* 113:383, 1972.

[90]Pfeffer R. Estrogen use and stroke risk in postmenopausal women. *Am J Epidemiol* 103:445, 1976.

[91]Pollner F. Osteoporosis: Looking at the whole picture. *Med World News* Jan 14, 1985. p. 38-58.

[92]Whitehead M. Effects of estrogens and progestins on the biochemistry and morphology of the postmenopausal endometrium *N Engl J Med* 305:1599, 1981.

[93]Silverberg S. Endometrial carcinoma in young women taking oral contraceptive agents. *Obstet Gynecol* 46:503, 1975.

[94]Krauss R. Effects of progestational agents on serum lipids and lipoproteins. *J Reprod Med* 27:503, 1982.

[95]Johansson B. On some late effects of bilateral oophorectomy in the age range 15-30 years. *Acta Obstet Gynecol Scand* 54:449, 1975.

[96]Horwitz R. Intravaginal estrogen creams and endometrial cancer: no causal association found. *JAMA* 241:1266, 1979.

[97]Deitrick J. Effects of immobilization upon various metabolic and physiologic functions of normal men. *Am J Med* 4:3, 1948.

[98]Hantman D. Attempts to prevent disuse osteoporosis by treatment with calcitonin, longitudinal compression and supplementary calcium and phosphate. *J Clin Endocrinol Metab* 36:845, 1973.

[99]Aloia J. Exercise and skeletal health. *J Am Geriatr Soc* 29:104, 1981.

[100]Smith E. Physical activity and calcium modalities for bone mineral increase in aged women. *Med Sci Sports Exercise* 13:60, 1981.

[101]Licata A. Acute effects of dietary protein on calcium metabolism in patients with osteoporosis. *J Gerontol* 36:14, 1982.

[102]Tiegs R. Calcitonin secretion in postmenopausal osteoporosis. *N Engl J Med* 312:1097, 1985.

[103]Gruber H. Long-term calcitonin therapy in postmenopausal osteoporosis. *Metabolism* 33:295, 1984.

[104]Synthetic calcitonin for postmenopausal osteoporosis. *Med Lett Drug Ther* 27:53, 1985.

[105]Marcus R. Menstrual function and bone mass in elite women distance runners. Endocrine and metabolic features. *Ann Intern Med* 102:158, 1985.

[106]MacDonald P. Effect of obesity on conversion of plasma androstenedione to estrone in postmenopausal women with and without endometrial cancer. *Am J Obstet Gynecol* 130:448, 1978.

[107]Dalen N. Bone mass in obese subjects. *Acta Med Scand* 197:353, 1975.

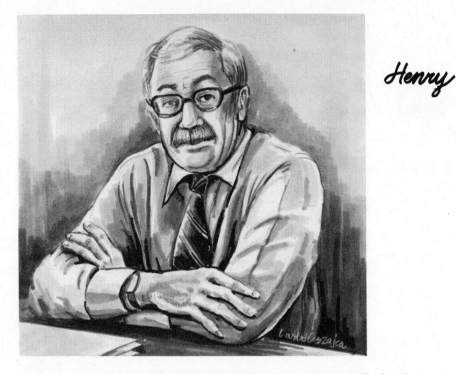

Henry

Two years ago I began having pains in my legs when I walked only one city block. My doctor told me the problem was my circulation. Last year I had the arteries in my neck cleaned out; they were so plugged up with cholesterol that I was having a number of little strokes. Now the same surgeon has diagnosed an enlarged blood vessel in my belly that he says will burst if it gets any bigger; for this, more surgery will be necessary soon, he predicts. Well, it's not his artery that's going to be replaced with a plastic hose. If there is any way to make my arteries healthier, I've got to find it. Every doctor I've seen tells me that hardening of the arteries is something everybody gets along with age and that it can't be prevented, much less made better. What have I done to myself to be stuck with such rotten arteries? I never smoked and I hardly touch alcohol. Coffee is about my only "bad habit." And I've never thought it was bad. I must have a thousand miles of blood vessels that are all plugged up. One surgeon could retire just on the income from the repair jobs I need.

4

ATHEROSCLEROSIS

What is this disease that is destroying my arteries?

The trouble you call hardening of the arteries is known medically as *atherosclerosis*. You should think of it as being something like a lot of sores forming on the insides of your arteries that eventually grow into the walls of the arteries. Atherosclerosis actually begins as little wounds that produce tiny changes in the cells that line the innermost layer of the arteries.[1,2] Initially these cells are injured by high levels of fat and cholesterol that are present in the circulating blood of most people who eat the foods provided by the rich American diet.[2] Other sources of injury to the linings of the blood vessel are mechanical such as surgery and high blood pressure, chemical such as carbon monoxide and other by-products of tobacco smoke, and antigen-antibody complexes derived from food proteins that pass through the intestinal wall.[1-3]

If the injury occurs for only a short time and is not too severe, then the lining of the artery will heal. If, however, the cause of injury continues, as it usually does because of our daily eating and living habits, then permanent changes will take place.

These permanent changes consist of an overgrowth of the muscle cells that normally make up the central layer in an artery wall. Blood clotting elements, called *platelets,* and *white blood cells* that are attracted to the site of injury stimulate the growth of these muscle cells, thus playing an important part in the development of atherosclerosis.[1,2] As a result of the body's attempts to heal these wounds, scar tissue is deposited at the sites of injury, causing a condition known as *fibrosis*. Because the sores are open at all times to blood containing high levels of fat and cholesterol, these two substances can enter the artery and accumulate within the arterial wall. This mixture of muscle cells, scar tissue, fats, and cholesterol forms a swelling on the inner surface of the artery. A single such swelling is called a *plaque*.[1]

In the early stages of plaque formation, the process of fat accumulation is most evident and the areas of atherosclerosis are known as *fatty streak deposits*. Later, scar tissue predominates, and the disease consists of many hard fibrous plaques. This is when the condition is known as hardening of the arteries. All stages of the disease, from fatty streaks to plaques, are present in the arteries of most adults. Even in later years of life and more advanced stages of disease, atherosclerosis is a dynamic process of deterioration and repair within the arterial wall rather than permanent progression toward a catastrophic event.[4,5]

Atherosclerosis affects the arteries in two ways that can threaten your health and your life. First, the plaques accumulate within the passageway in the artery, interfering with the normal flow of blood. Eventually the blockages become so severe that insufficient blood reaches the tissues. Then troubles like pain or death of the starved tissues occur. Second, atherosclerosis causes degeneration of the artery wall so that the walls lose their strength and elasticity. An eventual outcome of weakened arteries can be rupture of the wall. Some strokes are caused when a blood vessel in the brain leaks or bursts wide open. The bulging artery in your belly is caused by loss of strength in the walls of the largest blood vessel in your body, the condition is called an abdominal aortic *aneurysm*. When the aneurysm reaches a certain size, the chances of its rupturing become very likely.

I really have felt great all my life, until only a couple of years ago. How long did it actually take for my arteries to get into this awful condition?

This disease of the blood vessels develops without any symptoms until most of the damage is already done. Tragically, blood vessels begin to clog up and suffer damage soon after the first bite we take from a "well balanced" meal plan arranged around the basic four food groups. Children as young as nine months of age can show the beginnings of atherosclerosis by the fatty streak deposits found along the walls of their large arteries.[6] Every child who has been raised on the high fat, high cholesterol American diet, which offers plentiful amounts of cow's milk, cheese, hot dogs, hamburgers, milk shakes, and french fries has signs of this disease by the tender age of three.[6] By the teenage years the degree of damage has advanced to the stage where the soft deposits of fats in the arteries are joined by hard fibrous scar tissue to form the larger sores inside the artery wall, which are referred to as *hard fibrous plaques*.

And all these years I thought I was healthy. I am amazed that this disease gets started when we're so young. How do doctors know this?

Arteries can be examined during life, by an X-ray technique called *angiography*, or after death at autopsy. One study which shows how severe and frequent this disease is in youth was done on American battle victims during the Korean conflict.[7] The average age of those physically conditioned fighting men was twenty-two years. On autopsy examination, 77 percent of the hearts showed atherosclerotic disease in the arteries that supplied their heart muscle, known as the *coronary arteries*. The hard fibrous variety of plaques were evident in 35 percent of the autopsy specimens. Of the 300 men examined, eight actually had nearly complete or complete blockage of at least one of the essential arteries that had kept their hearts beating long enough to allow them to be killed in action.

This epidemic disease really gets out of control as people approach their middle years. By then the atherosclerotic plaques in the arteries have grown so much that the majority of the hearts of men at high risk, often because they already suffer with some chest pains, have serious disease. For example, when examined by angiography, studies show that at least one out of the three major coronary arteries is narrowed by 50 percent or more in approximately half of the high-risk men below the age of forty.[8,9] With each year of life atherosclerosis affects more people and the disease becomes more severe in each person.[9]

Most of the people I know seem to be doing just fine, and many are quite old. I seem to be the only one with atherosclerosis. What are some of the problems that people get when their arteries become clogged up?

Most of the complications of atherosclerosis are regarded as problems with the organs that depend upon their supply of blood from a severely diseased artery. Because the entire blood vessel system suffers from poor health, people with extensive atherosclerosis usually have a number of problems that, in fact, are all explained by the poor condition of their arteries.

In the United States, the most common problems from atherosclerosis are seen when the blood vessels to the heart are affected. Heart victims

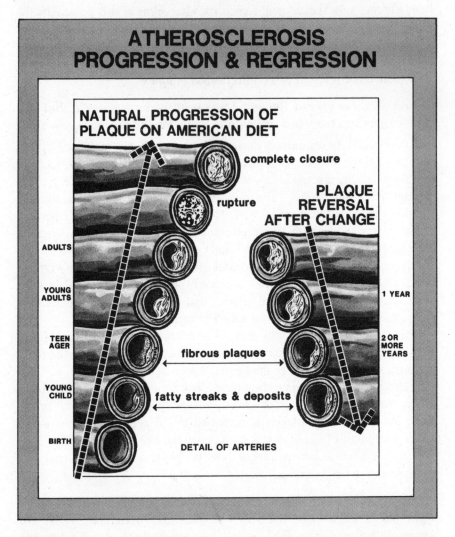

The development of atherosclerosis is a dynamic process with progression and regression occurring simultaneously.[2] Because of the diet and lifestyle of most people in affluent countries, progression is favored. However, a change in diet and lifestyle can result in substantial healing of the diseased arteries and a regression of atherosclerosis.

may develop chest pains, called *angina,* from partial blockage resulting in inadequate circulation to the heart muscle. When this ''silent disease'' progresses to a complete blockage of a coronary artery, the piece of heart muscle then deprived of blood dies. This event, no longer silent, is known as a *heart attack.* Interestingly enough, heart attacks can first start to appear in teenagers.[10] And as people get older this cause of death and disability increases in magnitude until it becomes epidemic. More than a million heart attacks are reported each year in this country. Coronary heart disease accounts for nearly 700,000 deaths annually, which is more deaths than are caused by any other disease, including all forms of cancer.[11] Men are more susceptible to coronary artery disease and heart attacks than women. However, as women pass through menopause the protective advantage of their gender disappears.[12] Often, events caused by artery blockage are sudden and unexpected and approximately half the victims dying from heart attacks never knew they were at risk because they had no previous warning symptoms.[13,14] Heart attacks are highly lethal; half the people suffering from an attack never reach a hospital alive.[13,14]

As you have become aware all too painfully, all the arteries in the body are equally susceptible to atherosclerosis. Clogged and damaged arteries to the brain lead to *strokes, hemorrhages,* and temporary losses of brain function called *transient ischemic attacks,* or *TIAs.*[4,5] Even *senility* is caused in many people by deterioration of the blood vessels that supply the brain.[15] Lowered supply of blood to the kidneys from narrowed arteries causes high blood pressure and kidney failure. When the legs are deprived of essential nutrients, walking becomes painful, as has happened in your case. Eventually the foot or the entire leg may die from lack of blood, and gangrene may develop, which, of course, requires amputation.

Hearing loss is an expected part of growing old in our country. However, in many other parts of the world people keep this important function until they die at an old age.[15,16] Common to societies where hearing is preserved is a low incidence of atherosclerosis.[15,16] As atherosclerosis develops throughout the body, the arteries that supply blood to the hearing apparatus become plugged and deafness begins. Close to the hearing organs are the organs regulating balance. Poor circulation to those organs can cause dizziness and loss of balance or *vertigo.*

Recent evidence shows that many cases of *impotence,* failure of sexual performance in men, are the result of atherosclerotic disease of the vessels that supply blood to the penis and nerves that enable erection along with sexual arousal.[18] Thirty-four percent of middle-aged men suffer from impotence.[19] How many of these cases are the result of artery disease has yet to be determined. For many men the threat of this dismaying problem may be a greater motivation for taking better care of their health than is the risk of a stroke or heart attack.

Now that you mention some of the diseases caused by atherosclerosis, I can see that this problem has affected many people I know. Do the arteries just slowly close up until the blood stops flowing? It seems like the people I've known who have had heart attacks had trouble all of a sudden.

Even though for most of us atherosclerosis develops over a lifetime, in some people this disease can progress quite rapidly, closing off arteries in a matter of months.[20] However, the sudden event that ends in a heart attack is not usually caused by the eventual closure of a coronary artery by plaque material, but is rather the result of the rupture of a plaque.[21]

Plaques are filled with fat. When they reach a large enough size they become "ripe," and can easily break open, spilling their fatty contents into the bloodstream. This triggers the formation of a clot, called a *thrombosis,* which suddenly plugs the artery completely.[21] Along with the clot formation, strong spasms of the muscles in the artery wall occur. These spasms cause damage by further decreasing the flow of blood to the heart muscle or other vital tissues.[21] Plaque rupture and clot formation are more likely to happen as atherosclerosis progresses while one grows older and becomes poorer in general health.

You said that the typical American diet causes our arteries to become diseased. What exactly in my diet causes atherosclerosis?

Cholesterol in your diet and in your body should be the central focus of your understanding of the cause, prevention, and treatment of atherosclerosis. Cholesterol is a waxy substance that is synthesized by all animals as an important part of their tissues. It is used in the body for the production of certain hormones and for the synthesis of bile acids and vitamin D. Being highly efficient human beings, we make all the cholesterol we need. No additional cholesterol is required from our diet. On the other hand, no plant produces or contains any cholesterol at all.

In addition to making all the cholesterol that their bodies need, most people in our affluent society eat large quantities of this substance in the flesh of other animals and the by-products of animals, such as milk, ice cream, cheese, and eggs.[22] Cholesterol is easily absorbed through the intestines, but unfortunately the body eliminates it with difficulty. Approximately half of the amount we consume passes through the intestinal wall directly into the the blood stream.[23] In an attempt to get rid of this excess, cholesterol is excreted by the liver into the gallbladder and then out into the intestinal contents. Unfortunately, the liver's capacity to excrete this waxy substance is very limited and the liver, working overtime, cannot keep up with the intake of most people who are eating the usual American diet. As a result, large amounts of this substance accumulate in the tissues, including the lining of the arteries. Examination of the makeup of the atherosclerotic plaque shows that cholesterol is a major component.[24,25]

Cholesterol that has been exposed to air and heat is changed into an oxidized form that is believed to be especially damaging to the blood vessels.[26] Dried, powdered, aged, smoked, and cooked meats, dairy, and egg products contain the greatest amounts of this oxidized, highly toxic cholesterol.[26]

How can I find out how much cholesterol is in my body? And more important, how much damage has already been done to my arteries?

An almost painless, inexpensive test your doctor can order will determine the amount of cholesterol in your blood. This blood cholesterol value is usually an accurate indication of the amount of cholesterol deposited throughout your body.

Studies at the Cleveland Clinic using coronary angiography have shown that nearly half of all men under the age of forty who are evaluated for chest pains have extensive arterial disease.[8] Most important, the chance of finding serious artery disease was directly related to the cholesterol level in the blood.[8,9] Many other studies have confirmed the importance of the blood cholesterol level in predicting the condition of the arteries as determined by angiography.[27-30]

This chart shows the results of angiograms performed on young men, as compared with their blood cholesterol values.

CHANCE OF 50% OR GREATER CLOSURE OF ONE OR MORE CORONARY ARTERIES IN MEN UNDER THE AGE OF FORTY[8]

CHOLESTEROL (milligram percent)	SIGNIFICANT CLOSURE 50% OR GREATER (percent of angiograms)
less than 200	20
201-225	38
226-250	48
251-275	60
276-300	77
301-350	80
greater than 350	91

The relationship is clear: the higher the cholesterol level, the worse the condition of the arteries.

Another important possibility that a blood cholesterol level can predict is the chance of a person's dying from heart disease. The average cholesterol level in Americans is 210 to 220 milligram percent; the average American has almost a 50 percent chance of dying from heart disease. An important concept to understand is that what is considered to be "average health" among Americans is not desirable health. Comparing cholesterol levels with the eventual causes of death has demonstrated that those people with levels of cholesterol of 200 milligram percent or less have only one-fifth the chance of dying from heart disease, as compared with persons having a cholesterol level of 260 milligram percent or greater.[31] People who maintain

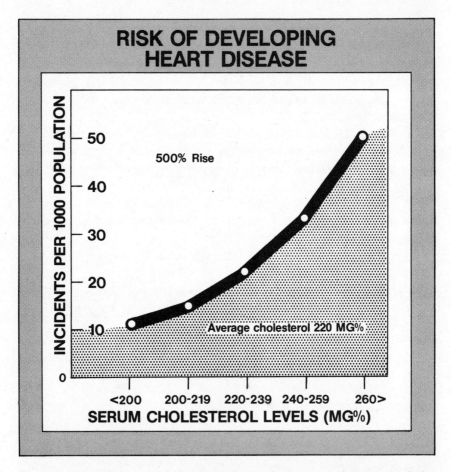

The serum (blood) cholesterol level is highly predictive for the chance of a person developing and dying from heart disease.[31] The risk is increased by 500 percent with a rise in cholesterol levels of only 60 milligram percent. An average cholesterol for Americans of 210 to 220 milligram percent is associated with approximately a 50 percent chance of dying from heart disease. Heart disease is very rare when cholesterol levels are maintained below 180 milligram percent for a lifetime.[22] Our goal should be to attain and maintain a level of 160 milligram percent or lower in order to improve the health of our already damaged blood vessels.

cholesterol levels of 180 milligram percent or less during their lifetime have little risk of developing a heart attack.[22]

The cholesterol level falls to a new and lower level about three weeks after a person changes his or her diet and the other habits that otherwise raise cholesterol levels.

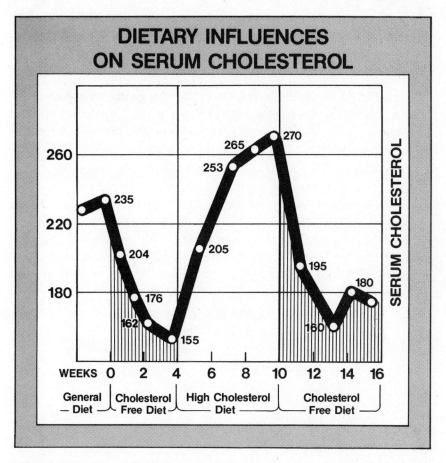

The cholesterol rises and falls by significant amounts depending on the foods chosen. In only three weeks the effects of a dietary change are evident by blood tests. The lowest possible level of cholesterol is maintained by consuming a no-cholesterol, low-fat, starch-based diet daily as your lifestyle.

A goal for most people who have had elevated cholesterol levels for many years should be to lower the level to 160 milligram percent or less. Actually, the lower the level the better. However, someone starting with a high level, for example 300 milligram percent or above, should be happy to lower his or her level to 200 milligram percent. When accumulation of cholesterol is great, as it would be in this instance, then the large deposits of cholesterol throughout the body serve to release it into the blood and in that way keep the level elevated for a long time. Eventually, after several years of eating proper foods, the cholesterol deposits may be depleted and the cholesterol levels for many of these sensible people will fall to 160 milligram percent or less. In the meantime, persons with such a very high cholesterol level should be consoled by the fact that their arteries are becoming healthier for the first time in their life, instead of being as fouled by atherosclerosis as a ship's bottom is by barnacles.

I tried to lower my cholesterol level once by giving up red meat for chicken and fish. My level didn't go down at all. The doctor and the dietitian I visited said I probably had some genetic problem. I feel I'm incurably ill.

Most likely, you don't have a genetic defect. Not many people do. Instead, what went wrong were the ineffective dietary changes you made, based on incorrect information. Actually, all kinds of the meats you've mentioned are muscles from different animals: some move tails, others limbs. If you lay pieces of those meats side by side on a tabletop, you will see that they look quite similar and are distinctly different from an ear of corn or a head of cabbage. When evaluated by size of portions, the cholesterol content of each of those meats is about the same.

CHOLESTEROL CONTENT
(based on portion size)

FOOD	milligrams/100 grams
beef	70
pork	70
lamb	70
chicken (skinned)	60
turkey (skinned)	82
halibut	50
haddock	60
tuna	63
mackerel	95
crab	100
shrimp	150
lobster	200

cheese (cheddar)	106
liver	300
egg	550
all plant foods	0

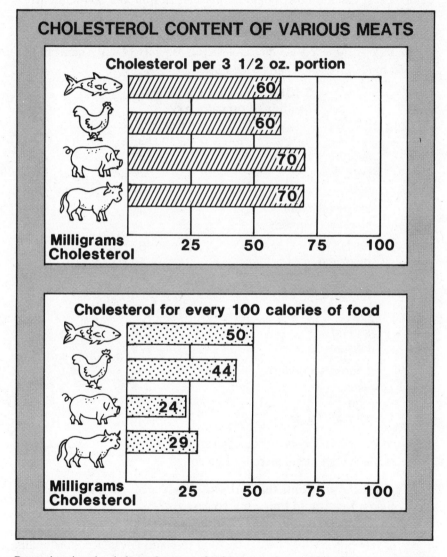

CHOLESTEROL CONTENT OF VARIOUS MEATS

Cholesterol per 3 1/2 oz. portion

Fish: 60
Chicken: 60
Pig: 70
Cow: 70

Milligrams Cholesterol: 25 50 75 100

Cholesterol for every 100 calories of food

Fish: 50
Chicken: 44
Pig: 24
Cow: 29

Milligrams Cholesterol: 25 50 75 100

By portion size, the cholesterol content of red meat, poultry, and fish all are essentially the same. Based on calories consumed fish and poultry have approximately twice the amount of cholesterol as red meats.(source: Pennington J. Food Values of Portions Commonly Used. 14th ed. Harper & Row. New York. 1985)

A more valid comparison of the cholesterol content of different meats is one that measures the number of milligrams of cholesterol based on calories consumed. The reason why this is a better comparison is that each day a person must supply his or her body with a specific number of calories, or else lose weight. The foods chosen to provide those calories will contain other components such as iron and non-nutrients such as cholesterol. Thus, the caloric value serves as the common denominator when we compare the values of different foods.

On a per-calorie basis, the cholesterol contents of an American's favorite foods give some surprising figures.

CHOLESTEROL CONTENT
(based on calories)

FOOD	milligrams per 100 calories
lamb	21
pork	24
beef	29
turkey (skinned)	43
chicken (skinned)	44
halibut	50
mackerel	50
tuna	50
haddock	76
crab	108
shrimp	165
lobster	278
cheese (cheddar)	27
liver	214
egg	353
all plant foods	0

Based on calories consumed, chicken and fish have approximately twice as much cholesterol as red meats do.

Why did the dietitian think that if I replaced red meat with fish and chicken this would lower my cholesterol?

Dietitians and doctors have focused their attention on the quantity and types of fats present in a particular food to claim advantages for poultry and fish over red meats such as beef, pork and lamb. Red meats, and dairy products also, contain higher amounts of the saturated varieties of fats. These types of fats raise the blood cholesterol level.[32,33] Fish and chicken contain less saturated fats and more polyunsaturated fats. Polyunsaturated fats tend to lower cholesterol levels. These fats cause the body to excrete more cholesterol and thereby actually drive cholesterol out of the arteries and the body.[32,33] Gram for gram, saturated fats raise the cholesterol level about twice as much as polyunsaturated fats will lower the cholesterol.[34]

Ultimately, when fed as meats, however, these fats from different cholesterol-containing muscle foods cause little change in blood cholesterol levels. In other words, when beef, chicken, or fish is fed to volunteers, each kind of meat causes a similar rise in blood cholesterol level in the subjects.[35-39] The higher cholesterol content of chicken and fish cancels the effect of the lower content of saturated fats; the end result is a similar effect on the blood cholesterol. All of these muscle foods must be eliminated from your diet, or at the very least decreased considerably in amount, if you want to lower your cholesterol level and improve the health of your arteries.

I've heard that there is "good" cholesterol and "bad" cholesterol. Is this important for me to know about?

The types of cholesterol found in your blood are less important for you to know about than is the total amount of cholesterol.

Cholesterol in the blood is found in packages, called *lipoproteins,* that also contain proteins and fats.[40] The relative amounts of each of these three components in the package divides it into fractions, each of which contains some portion of the total cholesterol content. Each portion is recognized according to its compactness or density. Thus, there are very-low-density, low-density, intermediate-density, and high-density fractions of lipoproteins. Each fraction of lipoprotein represents stages of cholesterol metabolism from the entry of the cholesterol into the body to its eventual degradation in the liver. The low-density cholesterol, *LDL-cholesterol,* is found at the early stage of cholesterol metabolism where the cholesterol enters the tissues and does its damage; hence, its designation as "bad" cholesterol. The high-density cholesterol, called *HDL-cholesterol,* is known as the "good" cholesterol because it is the end product of cholesterol metabolism and represents a stage where the substance is being removed from the tissues.

People who rapidly and efficiently convert the low-density to the high-density cholesterol will be favoring the removal of cholesterol from the tissues. This will be reflected in a blood test that measures the amounts of each of these fractions of lipoproteins. Several factors influence the efficiency of cholesterol metabolism. Obesity, smoking, diabetes, and the use of birth control pills will decrease the amount of HDL-cholesterol.[41-44] Exercise, alcohol, and high-fiber diets will raise the HDL-cholesterol levels.[45-48].

The level of HDL-cholesterol provides valuable information in predicting the risk of developing complications from atherosclerosis, such as heart attacks, strokes, closure of the arteries in the legs, and senility.[15,49-51] This correlation, however, holds only when comparing people who all eat a similar diet, in this case a diet high in fats and cholesterol. Differences in the individuals' ability to metabolize the large amounts of cholesterol consumed are reflected in the levels of the various fractions of cholesterol and the extent of atherosclerosis that is present.

When people who eat different types of diets are compared, the relationship between the HDL-cholesterol level and lower risk of complications from atherosclerosis no longer holds. Populations living on low-cholesterol diets have low levels of all types of cholesterol, including the "bad" LDL-cholesterol and the "good" HDL-cholesterol, and low levels of athero-sclerosis.[52] This is because, as I've mentioned, HDL-cholesterol is the end product of cholesterol metabolism.[53] If less metabolism is occurring, because less is eaten, then less HDL-cholesterol will appear in the blood. In other words, the more cholesterol that is consumed, the more HDL-cholesterol will appear in the blood.[53]

If you want to be compared with a population that suffers from an epidemic of atherosclerosis, then HDL-cholesterol may have some meaning for you. However, a better choice would be for you to follow a diet that lowers all fractions of cholesterol and is associated with the least chance of suffering from all the complications of artery disease. This is a diet that contains no cholesterol and is also low in all types of fats.

I have a serious concern about the widespread use of tests for HDL-cholesterol in the general practice of medicine. People who have a high cholesterol level may be comforted into believing that everything is all right because their HDL-cholesterol is also elevated. They may fail to realize that in spite of the HDL-cholesterol level, they are still living under an unacceptable high risk for complications from atherosclerosis. Because of this false comfort, they fail to change both diet and lifestyle. I don't even bother to ask a laboratory to determine the fractions of cholesterol for my patients. For your purpose and mine, a value for total cholesterol is all the information we need to make effective decisions about diet and lifestyle.

If eating fish will make my cholesterol level stay elevated, then why have I heard that fish will prevent heart disease? Wouldn't it be a good idea to include a lot more fish in my diet?

As we have discussed, people who eat fish have much the same levels of blood cholesterol as people who eat other flesh foods.[39] However, the blood fats, called *triglycerides,* are lowered when more fish is eaten.[39] Lower levels of triglycerides do benefit health to some extent. Some investigators attribute a lower risk of heart disease to lower triglyceride levels. Yet others aren't quite convinced.[54] The oils in fish are the ingredients that seem to reduce the triglyceride levels.[55] The effect of fish oil on lowering blood triglycerides is not shared with polyunsaturated vegetable oils obtained from seeds such as corn and safflower.[55,56] These vegetable oils lead to a rise in triglycerides. The fats in fish oil have a special chemical structure that is also found in some parts of plant cells but not in their seeds.[56]

However, a diet low in all types of fats and based upon plant foods, is equally as effective as fish and fish oils in lowering blood triglycerides.[57,58] Pure fish oil not only will decrease the level of triglycerides in the blood, but, unlike fish meat, it will lower the cholesterol level as well.[55] Some health professionals believe that Americans with high blood levels of tri-glycerides and cholesterol will not accept a low-fat diet for their health problems. An easier alternative, these authorities suggest, would be to add high-fat fish or fish-oil to the diet each day.

The primary reason why eating fish, and probably fish oil, is associated with a lower risk from heart disease is not related to their effects upon cholesterol or triglycerides, but is rather because of the way they affect the tendency of blood to form clots in the arteries. Clots, of course, are involved in the development of most heart attacks.[21] Some fatty fish contain a considerable amount of a polyunsaturated fat called *eicosapentaenoic acid,* abbreviated as *EPA*. This fat has a tendency to "thin" the blood by decreasing the stickiness of the blood clotting elements called *platelets*. This property of fatty fish may be the best explanation for the low rate of heart attacks among the meat-eating Eskimos, who also eat a lot of fish.[59,60]

Some evidence suggests that fish oils, either in the pure form or in fatty fish, also may slow the development of atherosclerosis by decreasing the activity of platelets and white blood cells. These two components of blood are thought to promote the growth of muscle cells in the artery walls during the development of atherosclerosis.[2,56] Thus, fish fats may slow the process of plaque growth.[56]

So fish oil, without the cholesterol found in the fish, sounds like a great addition to my diet. Right?

Not exactly. As a result of these findings, capsules containing EPA have been promoted by the health food industry and some medical professionals, and fish has become America's newest "health food". However, the positive benefits of fish, as well as fish oil, for decreasing the risk of heart disease must be balanced against some negative effects. Eating large amounts of fish fat, even in the form of the fish that yield it, can cause serious bleeding problems because of its "blood-thinning" property.[60] Excess polyunsaturated fat from any source is also associated with increased chances for developing cancer and gallbladder disease.[61,62] Fish-oil is 100 percent fat, and high-fat fish is 60 percent fat. Fish, like other kinds of meats, consists principally of proteins and fats, with essentially no carbohydrates, fibers, or vitamin C. The body requires carbohydrates for energy and other metabolic needs. Excess amounts of proteins from the fish will cause loss of calcium from the bones and likely damage to the kidneys.[63,64] Furthermore, since fish occupy a position high in the food chain, they are heavily contaminated with pesticides, insecticides, and other environmental pollutants. Also, people who eat lots of high-fat fish can have oily skin and hair and can even smell like fish.[65] Therefore, for the sake of your general health, I suggest that you keep to a minimum all the flesh foods in your diet, including fish. Taking fish oil to prevent heart disease makes little nutritional sense.

I read a news story that said people can eat eggs every day and not raise their cholesterol level. How can that be?

Industries that market foods high in cholesterol want to play down its effects on our health, naturally; and they are willing to spend money to this end. A good example is the egg industry, which supports "research" to show that eggs will not raise our blood cholesterol levels and, therefore, that eating eggs every day does not threaten our lives.[66-70] But eggs, as most of us realize, are very high in cholesterol, containing ounce for ounce eight times as much as beef. They are also loaded with saturated fats, which are known to raise blood cholesterol levels. The egg industry has indulged in a considerable amount of ingenuity in order to "discover" results favorable to its product.

The "success" of their experiments was made possible because they selected human subjects for their studies who were already eating a high-cholesterol diet.[66-70] When people are consuming 400 to 800 milligrams of cholesterol a day, as most Americans do, swallowing additional amounts of cholesterol will have only a minor effect on their blood cholesterol levels.[71,72] Therefore, when the people under study are saturated first with cholesterol from other sources, such as chicken, fish, and beef, the addition of an egg or two makes little or no difference at all.[66-70] However, when people who eat a low-cholesterol diet are fed a single egg a day, LDL-cholesterol, the harmful portion of blood cholesterol, rises by 12 percent.[73] Many other well-designed studies by investigators working independent of the food industry clearly demonstrate the detrimental effects of eggs on blood cholesterol levels.[37,74-77]

I really get confused when I read about the cause of hardening of the arteries and heart disease. Are the people who write about these problems also confused?

At first glance, the several opinions expressed in the popular and the medical press about which component of our diet is most guilty of causing arterial disease can be somewhat confusing. One faction believes that cholesterol is enemy number one, and another group says that animal fats do the most damage. A researcher from England believes that cholesterol accumulates because of a deficiency of "cholesterol-removing" fiber in the American diet.

As smart consumers, we can assume that there is some truth in all of these theories; they're all based on the same observation that people living in affluent countries, eating rich foods, are suffering an epidemic of heart disease. We can resolve the apparent controversy by understanding the composition of different rich foods from the nutritional point of view.

All foods derived from animals are completely free of fiber and most are loaded with cholesterol. On the contrary, all plant products are free of cholesterol and all have plentiful amounts of fiber. With the exception of coconut, chocolate, and a few oils derived from vegetable sources, all plants are low in the saturated varieties of fats, and most are low in their total content of fats. With these thoughts in mind, we should have no trouble walking down the supermarket aisles and choosing the plant foods that will keep our arteries wide open.

Here is a simple list of the different components of food and their effects on cholesterol in your body:

Components of Foods That Affect Cholesterol Levels	
Raises Levels	**Lowers Levels**
Dietary cholesterol	Plant fibers
Animal (saturated) fats	Vegetable (polyunsaturated) fats
Animal proteins	Plant proteins
= Red meat, poultry, fish, dairy products, eggs	= Starches, vegetables, fruits

Even though I don't drink much alcohol, I do love coffee. How do these beverages affect my cholesterol and my chances of dying from arterial disease?

Alcohol provides calories and thereby displaces foods that otherwise would be eaten with their load of cholesterol and fats. In this way, alcoholic beverages do help to lower the total cholesterol content of the blood. Alcohol also causes changes in the metabolism of cholesterol and the body produces more HDL-cholesterol.[47] Many studies have shown a decreased risk of death from heart disease when alcohol is consumed in moderate amounts.[78,79] However, this benefit is offset by an increase in numbers of deaths from other causes, such as cirrhosis of the liver, malnutrition, and accidents among drinkers.[78,80]

I'm sorry to tell you this, but coffee raises the level of cholesterol in the blood.[81,82] On the other hand, people with high blood levels of cholesterol who give up this beverage show a significant drop in their cholesterol levels. The improvement can mean a 10 percent decrease in cholesterol levels, which could have a considerable impact on the danger of dying from heart disease while keeping your arteries in better general health.[81] Giving up coffee should be considered as an additional way to lower an elevated cholesterol value. People with already low cholesterol levels should not expect a further reduction in cholesterol when they stop drinking coffee.

There must be some easier way than changing my diet and giving up my morning coffee in order to lower my cholesterol and make my arteries healthier. How about lecithin or garlic capsules? The last time I was in a health food store the salesperson told me that all I had to do was take those pills and then I could eat anything. Should I believe her?

Don't believe her. *Lecithins* are waxy substances that contain phosphorus and fats. They are found in all kinds of plant and animal foods. When the fat component of lecithin is primarily the polyunsaturated variety, then the cholesterol will be lowered if enough lecithin is taken.[83] However, when the fat is of the saturated variety, then no such effect upon cholesterol is seen. As far as cholesterol levels are concerned, there appears to be nothing special about lecithin over the effects of any polyunsaturated fat, such as corn oil or safflower oil.

Garlic oil pills have been shown to decrease the cholesterol and triglyceride levels when they are compared with the effect of a placebo capsule containing no oil.[84] In one experiment garlic was administered to people daily as an oil corresponding to the amount expressed from one ounce of garlic cloves. Over an eight-month period the drop in cholesterol was about 5 percent for those individuals with average cholesterols. Those with higher cholesterol levels showed greater decreases. Other studies have shown that garlic keeps the blood from clotting by preventing the platelets from sticking together and by increasing factors that break down clots in the blood.[84] These three qualities of garlic oil may be benefits that help to decrease the risk of heart disease and atherosclerosis.

The question is how much of the cholesterol decrease was due to the special properties of garlic and how much from the the fact that this is another vegetable oil. As mentioned, polyunsaturated oils from fish and plants will lower the cholesterol level and prevent blood clotting. A comparison would make a good experiment.

A 5 percent drop in cholesterol over eight months is not much to brag about when a properly designed diet will drop the cholesterol levels by 25 percent in three weeks, at no added cost and with many more benefits than can be obtained from lecithin capsules or garlic oil in capsules or in odiferous cloves.[76] Do include garlic in your health-supporting diet as a flavoring, if you like it, but not for any medicinal benefits. Similarly, lecithin of the polyunsaturated variety will be plentiful enough in a diet of starchy foods, vegetables, and fruits.

Will taking large doses of vitamins lower my cholesterol?

In 1950, a Russian scientist reported that vitamin C retarded the growth of atherosclerotic plaques in rabbits.[85] This discovery brought up the possible relevance of vitamin C and cholesterol in people and the possible prevention of heart disease. Guinea pigs are similar to humans in that both species share a rare metabolic inability to synthesize vitamin C. Most other mammals make all of this vitamin that they need. Vitamin C deficiency in guinea pigs raises their cholesterol level. Experiments on people, using 1 to 4 grams of vitamin C per day, showed no lowering effect for those who did not have seriously elevated levels of cholesterol to begin with. However, people with high levels of cholesterol have been found to benefit from vitamin C, which does decrease their cholesterol content.[85] Vitamin C given to people with low vitamin C intakes has also had the additional benefit of lowering the levels of the "bad", LDL cholesterol. More study is needed before the role of vitamin C in lowering cholesterol levels and preventing heart disease is understood. However, I assure you that people who eat lots of fresh fruits and vegetables have no need for additional vitamin C from supplements. Nor need they worry about gaining additional protection from heart disease. This diet provides both. Much of the medical profession and the health food industry is dedicated to solving people's health problems by giving them plenty of pills to compensate for an improper diet and an unhealthy lifestyle, instead of dealing with the causes of disease. Such attempts are never satisfactory solutions, because they do not correct the underlying problems.

Large doses of vitamin B3 (or niacin), 3 to 6 grams a day, will effectively reduce cholesterol and triglyceride levels and have been used by doctors to treat people with elevated levels.[86] But the side effects of flushing are troublesome for many people. Also, vitamins A, D, and E, packed in vegetable oil, will lower the cholesterol level slightly, because of the effect of the polyunsaturated oil, not the vitamins.

Aren't there some powerful cholesterol-lowering drugs that doctors can prescribe? I recently read about a study that used a drug to reduce the chance of dying of heart disease and proved that cholesterol caused heart disease.

The day of reckoning for skeptics about the role of cholesterol finally arrived on January 20, 1984. Newspaper headlines across the country proclaimed: "CHOLESTEROL NOW PROVED TO CAUSE HEART DISEASE." This welcome news, long overdue, came from the National Heart, Lung, and Blood Institutes. Data from ten years of research on 3806 men with dangerously high levels of cholesterol convinced investigators to reach that momentous conclusion.[87,88]

The average cholesterol level of the subjects in this study was over 290 milligram percent. This high level predicted with a great degree of certainty that all too soon a subject's death certificate could read "Cause of death: HEART DISEASE." The study focused mostly on the benefit of using a drug, *cholestyramine,* to lower blood cholesterol. The subjects were placed on a relatively ineffective experimental diet containing 250 milligrams of cholesterol, only a 50 milligram reduction from their usual diet. As would be expected from such an insignificant change, the experimental diet had little effect on the subjects' blood cholesterol levels.

Did they find that cholestyramine is effective in lowering cholesterol? Maybe I should take this drug in addition to the other things you think I should do.

The drug is very effective, but, naturally, an unwelcome price is attached to it. It acts by binding cholesterol while it is still in the intestinal tract and thereby prevents it from being absorbed. Individuals who were able to stomach the six packages of cholestyramine powder a day had most of the cholesterol derived from their diet converted into the unabsorbable form. However, few subjects were willing to take all of the drug during the time of the experiment because of its unpleasant side effects: indigestion, constipation, and bloating. All these, incidentally, are problems easily controlled by a proper diet.

In those people who took the full dosage of the drug, blood cholesterol levels went down by 25 percent. These faithful persons, according to calculations based on data derived from the study, benefited by as much as a 50 percent reduction in their chance of dying from a heart attack.[88] They also made fewer trips to operating rooms for bypass surgery, and some evidence suggested also that their atherosclerotic plaques were being reversed.[87,88]

During this study the cost of the drug for each subject was $150 per month, for a total drug cost of $15 million. Ten "extra lives" were saved during the ten-year study period, bringing the cost per life saved to $1.5 million in the medication alone. I believe that a competent health educator, with equivalent funds and a decent cholesterol-lowering diet, would easily save many more lives then ten. An average reduction of 25 percent in cholesterol levels through diet change alone can be expected, as has been indicated by many studies on human subjects during the last forty years.[76] However, the real benefit is keeping people alive longer.

How about some of the medications I have heard about that "thin" the blood. I've heard that taking an aspirin a day will prevent heart attacks and strokes. Does aspirin really work?

Aspirin, like fish oil, suppresses the blood-clotting activity of platelets, but by a different mechanism. A portion of the aspirin binds irreversibly to the platelets, making them permanently useless.[89] Only after new platelets are produced can these components of the clotting system function as they should. The theory is that with less platelet activity the development of atherosclerosis should be slowed, and if the blood is "thinner"—from aspirin, say, or from fish oil—then the tendency for clots to form would be reduced, whenever plaques did rupture.[21]

Several big studies have tried to determine whether or not aspirin will reduce the risk of death in patients who have recently suffered a heart attack. Six studies showed a very small reduction in death rates, at a very high cost.[90] The recommended doses of three aspirin a day caused nausea, stomach pains, and vomiting in as many as 20% of the participants.[90] Other side effects from the aspirin were constipation, gout, and gastrointestinal bleeding.

Two other antiplatelet drugs are commonly prescribed: Persantine and Anturane. They must be taken three times a day and are much more expensive than aspirin. They are no more effective than aspirin in preventing death.[90]

Daily aspirin therapy has also been used in an attempt to reduce the complications of other blood vessel diseases. Sudden but temporary attacks that cause the loss of a variety of brain functions are called *transient ischemic attacks,* or *TIAs.* Temporary and partial loss of vision and weakness or numbness of a part of the body are common occurrences with TIAs. In many of these attacks the immediate cause is small blood clots and other debris, such as cholesterol crystals, that collect on the atherosclerotic plaques lining the insides of the arteries that provide blood for the brain.[91] The clots and debris break off and travel to the brain, where they lodge in a smaller blood vessel, causing the brain to malfunction. Aspirin has been used with some success in reducing the number of TIAs. When larger clumps and clots break off and travel to the brain, then death of brain tissue in local places can occur. This event is known as a *stroke*. Studies on the prevention of stroke with daily aspirin have been somewhat disappointing.[92,93] One study has shown some benefit of stroke prevention for men, but none for women.[93]

Attempts have been made to use aspirin to reduce the formation of blood clots in veins. This could be an important therapy, because blood clots in the leg veins and lungs are found in 30 to 50 percent of patients after surgery for any cause.[94] Aspirin has not been helpful in this respect.[95]

There is a much more effective, safe, and economical way to prevent platelet stickiness, clot formation, heart diseases, strokes, and other diseases of the blood vessels. A diet low in saturated fats and cholesterol provides all these benefits without any of the disadvantages found with drugs.[96-100]

Let me ask about one last quick-fix treatment. Chelation therapy works, I've heard, and it certainly sounds a lot better than surgery on my arteries.

Chelation therapy is popular, but not necessarily because it works to clean out the arteries. This is a highly profitable business for those who perform it, and the patient is happy to just lie back and get fixed, so to speak. Approximately 1000 chelationists perform chelation therapy on nearly a quarter of a million people. Centers have flourished amid claims that this therapy may be used as an alternative to bypass and other artery surgery. But claims for benefits on atherosclerosis with chelation have been as hard to substantiate as other claims made about curing rheumatoid arthritis, staving off old age and senility, reducing blood pressure, and improving diabetic conditions.[101] The cost of chelation therapy to each patient may be as high as $6000 for a series of treatments, with each infusion ranging from $70 to $110.[102]

According to the theory, a chelating agent, EDTA, combines with the calcium in the plaques.[102] This complex molecule leaves the plaques and is excreted through the kidneys. With this removal of calcium, the atherosclerotic disease is supposed to dissolve away. Patients are shown their urine with the calcium-EDTA sediment, and many are amazed by this demonstration of the marvels of physiological chemistry. People undergoing this treatment do report relief of chest pains and feelings of improved blood circulation.[102-104]

The medical profession is quite critical of doctors who use this treatment. But the profession has been slow to undertake studies to prove or disprove the chelationists' claims. One reason for lack of interest in testing is that EDTA is no longer controlled by patent rights, and therefore no drug company has a large enough financial stake in the dispute to be interested in determining the effectiveness of the therapy.[104]

The theory, however, is in contradiction to what is known about the physiology of the body, which protects very carefully the level of calcium in the blood. When EDTA removes some of the calcium from the blood, the bones must quickly release more calcium into the blood in order to keep the level constant. Calcium in plaque is less accessible than is calcium in bones, and is therefore less likely to be removed by EDTA. Actually, the amount of calcium in a plaque is quite small until very late stages of atherosclerosis.[105,106]

In a way, the supposed effects of "chelation" do work when the cholesterol in the blood is lowered by dieting for long periods of time. With a constant lower level of cholesterol in the blood, cholesterol is separated from the plaques, and the atherosclerosis is reduced without cost or risk to you.

Can I stop the damage if I stop eating these high-fat, high-cholesterol foods? Better yet, you mentioned reversal of the atherosclerosis. Can it really be reversed?

These are very important questions to answer for older people like you and me who have spent our entire lives eating high-cholesterol, high-fat foods. Undoubtedly our arteries have developed a considerable amount of plaque, some of which we're aware of, but much of which we are not. Atherosclerotic diseases of the blood vessels occur almost exclusively in parts of the world where the diet is centered around meats, dairy products, eggs, and refined and processed foods. People thriving on rice, potatoes, sweet potatoes, corn, beans, and wheat-based diets are almost immune from the complications of atherosclerosis. Most of us have had the misfortune of being raised according to the doctrine of the basic four food groups. As a result we have partly blocked arteries and arterial disease that is progressing. Fortunately, our bodies have the ability to stop this progression, correct much of the damage, and reverse some of the atherosclerosis—once we stop eating unhealthy foods.

Some very persuasive evidence that we can change the course of our lives comes from societies of people that were forced to change their diets during World War II.[107] In most of Western Europe the diets of people were greatly changed. Foods of all kinds became scarce and the shortages were primarily of foods high in fats and cholesterol. At the same time, incidentally, nervous stress and strain increased enormously because of the war. Studies show that up until 1940 the numbers of deaths from complications of atherosclerosis were rising. During the period of most food deprivation, 1943 to 1945, populations experienced the lowest death rates from blood vessel diseases, and the decline affected all age groups.[107] After the war years, as the rich foods returned, the death rates from complications of atherosclerosis increased to that of the prewar years. The people who experienced the decline in death rate were in their fifties, sixties, seventies, and eighties. They had spent many years eating rich foods and damaging their arteries. Yet when dietary change was forced upon entire nations, the people in these populations actually became healthier because of the reduction in arterial diseases. Many other disease conditions, including obesity, gout, diabetes, and multiple sclerosis improved during these times of stress and deprivation of rich foods.

Norway is an example of a country that experienced those dramatic changes in foods and mortality. The graphs on page 121 demonstrate the course of those changes during the war.

The war experiences have provided other valuable information about the effects of changes in food on the health of the arteries. After World Wars I and II, autopsies on people who suffered from malnutrition showed a reduction in the amount of atherosclerosis in their arteries, as compared with the smaller number of the population who were "well fed" and sometimes even obese.[108] A similar finding has been made with people who die from wasting diseases such as cancer.[108] During the last weeks of life, their appetite is depressed and their food intake is lowered. When their arteries are examined after death, the blood vessels appear much healthier. In other words, less atherosclerosis is present. The fat and cholesterol deposits apparently left the artery walls and provided calories for the body's metabolic needs during the patients' terminal weeks.

Have there been any scientific experiments that show that athero-sclerosis is reversible?

Animal experiments have been carried out for years, and they show that a high level of blood cholesterol and atherosclerosis can be caused by feeding high-fat, high-cholesterol diets to primates, such as the rhesus monkey.[108,109] Later, when these monkeys are put back on their natural, almost vegetarian diet, a reduction in cholesterol levels is gained in about three weeks, and much of the atherosclerosis is reversed in several months.[109]

Many studies on people have also shown that the progression of arterial

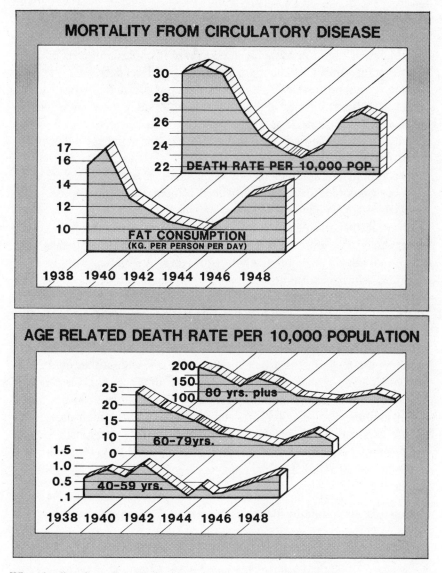

MORTALITY FROM CIRCULATORY DISEASE

DEATH RATE PER 10,000 POP.

FAT CONSUMPTION
(KG. PER PERSON PER DAY)

1938 1940 1942 1944 1946 1948

AGE RELATED DEATH RATE PER 10,000 POPULATION

80 yrs. plus

60-79yrs.

40-59 yrs.

1938 1940 1942 1944 1946 1948

When the diet of people in Norway changed as a result of World War II the death rate from heart disease decreased dramatically.[107] This decrease in disease occurred in all age groups; thus demonstrating that even in people with established artery disease, forty to eighty plus years old, death from heart disease decreases as health improves shortly after a change from a high fat, high cholesterol diet to a low-fat, low cholesterol diet.

disease can be slowed or stopped after decreasing blood cholesterol by diet and medications.[110-114] If enough corrective measures can be made by lowering the cholesterol level, then the atherosclerotic disease is actually reversible.[113] The most important factor foretelling the reversal of this disease is the drop in blood cholesterol level.[113] On the average, people in the group that showed reversal had a decrease in cholesterol level of about 65 milligram percent.[113] The more the cholesterol level decreases, the more likely it is that reversal will be seen in the course of months or years. A recent study used high-resolution ultrasound to study forty-three plaques in the arteries of the neck in thirty-one patients over the course of eighteen months.[114] Regression of some of the plaques and repair of some of the ulcers in the artery linings were seen.

In addition to studies of groups of patients, many documented cases have been recorded of dramatic reversal of atherosclerotic disease in individuals.[115-119] No longer is the question whether or not the disease can be reversed. Rather, the questions are: to what degree can reversal be expected when cholesterol level is lowered, how long the process will take, and which individuals are most likely to show reversal. The answers to these questions will depend almost certainly upon the effectiveness of the cholesterol-lowering program the patient is maintained on. I recommend that people who are serious about improving their health should eat foods that contain no cholesterol and very little fat of all types.

For some people with elevated blood cholesterol levels who are not able to follow the recommended diet, or for those few who get an inadequate response from the change in diet alone, a powerful drug such as cholestyramine may be added. In rare families some members do suffer from a true genetic defect in cholesterol metabolism, and that leads to very high death rates from complications of atherosclerosis. These people are most likely to benefit from a combination of diet and drugs in order to lower cholesterol levels in the blood that often reach as high as 400 to 600 milligram percent.[120]

How will a change in diet cause reversal of atherosclerosis?

The cholesterol in atherosclerotic plaques is not set and immovable, like concrete, but it is actually involved in a dynamic exchange with the cholesterol in the blood. When radioactive cholesterol is fed to volunteers with advanced atherosclerotic lesions, this labeled cholesterol is incorporated into the atherosclerotic plaque.[121] When it is measured later, however, the radioactive cholesterol has reentered the blood. We can conclude that the cholesterol does come out of the plaque. Simple principles of physical chemistry show that the flow of cholesterol is in the direction of achieving an equilibrium between higher concentrations and lower concentrations. The proper conditions for reversal of atherosclerosis will lower the concentration of cholesterol in the blood to enable excessive amounts of it to leave the arterial walls. As blood with lower cholesterol and lower fat levels bathes the damaged artery walls, the fixed cholesterol and fat components are drawn out of the plaques. These plaques in turn grow smaller, opening up the arterial channel to the flow of blood needed by vital organs. The overall effect is improved health of the arteries and larger openings for the passage of nurturing blood.

Do people with poor circulation have to wait for years before gaining any improvement? I might give up if I didn't get some rewards pretty soon after I've begun all my efforts.

Studies have shown very rapid improvement in the health of people with atherosclerosis who have made dietary and lifestyle changes. Patients suffering from angina have benefited in about three weeks, with a 91 percent reduction in chest pains.[122] Walking that is limited by pain caused by poor circulation in the legs, a condition called *intermittent claudication,* begins to improve within five days after a patient starts on a low-fat diet.[123] After four months a patient may be able to walk twice as far because of improved circulation gained by the improved diet. Recovering from hearing loss and vertigo also follows upon a change to a cholesterol-lowering, low-fat diet.[124] In all of these instances of improved circulation, the benefits come not simply from a reversal of atherosclerosis, which takes from months to years to achieve, but also from the improved circulation that is the result of the low-fat content of a healthier diet.[125-127]

Fat causes the red blood cells to form clumps that clog the circulation.[125-127] The blood cell walls become relatively rigid in the presence of fat in the blood stream, and as a result they will not pass through the smaller blood vessels. Whereas vegetable fats cause platelets to become less sticky, animal fats cause them to stick together more easily.[128-132] When the platelets stick together, substances are released that cause spasms of the blood vessels, decreasing circulation even further.[21] Also, a considerable drop in the oxygen content of the blood occurs after eating fatty foods.[123] An immediate improvement in circulation can be expected because of the effects of low amounts of fats in the diet, and long-term improvements are gained in time with the reversal of atherosclerosis.

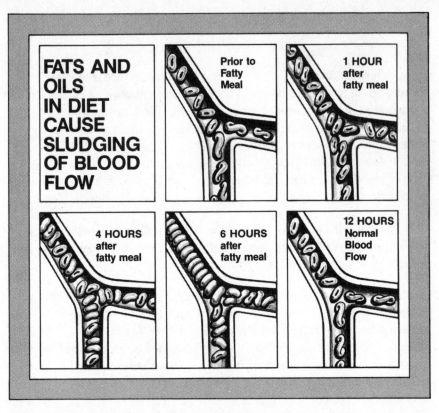

FATS AND OILS IN DIET CAUSE SLUDGING OF BLOOD FLOW

Prior to Fatty Meal

1 HOUR after fatty meal

4 HOURS after fatty meal

6 HOURS after fatty meal

12 HOURS Normal Blood Flow

Blood cells within the blood vessels flow freely and bounce off one another prior to a meal high in fat. Approximately one hour after a fatty meal, the cells begin to stick together upon contact and form small clumps. As this clump formation progresses, the flow of blood slows (sludging). Six hours after the meal the clumping becomes so severe that blood flow actually stops in many small vessels. Several hours later the clumps break up and the blood flow returns to the tissues.[125-127] In addition to reducing the flow of blood to the tissues, this effect of fatty foods on circulation decreases the oxygen content of the blood by over 20%.[123] No wonder people feel tired after eating.

The levels of fats that cause important changes in the circulation are not unusual for people eating the American diet to consume every day—often three, four or more times. When 67 percent of the calories (and probably even fewer calories) are derived from fat in the diet, the blood sludges, small blood vessels become blocked and the tissues are deprived of nutrients and oxygen.[126] Consider the fat content of some favorite ingredients of culinary delights:

FOOD	percent calories of fat
Avocado	88
Bacon	94
Beef (T-bone steak)	82
Butter	100
Cashews	73

Cheddar cheese	73
Cream cheese	91
Eggs	65
Lamb	76
Mackerel	60
Milk	49
Margarine	100
Pork	75
Sunflower seeds	76

The effects of the fat from each meal last twelve or more hours. With little effort, and less thought, most people hinder their circulation all day long.

I can see that my diet and lifestyle are very important in reducing my risk of complications from atherosclerosis and in improving my health. I have full control over these factors, and I'm going to do something about them, starting today. But one thing troubles me that I don't feel I have control over. What do I do about stress?

There is some evidence that people who are under stress suffer more from heart disease.[133-134] However, there is also evidence to the contrary.[135] I believe that for most people stress is a normal and necessary part of life. Stress gets us motivated to get jobs done and problems solved. I don't look at stress as an important hazard to health—unless, of course, stress drives you to eat more high-cholesterol foods, drink more cups of coffee, and smoke more packs of cigarettes per day. I encourage you to focus first and foremost on the health factors that are manageable, such as what you eat and drink. Not that you should neglect efforts that will bring you mental and emotional tranquility, but don't use stress as an excuse for your health problems when other things—like fats and cholesterol—are more certain to be the culprits.

There seems to be so much resistance to changing the diet that is served in schools, in the military services, in almost every restaurant and every family dinner table. Why does it take so long for the right dietary advice to reach the public?

Personal bias of our health professionals is one important factor. Most dietitians, doctors, and other health professionals themselves still eat foods that are high in cholesterol and fats—the very same diet that is condemned by so much evidence. Consider the fact that members of the Heart Association still serve beef, butter, cheese, and ice cream at their annual meetings and fund-raising functions. Here is proof that they don't take seriously their own recommendations—and the last eighty years of scientific research concerning heart problems. Imagine a meeting of the Lung Association that provided complimentary packs of cigarettes and an ashtray for each guest at the banquet table! This kind of contradictory behavior has serious effects upon the policies that shape our national health.

Only after considerable time and effort are spent on general education will this situation improve. But, more important, real progress will be held up until the diets and lifestyles of health authorities and policy makers, as individuals, change for the better. Back in the 1950s, before the Surgeon General's Report on Smoking, only 48 percent of the population smoked. That left half the people in a position to see the harmful effects of smoking from an unbiased point of view. Today, almost everyone in America follows the rich, high-fat, high-cholesterol diet. For this reason alone, all but a few people cannot perceive the serious consequences of these foolish eating habits or realize that an enjoyable alternative exists. Also, we must realize that the food industry is many times larger and more powerful and pervasive in our society than the tobacco industry. All you can do for now is be satisfied that you see the issues correctly, and all by yourself, if need be, make effective changes in diet for your family and yourself.

For more than eighty years scientific research has been pointing the accusing finger at the rich American diet. But the industries that provide us with all these tasty goodies continue to deny the evidence. Many of us are beginning to accept the evidence, because we really do want to be healthier and are willing to work toward that goal. We are learning that there are no quick fixes in the form of pills, infusions, or surgeries to safeguard our health. Sensible Americans want to keep their health by changing to better practices of eating and living. Exercise has been walking, jogging and even dancing into our consciousness. Notice how many people are eating at salad bars and asking for whole-wheat buns. And observe how the fast-food industry has responded. The industry has discovered that it can profit by selling things that will help people to live healthier and more productive lives. The dollar may triumph again, but this time it may do so for the benefit of health.

℞

• The prevention of atherosclerosis is based on a low-fat, no-cholesterol high fiber diet. This disease is preventable if proper diet is started early enough in life. And it can be corrected if treatment is begun before serious damage is done to the heart or the major blood vessels.

• Treatment of atherosclerosis is based on a low-fat, no-cholesterol high-fiber diet. Circulation improves and atherosclerosis is reversed with the proper diet and change in lifestyle.

• Blood cholesterol levels should be relied upon to follow progress of changes in diet and lifestyle. Other laboratory tests should also be made, at least initially. These should include levels of triglycerides, blood sugar, and uric acid. Levels of abnormal tests should be rechecked every three weeks until the values stabilize, then check them much less often.

• Drugs taken to lower cholesterol and triglycerides may be stopped under doctor's supervision shortly after starting the diet. Recheck blood tests in about three weeks. People often forget to limit their fruit intake and the triglycerides remain elevated.

• Polyunsaturated vegetable oils in the diet will lower blood levels of cholesterol and decrease the risk of complications from atherosclerosis. But those same polyunsaturated oils introduce other risks to health, such as obesity, gallstones, and cancer. Keep all oils in your diet at a minimum.

• Smoking tobacco, and drinking coffee will hasten the development of atherosclerosis in people who eat high-fat, high-cholesterol foods.

• Drinking alcohol in small amounts may reduce the risk of athero-sclerosis, but it also introduces other health hazards.

• Moderate physical exercise will benefit circulation but will not compensate for abuses in diet and lifestyle.

• Quick fixes in the form of lecithin, garlic, or vitamin pills will offer little or nothing toward the health of your arteries. Don't waste your money!

• Chelation therapy likewise is not helpful. Don't waste your money on this either.

• Aspirin and cholestyramine therapy will add little or nothing for the prevention and treatment of arterial disease gained by a health-supporting diet, and the side effects and costs of these drugs are significant. Use them only under special conditions, where diet and lifestyle changes alone will not suffice.

• Surgery for arterial disease should be reserved for a last effort, when atherosclerosis is threatening your circulatory functions and your life.

REFERENCES

[1]McGill H. Persistent problems in the pathogenesis of atherosclerosis. *Arteriosclerosis* 4:443, 1984.

[2]Ross R. The role of endothelial injury and platelet and macrophage interactions in atherosclerosis. *Circulation 70* (suppl III), III-77, 1984.

[3]Fust G. Circulating immune complexes in vascular diseases. *Lancet* 1:193, 1977.

[4]Imparato A. The carotid bifurcation plaque: pathologic findings associated with cerebral ischemia. *Stroke* 10:238, 1979.

[5]Lusby R. Carotid plaque hemorrhage. Its role in production of cerebral ischemia. *Arch Surg* 117:1479, 1982.

[6]Holman R. The natural history of atherosclerosis. The early aortic lesions as seen in New Orleans in the middle of the 20th century. *Am J Pathol* 34:209, 1958.

[7]Enos W. Pathogenesis of coronary disease in American soldiers killed in Korea. *JAMA* 158:912, 1955.

[8]Welch C. Cinecoronary arteriography in young men. *Circulation* 42:647, 1970.

[9]Page I. Prediction of coronary heart disease based on clinical suspicion, age, total cholesterol, and triglycerides. *Circulation* 42:625, 1970.

[10]Virmani R. Coronary heart disease at young age: a report of 187 autopsy patients who died of severe coronary atherosclerosis. *Cardiovasc Rev Rept* 5:799, 1984.

[11]Pooling Project Research Group: Relationship of blood pressure, serum cholesterol, smoking habit, relative weight and ECG abnormalities to incidence of major coronary events: Final report of the Pooling Project. *J Chronic Dis* 31:201, 1978.

[12]Barr D. Influence of sex and sex hormones upon the developement of atherosclerosis and upon the lipoproteins of plasma. *J Chronic Dis* 1:63, 1955.

[13]Bainton C. Deaths from coronary heart disease in persons fifty years of age and younger: a community-wide study. *N Engl J Med* 268:569, 1963.

[14]Gordon T. Premature mortality from coronary heart disease: the Framingham study. *JAMA* 215:1617, 1971.

[15]Muckle T. High-density lipoprotein cholesterol in differential diagnosis of senile dementia. *Lancet* 1:1191, 1985.

[16]Rosen S. Epidemiologic hearing studies in the USSR. *Arch Otolaryng* 91:424, 1970.

[17]Rosen S. Dietary prevention of hearing loss. *Arch Otolaryng* 70:242, 1970.

[18]Virag R. Is impotence an arterial disorder? A study of arterial risk factors in 440 impotent men. *Lancet* 1:181, 1985.

[19]Slag M. Impotence in medical clinic outpatients. *JAMA* 249:1736, 1983.

[20]Editorial: The progression of atherosclerosis. *Lancet* 1:791, 1985.

[21]Oliva P. Pathophysiology of acute myocardial infarction, 1981. *Ann Intern Med* 94:236, 1981.

[22]Connor W. The key role of nutritional factors in the prevention of coronary heart disease. *Prev Med* 1:49, 1972.

[23]Samuel P. Further validation of the plasma isotope ratio method for measurement of cholesterol absorption in man. *J Lipid Res* 23:480, 1982.

[24]Insull W. Cholesterol, triglyceride, and phospholipid content of intima, media and atherosclerotic fatty streak in human thoracic aorta. *J Clin Invest* 45:513, 1966.

[25]Katz S. Physical chemistry of the lipids of human atherosclerotic lesions: demonstration of a lesion intermediate between fatty streaks and advanced plaques. *J Clin Invest* 58:200,1976.

[26]Taylor C. Spontaneously occurring angiotoxic derivatives of cholesterol. *Am J Clin Nutr* 32:40, 1979.

[27]Zampogna A. Relationship between lipids and occlusive coronary artery disease. *Arch Intern Med* 140:1067, 1980.

[28]Cohn P. Serum lipid levels in angiographically defined coronary artery disease. *Ann Intern Med* 84:241, 1976.

[29]Jenkins P. Severity of coronary atherosclerosis related to lipoprotein concentration. *Br Med J* 2:388, 1978.

[30]Proudfit W. Selective cine coronary arteriography: correlation with clinical findings in 1,000 patients. *Circulation* 33:901, 1966.

[31]Kannel W. Cholesterol in the prediction of atherosclerotic disease: new perspectives based on the Framingham study. *Ann Intern Med* 90:85, 1979.

[32]Anderson J. The dependence of the effects of cholesterol and degree of saturation of the fat in the diet on serum cholesterol in man. *Am J Clin Nutr* 29:1784, 1976.

[33]Jackson R. Influence of polyunsaturated and saturated fats on plasma lipids and lipoproteins in man. *Am J Clin Nutr* 39:589, 1984.

[34]Keys A. Effect on serum cholesterol in man of mono-ene fatty acid (oleic acid) in the diet. *Proc Soc Exp Biol Med* 98:387, 1958.

[35]Flynn M. Serum lipids in humans fed diets containing beef or fish and poultry. *Am J Clin Nutr* 34:2734, 1981.

[36]Flynn M. Dietary "meats" and serum lipids. *Am J Clin Nutr* 35:935, 1982.

[37]O'Brien B. Human plasma lipid responses to red meat, poultry, fish, and eggs. *Am J Clin Nutr* 33:2573, 1980.

[38]Fehily A. The effect of fatty fish on plasma lipid and lipoprotein concentrations. *Am J Clin Nutr* 38:349, 1983.

[39]Kromhout D. The inverse relation between fish consumption and 20-year mortality from coronary heart disease. *N Engl J Med* 312:1205, 1985.

[40]Tall A. Current concepts. Plasma high-density lipoproteins. *N Engl J Med* 299:1232, 1978.

[41]Gordon T. Diabetes, blood lipids, and the role of obesity in coronary heart disease risk in women. The Framingham study. *Ann Intern Med* 87:393, 1977.

[42]Garrison R. Cigarette smoking and HDL cholesterol: the Framingham offspring study. *Atherosclerosis* 30:17, 1978.

[43]Chase H. Juvenile diabetes mellitus and serum lipids and lipoprotein levels. *Am J Dis Child* 130:1113, 1976.

[44]Arntzenius A. Reduced high-density lipoprotein in women aged 40-41 using oral contraceptives. Consultation Bureau Heart Project. *Lancet* 1:1221, 1978.

[45]Wood P. Plasma lipoprotein distributions in male and female runners. *Ann N Y Acad Sci* 301:748, 1977.

[46]Hulley S. Plasma high-density lipoprotein cholesterol level. Influence of risk factor intervention. *JAMA* 238,2269, 1977.

[47]Castelli W. Alcohol and blood lipids. The Cooperative Lipoprotein Phenotyping Study. *Lancet* 2:153, 1977.

[48]Flanagan M. The effects of diet on high density lipoprotein cholesterol. *J Hum Nutr* 34:43, 1980.

[49]Streja D. Plasma high-density lipoproteins and ischemic heart disease. Studies in a large kindred with familial hypercholesterolemia. *Ann Intern Med* 89:871, 1978.

[50]Rossner S. Normal serum-cholesterol but low HDL-cholesterol concentration in young patients with ischaemic cerebrovascular disease. *Lancet* 1:577, 1978.

[51]Bradby G. Serum high-density lipoproteins in peripheral vascular disease. *Lancet* 2:1271, 1978.

[52]Knuiman J. HDL-cholesterol in men from thirteen countries. *Lancet* 2:367, 1981.

[53]Mistry P. Cholesterol feeding revisited. *Circulation* 53 & 54 (suppl II): II-178, 1976.

[54]Hulley S. Epidemiology as a guide to clinical decisions. The association between triglyceride and coronary heart disease. *N Engl J Med* 302:1383, 1980.

[55]Phillipson B. Reduction of plasma lipids, lipoproteins, and apoproteins by dietary fish oils in patients with hypertriglyceridemia. *N Engl J Med* 312:1210, 1985.

[56]Glomset J. Editorial: Fish, fatty acids, and human health. *N Engl J Med* 312:1253, 1985.

[57]Connor W. The dietary treatment of hyperlipidemia: rationale, technique, and efficacy. *Med Clin North Am* 66:485, 1982.

[58]Fraser G. The effect of various vegetable supplements on serum cholesterol. *Am J Clin Nutr* 34:1272, 1981.

[59]Siess W. Platelet-membrane fatty acids, platelet aggregation, and thromboxane formation during a mackerel diet. *Lancet* 1:441, 1980.

[60]Dyerberg J. Haemostatic function and platelet polyunsaturated fatty acids in Eskimos. *Lancet* 2:433, 1979.

[61]Committee on Diet, Nutrition, and Cancer, Assembly of Life Sciences, National Research Council, *Diet, Nutrition and Cancer,* Washington D. C.: National Academy Press, 1982.

[62]Bennion L. Risk factors for the developement of cholelithiasis in man, (second of two parts). *N Engl J Med* 299:1221, 1978.

[63]Robertson W. The effect of high animal protein intake on the risk of calcium stone-formation in the urinary tract. *Clin Sci* 57:285, 1979.

[64]Brenner B. Dietary protein intake and the progressive nature of kidney disease: the role of hemodynamically mediated glomerular injury in the pathogenesis of progressive glomerular sclerosis in aging, renal ablation, and intrinsic renal disease. *N Engl J Med* 307:652, 1982.

[65]Smith M. The use of smell in differential diagnosis. *Lancet* 2:1452, 1982.

[66]Flynn M. Effect of dietary egg on human serum cholesterol and triglycerides. *Am J Clin Nutr* 32:1051, 1979.

[67]Dawber T. Eggs, Serum cholesterol, and coronary heart disease. *Am J Clin Nutr* 36:617, 1982.

[68]Flaim E. Plasma lipid and lipoprotein cholesterol concentrations in adult males consuming normal and high cholesterol diets under controlled conditions. *Am J Clin Nutr* 34:1103, 1981.

[69]Porter M. Effect of dietary egg on serum cholesterol and triglyceride of human males. *Am J Clin Nutr* 30:490, 1977.

[70]Slater G. Plasma cholesterol and triglycerides in men with added eggs in the diet. *Nutr Rep Int* 14:249, 1976.

[71]Liebman B. Poor design undercuts cholesterol study results (letter). *Am J Clin Nutr* 35:1041, 1982.

[72]Connor W. Reply to letter by Oster (letter). *Am J Clin Nutr* 36:1261, 1982.

[73]Sacks F. Ingestion of egg raises plasma low density lipoproteins in free-living subjects. *Lancet* 1:647, 1984.

[74]Roberts S. Does egg feeding (i.e., dietary cholesterol) affect plasma cholesterol levels in humans? The results of a double-blind study. *Am J Clin Nutr* 34:2092, 1981.

[75]McMurry M. Dietary cholesterol and the plasma lipids and lipoproteins in the Tarahumara Indians: a people habituated to a low cholesterol diet after weaning. *Am J. Clin Nutr* 35:741, 1982.

[76]Mattson F. Effect of dietary cholesterol on serum cholesterol in man. *Am J. Clin Nutr* 25:589, 1972.

[77]Connor W. The interrelated effects of dietary cholesterol and fat upon human serum lipid levels. *J Clin Invest* 43: 1691, 1964.

[78]Kozararevic D. Frequency of alcohol consumption and morbidity and mortality: The Yugoslavia Cardiovascular Disease Study. *Lancet* 1:613, 1980.

[79]Yano K. Coffee, alcohol and risk of coronary heart disease among Japanese men living in Hawaii. *N Engl J Med* 297:405, 1977.

[80]Blackwelder W. Alcohol and mortality: the Honolulu Heart Study. *Am J Med* 68:164, 1980.

[81]Forde O. The Tromso heart study: coffee consumption and serum lipid concentrations in men with hypercholesterolaemia: a randomised intervention study. *Br Med J* 290:893, 1985.

[82]Little J. Coffee and serum-lipids in coronary heart disease. *Lancet* 1:732, 1966.

[83]ter Welle H. The effect of soya lecithin on serum lipid values in type II hyperlipoproteinemia. *Acta Med Scand* 195:267, 1974.

[84]Bordia A. Effect of garlic on blood lipids in patients with coronary heart disease. *Am J Clin Nutr* 34:2100, 1981.

[85]Editorial: Vitamin C and plasma cholesterol. *Lancet* 2:907, 1984.

[86]Miller O. Investigation of the mechanism of action of nicotinic acid on serum lipid levels in man. *Am J Clin Nutr* 8:480, 1960.

[87]Lipid Research Clinics Program. The Lipid Research Clinics Coronary Primary Prevention Trial results. I. Reduction in incidence of coronary heart disease. *JAMA* 251:351, 1984.

[88]Lipid Research Clinics Program. The Lipid Research Clinics Coronary Primary Prevention Trial results. II. The relationship of reduction in incidence of coronary heart disease to cholesterol lowering. *JAMA* 251:365, 1984.

[89]Rome L. Aspirin as a quantitative acetylating reagent for the fatty acid oxygenase that forms prostaglandins. *Prostaglandins* 11:23, 1976.

[90]Editorial: Aspirin after myocardial infarction. *Lancet* 1:1172, 1980.

[91]Pfaffenbach D. Morbidity and survivorship of patients with embolic cholesterol crystals in the ocular fundus. *Am J Opthalmol* 75:66, 1973.

[92]Whisnant J. The Canadian trial of aspirin and sulfinpyrazone in threatened stroke. *N Engl J Med* 299:953, 1978.

[93]The Coronary Drug Project Research Group. Aspirin in coronary heart disease. *J Chronic Dis* 29:625, 1976.

[94]Le Quesne L. Diagnosis and prevention of postoperative deep-vein thrombosis. *Ann Rev Med* 26:63, 1975.

[95]Medical Research Council (Report of the Steering Committee): Effect of Aspirin on postoperative venous thrombosis. *Lancet* 2:441, 1972.

[96]Acheson R. Does consumption of fruit and vegetables protect against stroke? *Lancet* 1:1191, 1983.

[97]Shekelle R. Diet, serum cholesterol, and death from coronary heart disease. The Western Electric Study. *N Engl J Med* 304:65, 1981.

[98]Burkitt D. Some diseases characteristic of modern Western civilization. Occasional review. *Br Med J* 1:274, 1973.

[99]Stamler J. Lifestyles, major risk factors, proof and public policy. *Circulation* 58:3, 1978.

[100]Barnard R. Effects of an intensive, short-term exercise and nutrition program on patients with coronary heart disease. *JCR* 1:99, 1981.

[101]Stevenson J. Chelation therapy in atherosclerosis. *Ann Intern Med* 97:789, 1982.

[102]Chelation therapy: a second look. *Harvard Medical School Health Letter* 9:1, 1984.

[103]Pentel P. Chelation therapy for the treatment of atherosclerosis. An appraisal. *Minn Med* 67:101, 1984.

[104]Bruni P. Chelation therapy: Opposition stymied by lack of definitive studies. *Patient Care,* May 30, 1985. p-20.

[105]Rathmann K. Chelation therapy of atherosclerosis: an opinion. *Drug Intell Clin Pharm* 18:1000, 1984.

[106]Gotto A. Chelation therapy in 1984. *Texas Med* 80:36, 1984.

[107]Strom A. Mortality from circulatory diseases in Norway 1940-1945. *Lancet* 1:126, 1951.

[108]Wissler R. Studies of regression of advanced atherosclerosis in experimental animals and man. *Ann NY Acad Sci* 275:363, 1976.

[109]Armstrong M. Regression of coronary atheromatosis in Rhesus monkeys. *Circ Res* 27:59, 1970.

[110]Duffield R. Treatment of hyperlipidaemia retards progression of symptomatic femoral atherosclerosis. A randomised controlled trial. *Lancet* 2:639, 1983.

[111]Nikkila E. Prevention of progression of coronary atherosclerosis by treatment of hyperlipidaemia: a seven year prospective angiographic study. *Br Med J* 289:220, 1984.

[112]Ost C. Regression of peripheral atherosclerosis during therapy with high doses of nicotinic acid. *Scand J Clin Lab Invest Suppl* 99:241, 1967.

[113]Barndt R. Regression and progression of early femoral atherosclerosis in treated hyperlipoproteinemic patients. *Ann Intern Med* 86:139, 1977.

[114]Hennerici M. Spontaneous progression and regression of small carotid atheroma. *Lancet* 1:1415, 1985.

[115]Basta L. Regression of atherosclerotic stenosing lesions of the renal arteries and spontaneous cure of systemic hypertension through control of hyperlipidemia. *Am J Med* 61:420, 1976.

[116]Bassler T. Regression of atheroma. *Western J Med* 132:474, 1980.

[117]Roth D. Noninvasive and invasive demonstration of spontaneous regression of coronary artery disease. *Circulation* 62:888, 1980.

[118]Sanmarco M. Arteriosclerosis: Its progression...and regression. *Prim Cardiol* July/Aug 1978, p-51.

[119]Hubbard J. Nathan Pritikin's heart. *N Engl J Med* 313:52, 1985.

[120]Glueck C. Therapy of familial hypercholesterolemia in childhood: Diet and cholestyramine resin for 24 to 36 months. *Pediatrics* 59:433, 1977.

[121]Jagannathan S. The turnover of cholesterol in human atherosclerotic arteries. *J Clin Invest* 54:366, 1974.

[122]Ornish D. Effects of stress management training and dietary changes in treating ischemic heart disease. *JAMA* 249:54, 1983.

[123]Kuo. P. The effect of lipemia upon coronary and peripheral arterial circulation in patients with essential hyperlipemia. *Am J Med* 26:68, 1959.

[124]Spencer J. Hyperlipoproteinemias in the etiology of inner ear disease. *Laryngoscope* 85:639,1973.

[125]Cullen C. Intravascular aggregation and adhesiveness of the blood elements associated with alimentary lipemia and injections of large molecular substances. Effect on blood-brain barrier. *Circulation* 9:335, 1954.

[126]Friedman M. Serum lipids and conjunctival circulation after fat ingestion in men exhibiting type-A behavior pattern. *Circulation* 29:874, 1964.

[127]Friedman M. Effect of unsaturated fats upon lipemia and conjunctival circulation. A study of coronary-prone (pattern A) men. *JAMA* 193:882, 1965.

[128]Greig H. Inhibition of fibrinolysis by alimentary lipaemia. *Lancet* 2:16, 1956.

[129]Mustard J. Effect of different dietary fats on blood coagulation, platelet economy, and blood lipids. *Br Med J* 1:1651, 1962.

[130]Hornstra G. Influence of dietary fat on platelet function in men. *Lancet* 1:1155, 1973.

[131]O'Brien J. Acute platelet changes after large meals of saturated and unsaturated fats. *Lancet* 1:878, 1976.

[132]Simpson H. Hypertriglyceridaemia and hypercoagulability. *Lancet* 1:786, 1983.

[133]Patel C. Trial of relaxation in reducing coronary risk: four year follow up. *Br Med J* 290:1103, 1985.

[134]Friedman M. Coronary-prone individuals (type A behavior pattern). Some biochemical characteristics. *JAMA* 212:1030, 1970.

[135]Case R. Type A behavior and survival after acute myocardial infarction. *N Engl J Med* 312:737, 1985.

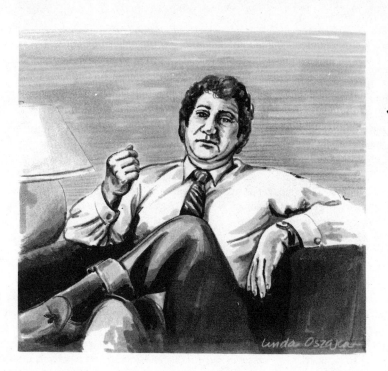

George

I know a lot of guys at work who have had heart surgery. It has become, like they say, a kind of status symbol around the office to brag about the number of bypass grafts some doctor or other has plugged into your heart. Me, I've had chest pains for only a couple of months now, but they're getting worse all the time, and the medicine my doctor has given me isn't making much difference anymore. I saw him the other day, and he said it's about time to operate.

It's really terrific, when you think what modern medical doctors are doing these days. I hear they can stop your heart for hours, keep your blood circulating through a machine, and, when they're ready, bring you back to life. So in my case I don't see much reason for delaying things. However, I've read a few newspaper articles that say bypass surgery is being overused. Maybe getting a second opinion would be smart. I trust my doctor, but still, if there is any safe alternative to getting my chest cracked open, I'm all for finding it. Frankly, I'm scared.

5

HEART DISEASE

My other doctor is always so vague with his answers to my questions. I really know very little about my condition and about the tests and treatments he says I should have. First off, I'd like to know why a person at my young age, only forty-two, would have these chest pains.

There are many causes for pains in and around the chest; some are serious, and others are only minor problems. The outer layers of the chest are made of skin, bones, and muscles. Within the chest lie the trachea (windpipe), esophagus (gullet), heart, lungs, and the membranes that line the heart and lungs. Any of these can be a source of chest pain. Sometimes the cause is clear, but at other times a thorough investigation is required to solve the mystery. Often, clues to the cause of the pain can be found. Especially helpful is information about any activity that brings on or increases the pain. For example, pain on swallowing suggests that the esophagus is the source. If moving your shoulders, taking a deep breath, or pressing on your chest makes the pain worse, then these movements suggest that the trouble is in the ribs or the chest muscles. A common source of chest pain is the rib joints, located about two inches from either side of the breast bone. They often become sore from hard physical work, but even something as ordinary as carrying a couple of heavy grocery bags can start this kind of chest pain. This condition, called *costochondritis,* can be very painful, but the fact that chest motion and pressing on the area of tenderness makes the pain worse should help to assure one that the source is not the heart. There are many variations to the patterns of pain and the causes; for example, pain on swallowing and deep breathing can also be an indication of inflammation of the linings surrounding the heart called *pericarditis.* You will certainly need the skills of your doctor to sort out the possible causes of chest pains.

Pain from heart disease is most often described as a dull pressure located in the front, at the center or just left of the center of the chest. Sometimes the pain travels to the inside of the left arm or up into the jaw. Often, when an actual heart attack has occurred, the victim will describe the pain as the worst feeling he or she has ever experienced: "It was like an elephant sat on my chest. I thought I was going to die." Heart attack pain usually lasts for several hours. Yet, surprisingly, you cannot always count on pain to warn you that the heart is in trouble: about 12 percent of people who have heart attacks feel little or no pain at all.[1] But these silent heart attacks are just as deadly as the painful ones.[1]

Your description of your kind of pain is what I would consider typical of someone suffering with heart disease that has not yet caused serious, permanent damage or, in other words, a real heart attack. This type of chest pain is called *angina pectoris,* which actually means pain in the chest, or more simply, angina. The chest discomfort is similar to that of a heart attack: dull and in the front central part of the chest. Unlike a heart attack, the pain can often be brought on repeatedly by physical activity, such as climbing stairs, and sometimes by emotional upset. Relief follows a short period of rest, and the fact that the pain is less intense also distinguishes angina from a true heart attack. Whenever you have strong or repeated chest pain, you should consult a qualified physician to make the correct diagnosis and offer recommendations for treatment.

A session of angina can be almost as serious as a heart attack. The chance of dying for a person who has suffered a heart attack averages about 5 percent each year, after the first year.[2] For a person with angina the chance is only slightly less, every year 4 percent of these people with heart disease will die.[3] Within five years the chance that a person with angina will suffer a nonfatal heart attack is 12 to 16 percent, depending on the severity of the heart condition.[4] You should take your chest pains as a serious warning. And you should not be satisfied with any treatment that simply relieves the pain rather than correcting the cause of the problem. The medications your doctor prescribed are intended primarily for the relief of symptoms that are telling you that your life is in danger.

Fine, that's all well and good. But what is wrong inside my heart to cause this pain every time I try to do something?

Your pain is the result of an insufficient blood supply reaching the tissues of your heart in order to meet the needs of this powerful muscle for oxygen and the other nutrients it must have in order to do its work. The exact way in which the pain begins is still unknown but probably is related to the accumulation of products of metabolism within the heart muscle because of sluggish blood flow.

The arteries that carry blood to the heart muscle are called *coronary arteries*. In most cases the flow of blood is slowed down by narrowings in the central openings of these arteries. These narrowings are the result of a slowly developing and lifelong disease known as *atherosclerosis*. With atherosclerosis, plaques made of cholesterol, fats, muscle cells, and scar tissue fill the insides of the arteries, hindering the normal flow of blood. This formation of plaque begins in early childhood and in most people continues as long as they live. Eventually, this disease process becomes a threat to useful function, as well as to life, for the majority of Americans.

During times of physical activity or emotional upset, the heart rate increases and the heart muscle pumps harder. As a result, these tissues of the heart demand more blood. Because the arterial channels are too small to meet the demand for increased flow of blood, the deprived muscle begins to hurt, which is its message to you to stop whatever you are doing. Unfortunately, many people who have diseased coronary arteries are given no such warning. Low blood supply to the heart is present without symptoms of chest pain, in 25 to 40 percent of cases of the people who are already known to suffer from heart disease.[5] In 2 to 4 percent of middle-aged men without any history of heart trouble, serious narrowings of the coronary arteries causing low blood supply to the heart muscle are present, but without any warning of chest pain.[5] Therefore, as in the case of a silent heart attack, a person with silent angina may not realize that anything is wrong until it is too late, when he or she is already a victim of a complication, such as a heart attack or death, of this sinister disease.

You should understand that two ways are available to stop chest pains: either keep your physical and heart activity within the limits of your poor circulation, or improve the circulation to your heart. Drugs, surgeries, and diet and lifestyle changes approach the problem of chest pain from both directions.

I have noticed with exercise that I feel the most pain when I first start off. Is this a warning that I shouldn't exercise?

Pain commonly occurs during the first few minutes after beginning vigorous physical activity such as walking, jogging, bicycling, or swimming. However, after this initial discomfort, many heart patients can perform physical activities for prolonged periods without further pain. This is called the *warm-up phenomenon,* and it is the result of an increase in blood flow to the heart muscle after the initial period of exercise.[6]

You must be careful about beginning any kind of exercise program, because the risk of sudden death while performing vigorous physical activities without adequate preparation is greater than during quieter activities.[7] In someone suffering from severe atherosclerosis, the added demand for blood by a hard working heart muscle during vigorous exercise sometimes can tip the balance toward a fatal event, such as a heart arrythmia or a heart attack. Many people who die suddenly while exercising have previous symptoms of heart disease, but others do not.[8] In the general population, the risk of sudden death is small and should not keep people with heart disease from using exercise as a means of improving their general health and reducing their risk of heart attacks.[9] But, exercise with caution! Start with relatively mild activities; then gradually build up to more demanding work. At the same time, attention must be paid to other factors that affect risk of heart attacks and sudden death, especially diet.

But I also feel chest pains at night when I'm lying down doing nothing. Can I do anything about this pain?

Fluids that have been accumulating throughout the day in your legs seep back into your blood vessels when you lie down, and as a result, the heart has more blood to pump. Also, while lying down, the return of blood to the heart is unimpeded by the forces of gravity. The extra return of blood to the heart causes the heart to pump harder. This in turn increases the heart muscle's demand for oxygen and nutrients; chest pains may occur when the coronary arteries are severely narrowed and adequate flow of blood to the heart muscle is impeded. People who experience chest pain at night can find relief by raising the head of the bed about 10 degrees so that the heart is higher than the legs.[10] In this position, you sleep while gravity helps to pull fluids away from the heart. Even after you get out of bed in the morning, considerable time may be needed for the excess fluids to leave the blood vessels and accumulate again in the leg tissues. For this reason, some people feel more angina in the mornings. A diet low in salt and fats is very important to lower the demand on the heart by keeping excess fluids from accumulating in the body and blood vessels.

On occasion, I've noticed a few skips in my heartbeat. Should I be taking some kind of medicine for that?

Irregular beats of the heart are called arrhythmias. They can be dangerous when they are associated with such symptoms as chest pains or fainting. Extra beats that originate from the greater portion of the heart muscle are called *ectopic ventricular beats*. These arrhythmias are common in apparently healthy people and most of the time are not serious.[11] Antiarrhythmic drugs are generally ineffective.[11] In fact, sometimes the drug therapy is more dangerous than the irregular beats. However, you will need medical evaluation to determine the kind of irregularity your heart is having and the need versus the hazard of drug therapy.

Arrhythmias can be the result of a poor blood supply to the heart muscle and to other specialized tissues that conduct electrical charges through the heart muscle.[11] Improvement in circulation can improve the heart's rhythm. Stimulating drugs, such as caffeine in coffee, tea, and chocolate, commonly cause irritability of the heart tissues. Prescription drugs, such as medications for heart conditions and asthma, antidepressants and stimulants, can also have the same effect.

Will the tests my doctor has planned for me tell how severely my arteries are affected by atherosclerosis?

Many different testing procedures are available to help your doctor determine the extent to which your coronary arteries are diseased. In most cases, testing begins with the safe and inexpensive ones first and then progresses to more expensive and riskier tests. The initial evaluation of a person like yourself with chest pain includes taking a history and having a physical examination, which includes an EKG while you are resting and tests of your blood for its content of cholesterol, triglycerides, sugar, uric acid, and thyroid hormones.

Often the next test a doctor orders for a patient with chest pains is a treadmill stress test, usually called simply a *treadmill* or a *stress test*. Essentially, this is an EKG performed while the patient is exercising, usually by walking on a moving belt. The treadmill stress tests are not very helpful in diagnosing coronary artery disease, because they add little to the physician's ability to pinpoint the cause of the condition by other means and because the results are frequently inaccurate. In most cases a person suspected of having heart disease can be diagnosed by evidence from his or her history and a resting EKG. The treadmill rarely makes the diagnosis any more definite, and this test adds a couple of hundred dollars to the cost of medical care.[12-16] When heart disease is unlikely according to the patient's history and EKG, then the treadmill test provides little additional information and a positive test may introduce some new problems including missing the real cause of the patient's distress. Another serious concern is that when the test is read as positive in someone without heart disease, in other words a false positive test result, this person may become psychologically upset from worrying about a condition he or she probably does not have, based on the history and EKG. Worse yet, a positive diagnosis frequently leads to more dangerous and expensive tests.[15] False positive results are much more common in women than in men. In one large study 54 percent of the results in women were false positives compared to 12 percent of those in men.[12] The detection and treatment of coronary artery disease by treadmill stress testing in someone without symptoms has not been shown to decrease the risk of sudden death from heart attacks or even heart attacks that are not fatal.[16] Therefore, the stress test should be avoided by people who feel relatively healthy and have otherwise a low risk of having heart disease.[12-16]

Some physicians feel that stress tests should be performed on men without symptoms of coronary artery disease if they are likely to have disease based on presence of risk factors for atherosclerosis and complications of coronary artery disease.[14] These risk factors include positive family history for heart disease, hypertension, smoking, and elevated cholesterol. The number and severity of the risk factors that physicians feel warrants further examination with a treadmill stress tests varies considerably. Some physicians recommend this test to almost everyone as a screening procedure, while others reserve it for those who are at very high risk for heart disease. A study has not yet been done to determine if any correlation exists between the ease with which a doctor orders a stress test for the patient and the number of payments that are left on the $20,000 office treadmill equipment. Regardless of the results of a stress test, risk factors should be treated vigorously and no consolation should be gained by a negative test result.[13]

Although treadmill stress testing may provide only marginal help in detecting significant coronary artery disease in patients with or without symptoms, the test does provide important information on the prognosis of the disease that could influence the course of treatment.[16-18] A result that shows profound changes with only a little exercise may be an indication of the presence of severe coronary artery disease and will suggest that further tests should be done.[15-18] A relatively normal stress test in someone having typical chest pains would be one indication that the arterial disease is not yet severe, and that further testing can be delayed.[15-18] Furthermore, many doctors agree that patients with few treadmill stress test changes can be treated quite confidently without surgery.[15-18]

What is the next test I should have if the treadmill is abnormal?

In an attempt to improve the usefulness of the treadmill test, a radioactive solution can be injected into the bloodstream. A picture is taken by a specialized scanning camera in order to observe the flow of blood with its content of radioactive solution to the heart muscle.[16] This procedure, called a *radionuclide scan*, costs several more hundred dollars and adds more information in the search for the cause of the chest pain. In one test the scanning is performed soon after the patient has finished running on the treadmill. The camera shows areas that are receiving too little blood for the amount of exercise being performed. Another kind of radionuclide scan is performed while the patient is still exercising. This procedure gives valuable information about the strength and motion of the heart muscle. A negative exercise radionuclide scan of either kind virtually excludes serious disease of the coronary arteries and puts a halt to further testing.[15] In patients with known coronary artery disease a normal treadmill stress test and exercise radionuclide scan indicate a good prognosis for a hopeful future regardless of what the arteries would look like on more detailed studies.[15] In 1981, an estimated 1.5 million cardiac radionuclide scans were done at a cost of $400- to-600 million.[19]

What further testing might be needed if the treadmill and radionuclide scan indicate I have serious heart disease?

The next step in discovering the extent of coronary artery disease, *the coronary angiography*, is a serious one with significant costs and risks. The indications for an angiogram depend a lot upon the symptoms of the patients.[15] Both a positive treadmill stress test and a positive radionuclide scan are required before making a diagnosis of serious coronary artery disease and performing coronary angiography in a person with atypical chest pains or no pain at all.[15] Because a normal treadmill stress test and radionuclide scan in someone with known coronary artery disease is such a favorable sign there is rarely an indication to procede with a angiogram with these findings.[15] An angiogram should be done in the patient who is known to have coronary artery disease—because of typical chest pains, positive findings from an EKG, a treadmill, and/or a radionuclide scan— when symptoms are unacceptable despite medical treatment or the tests indicate that a large amount of heart muscle would be lost, and life would be in serious jeopardy, if the diseased artery in question closed completely.[15] Angiograms are done in preparation for bypass or angioplasty surgery when the possibilities of such surgeries are likely.

A small-bore plastic tube is inserted into an artery of the leg or arm and is threaded through the vessel up to the heart. Then contrast material that can be detected by an X-ray machine is introduced through the catheter into the coronary arteries that feed the heart muscle and the pumping chambers of the heart. X-ray pictures reveal in detail the extent of arterial closure by showing shadows of the plaques that line the insides of the arteries. The X-ray also provides some information about the movement and strength of the heart muscle itself. The risk of a person dying from heart disease is related to the number of blood vessels whose passageways are closed by more than 50 percent with atherosclerotic plaques. Blockage of each of the three major vessels that supply the heart muscle means a different kind of risk to the patient's life and health, depending on the extent to which it supplies the heart muscle.[20-22] In addition, the more coronary arteries with serious disease, the greater the risks. Also, detecting abnormal motions of the heart gives evidence of poor muscle function and is a sign of poor outcome for the patient.[15,22]

Complications of bleeding, strokes, and heart attacks are possible consequences of coronary angiography.[23] Generally, the risk of death is much less than 1 percent and for serious complications less than 5 percent.[23] However, estimates have been reported that are as bad as an 18 percent risk of developing serious complications and a 2 percent risk of death from this test.[24] Your decision to submit to the procedure should not be made lightly. As the consumer patient, before you agree to the test you should clearly understand how its results will be used in making decisions about future treatment. Generally, the angiography should be reserved for patients who are really serious candidates for bypass surgery or a newer procedure called angioplasty.[15,20] Cardiologists who perform this angiography make $800 on the average for each patient. In 1980 alone, more than $600 million was spent on coronary angiographies.[19]

How often does the angiogram find serious disease?

In over half of the cases for whom coronary angiography is performed it leads to surgery. This is in part because the physicians who perform this procedure are careful to limit angiography to those likely to have disease and in part because advanced atherosclerotic coronary artery disease is almost the norm in the adult population in the United States. Studies at Cleveland Clinic using coronary angiography showed that nearly half of all men under the age of forty who underwent angiography for chest pains had extensive arterial disease.[25]

For an individual patient with advancing years, the number of arteries involved and the number of plaques that are formed in each artery becomes greater, and the passageways through which blood is supposed to flow freely become smaller and narrower.[26] And all the while our knives and forks are pitching cholesterol and fats into the arterial walls! Here are the probabilities of finding serious atherosclerosis in one or more heart arteries of a man with an average blood cholesterol level of 210 milligram percent and a low level of triglycerides who has had angiography performed. An increase in cholesterol or triglycerides will increase the probability of finding disease. These values are even more meaningful when you realize that for nearly 25 percent of the cases the atherosclerosis was described as moderate, and for over 60 percent the disease was said to be severe.[26] Severe and moderate atherosclerosis are the conditions that cause heart attacks and death. They are also the conditions for which surgeons operate.

AGE (years)	PROBABILITY OF FINDING CORONARY ARTERY DISEASE (%)
28	21.8
30	26.0
32	30.7
34	35.9
36	41.3
38	47.0
40	52.8
42	58.5
44	64.7
46	68.5
48	70.8
50	73.4
55	79.3
60	84.1
65	88.0
70	91.0

I'm not ready to give up my usual activities. Isn't there some way to improve the circulation to my heart muscle, so that when I walk, the pain will not come so often or so strong?

Basic plumbing principles suggest several ways to deal with your clogged pipes. In 1967, coronary artery bypass grafting, usually abbreviated as *bypass surgery,* was introduced by doctors from the Cleveland Clinic.[27] This technique removes dispensable veins from one of the patient's legs and connects these vessels above and below the clogged sections of the heart's arteries. These are detours, carrying blood past the narrow places in the arteries. When the vein from the leg, called the *saphenous vein,* is used, generally the upstream connection is made at the base of the *aorta,* the main artery leading from the heart. Then the blood vessel used for bypassing is attached downstream, past a blocked section in the artery. In this way, during a single operation, from one to eight (rarely more) bypasses can be performed on partially blocked coronary arteries and branches of these arteries in order to provide a greater supply of blood to the heart muscle.

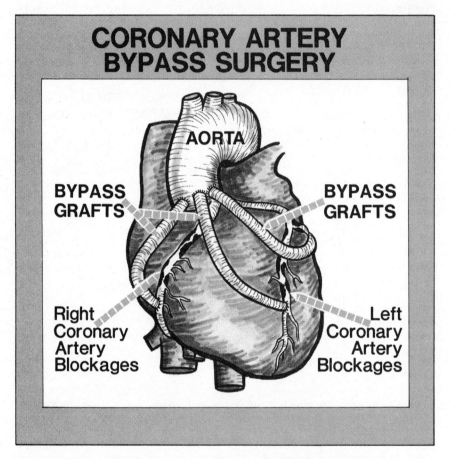

Bypass grafts from the saphenous vein in the leg or the internal mammary artery found along the breast bone are used to detour the blood around partial atherosclerotic blockages in the coronary arteries.

Sometimes the *internal mammary artery,* which lies along the inside of the breastbone, will be used instead of a leg vein in order to bypass the constricted length of a coronary vessel. At present this artery is being used more often as the graft instead of the leg vein, because it seems to last longer.[28]

Tell me more about the bypass operation. This is what they refer to as major-major surgery, I've heard.

The operation begins with an incision in the skin, followed by splitting of the breastbone lengthwise with a bone saw. Then the chest is pried open and the sack enclosing the heart is opened to expose the beating heart. One tube from the "heart-lung" machine is inserted into the right atrium, or the right upper chamber of the heart. This tube serves to remove the blood from the body and deliver it to the heart-lung machine. Another tube is inserted into the aorta in order to return the blood from the machine to the body. The heart-lung machine performs the functions of the patient's heart and lungs during the course of the operation, which may last several hours. While one group of surgeons is working over the organs in the chest, another surgical team is removing the saphenous vein from the leg.

In order to sew the vessels to the heart's arteries, the heart muscle must be stopped for a very short while. A muscle-paralyzing, very cold, high potassium solution is infused throughout the coronary arteries. Meanwhile the heart-lung machine cools the blood which in turn cools the entire body with a refrigeration unit. After the necessary bypasses are sewn in place, refrigeration is stopped, the heart muscle and blood are warmed, and the life-giving natural beat is allowed to resume. Sometimes the heart muscle must be given an electrical shock to restart a normal rhythm. The chest wall tissues are sewn closed and the patient is moved to the recovery room.

The surgeon needs delicate skills for sewing the fine blood vessels in place so that blood will flow freely without even the smallest of leaks. For this exquisite control of techniques, the bypass surgeon receives from $3000 to $6000 for each operation, which in some cases may require only a few minutes of actual operating time for the head-surgeon.[29] Bypass surgery is a $5-billion-a-year business that earns many surgeons $1 million and more annually. Acting almost by reflex, physicians send more than 200,000 trusting patients each year to such surgeons, asking to have their clogged arteries bypassed.[29]

Sounds like a terrible way to spend an afternoon! I'm surprised people can live through such an operation.

Bypass surgery is a strenuous ordeal, even for patients in top shape. All too often, people submitting to this surgery are old and have been ill for a long time with heart, lung, and other diseases before such surgical intervention is tried. Death rates have been reported to be as high as 18 percent for people over the age of seventy.[23,30] Under the best of circumstances the risk of death is about 5 percent in the elderly.[23] On the other hand, modern medical technology must be credited with a death rate of only about 2 percent or less when skilled surgeons operate on relatively healthy younger patients.[31]

I've heard that at least half of all bypass surgeries are done unnecessarily. But I'm sure my doctor won't make such a mistake with me.

Your doctor probably is caring for you with the most honorable of intentions, but he may not be aware of the high risks and the low benefits from this kind of surgery, much less about any alternatives for a patient with heart disease. On the other hand, a few doctors may not have the best intentions. Bypass surgery is big business, and physicians may have more to gain from it than you realize: increased income and fame, helping their hospital to keep its beds full, or supporting further personal or institutional expansion.[32] Furthermore, in these days of innumerable malpractice suits, some physicians find safety in going along with the crowd. A doctor can never be accused of failing to provide treatment or to do everything medically possible when his or her patient is advised to accept bypass surgery. Surgeons who perform this delicate operation are very well-educated and can be most intimidating to patients and to colleagues in other branches of medicine. Rare indeed is the family doctor who is willing and knowledgeable enough to recommend a more conservative approach for heart patients. These are only some of the reasons why too much unnecessary bypass surgery is performed in too many communities today.

I'd like to hear more about the risks involved.

Usually, on the surface, everything seems to go well for most patients who receive the care of this truly advanced science of surgery and life support. But in most cases the results are not really worth the $25,000 price tag, much less the pain and suffering that are attached.[29]

Many hazards are associated with any kind of extensive surgery. Major complications of one kind or another affect about 13 percent of patients.[33] Reoperation for bleeding, infections, blood clots reaching the lungs, heart attacks, strokes, kidney failure, lung failure, gastrointestinal bleeding, psychotic reactions, and death are only some of the unplanned consequences of bypass surgery.

The thought of having a stroke really scares me. If there is one thing I don't want to be, it is living as a helpless invalid dependent on my family.

A stroke isn't the only thing that threatens your mental functions. There is also a frequent form of damage to the brain that has appeared with the introduction of open-heart surgery. The heart-lung machine is far from being an ideal substitute for real hearts and lungs. Toxic chemicals, flakes of plastic from equipment, air bubbles, and clumps of fat and foreign material can be introduced into a patient's bloodstream during bypass surgery.[34-38] Injury to the blood cells also occurs as they pass through the tubes and oxygenating membranes of the machine. The relatively rough surfaces of plastic tubes and parts can damage many blood cells, and this injury causes the cells and other elements of the blood, especially platelets, to stick together in clumps.[36,37] After being returned to the patient's circulation, these damaged cells and clumps of blood elements, along with the flakes of foreign material and air bubbles, become stuck in the small blood vessels, and thereby block circulation of the blood. When that happens, blood with life-sustaining oxygen and nutrients is prevented from reaching the tissues, and injury and death of those tissues soon follows.

Studies show that nearly 100 percent of the patients who are placed on the heart-lung machine suffer some form of brain injury.[37-39] As a result of this injury and other complications that occur during the bypass operation, up to 100 percent of patients have dysfunction of their central nervous system immediately after surgery.[37] When examined at a later time, between 15 and 44 percent of people suffer detectable brain damage.[36,40-44] The persistent dysfunction tends to result in minor degrees of intellectual impairment, memory loss, sleep disturbances, and a degree of personality change, a feature often noticed by relatives.[40,44]

I think I've already got enough health problems. Now you're telling me I might get brain damage from the surgery. I certainly don't want that, but what choice do I have? This operation would save my life, wouldn't it?

The risk to life, the pain and expense of the operation, and the possiblity of permanent brain damage might be justified if bypass surgery led to a tremendous saving of lives. But unfortunately, the eighteen-year record for bypass surgery is nothing to brag about. Almost every review of the results of bypass surgery has concluded that this really heroic kind of surgery does not save lives when compared with simply giving patients drugs that relieve their angina.[31,32,45-47] Some evidence suggests that these drugs may have increased the survival rate in addition to relieving chest pains, but the success of drug therapy as a means of prolonging a patient's life with angina is small, at best.[48] The decline in the death rate from heart disease in recent years is attributed mostly to changes in diet and lifestyle and improved medical care rather than to bypass surgery, or even drugs.[49] Changes in diet and lifestyle are estimated to have accounted for 54 percent of the decrease in deaths from heart disease, while bypass surgery can be credited for only a 3.5 percent of the improvement. Drug therapy takes credit for 10 percent of the savings.[49]

Here are the results of the three largest and most important studies on bypass surgery that have been made since it was introduced more than eighteen years ago.[50]

STUDY REPORT	FIVE YEAR SURVIVAL RATES	
	SURGICAL	MEDICAL
Veteran's Study	82%	80%
European Study	93%	85%
CASS Study	95%	92%

The results of survival for the Veteran's Study and the CASS Study are interpreted as being statistically the same for the medical and surgical treatment groups. After five years the death rates in the surgically, but not in the medically treated group, have been found to accelerate, making this small and largely insignificant difference in the survivals of these two treatment approaches even more disappointing for surgical treatment.[50]

Why doesn't bypass surgery prolong life? It sounds like such a logical solution to the problems of clogged arteries.

Atherosclerosis is a disease of all the blood vessels in the heart, even though one site is usually more extensively involved than are other sites. Although this disease is usually thought of as involving only the large heart arteries, we have no reason to think that the smaller vessels are functioning normally. Impairment of blood flow through a small blood vessel can still cause angina and can lead to either fatal or nonfatal heart attacks. Bypass surgery is only a patch job for the areas that are most obviously affected.[46] Atherosclerosis continues to progress, unimpeded by bypass surgery, and the coronary arteries have the same or an even a worse tendency to get into trouble after the surgery. Add to this the number of deaths resulting from surgical procedures, and you have rates comparable to those from nonsurgical treatments. Another important reason why benefits from bypass surgery over medical treatment are hard to prove is that most people with atherosclerosis live a long time after diagnosis. Recently, death rates of less than 2 percent per year have been observed for patients who did not undergo surgery.[31] This low rate is tough to beat.

After your explanation, to believe that bypass surgery cures atherosclerosis certainly would be naive. Does atherosclerosis affect the new vein grafts also?

Unfortunately, yes. Grafts can become nonfunctional in two ways. Within the first few days to months after surgery, the transplanted vessels have a strong tendency to close up with blood clots, making them useless. About 10 percent of grafts are closed in two weeks and 20 percent are closed by the end of the first year after bypass surgery, and thereafter closure continues at a slow but steady rate.[32,51,52]

The other way in which the grafts can fail is by the slow but progressive development of atherosclerosis. Ten years after surgery, one-third of the grafts are narrowed and another one-third are totally blocked by athero-sclerosis.[53] This should not be surprising, since surgery has actually done nothing to correct the cause of atherosclerosis. This progressing disease is believed to be caused mostly by high levels of cholesterol in the diet and the resulting cholesterol in the circulating blood. As might be expected, the chances for the new grafts to close off are directly related to the levels of cholesterol in the blood.[53,54]

An alarming finding is that the progression of atherosclerosis is even more severe in coronary arteries that have had a bypass graft placed in them.[55] The rate of disease progression of atherosclerosis has been found to increase by tenfold in blood vessels that have received grafts compared to those that were left untouched by surgery.[55] This accelerated development of atherosclerosis may be due to changes in blood flow as a result of the bypasses.

This finding of accelerated atherosclerosis from placement of a graft should decrease the number of operations performed on blood vessels with small blockages, less than 50 percent narrowing. In the past, one reason that has been advanced for bypass surgery to minimally affected vessels is that it provides an auxiliary blood supply to the heart in the event of future growth of plaque in those vessels. However, because of the accelerated growth of plaque caused by the graft, a patient is much better off if a minimally affected vessel is left untouched.[55]

Return of chest pains is often related to closure of grafts by such processes as formation of clots or atherosclerosis.[51,56] However, when the heart is studied later by a repeat angiography, relief of chest pains is not always related to an open, functioning graft.[57,58] Some investigators also have found little correlation between open grafts and satisfactory capacity for exercise.[59,60] Even survival is not correlated with unblocked grafts.[57]. The lack of correlation between benefits and a successful operation puts into question the actual role of this specific surgery. If a patient reports that he or she is feeling better, even when the graft fails to function, then some factors other than improved circulation must account for these benefits subjectively felt.

Would it be possible to have another bypass if the first grafts closed off?

The problems are certainly not ended for the patients, once bypass surgery is finished. One-quarter of bypass patients return to the hospital within six months of their operation.[61] Nearly 60 percent of the readmissions are for chest pains and other heart-related events.[61] Repeat surgery accounts for from 2 to 6 percent (and more) of all bypass patients, and it is done in order to correct closed grafts and to do further bypass grafting of other untouched vessels.[62] However, this kind of repeat surgery is a hazard for the patient and can be technically difficult for the surgeon. Scar tissues from the previous operation surround the heart and many of the sites suitable for grafting have already been used.

Aren't there any situations where bypass surgery will keep the patient alive longer?

The largest coronary artery, which is called the left main coronary artery, is particularly dangerous when diseased.[52,63,64] This artery supplies a major part of the heart muscle, and if the blood flow to that part is suddenly closed off, a heart attack, and even death from the attack, usually follows. Death rates have been estimated to be as high as 10 percent per year for symptomatic patients with serious left main coronary artery disease treated without surgery.[52,63,64] Fortunately, dangerous blockages in this artery affect only about 5 percent of patients who undergo angiograms.[20,52] Most studies show better survival rates with surgical treatment than with medical treatment for this particular lesion in patients who have serious chest pains.[52,63,64] However, surgery for patients with disease of the left main coronary artery who have only mild distress or no symptoms of chest pain is not accepted as the only, or the best, approach to the problem by all investigators.[32,65-67]

Another situation that many doctors believe is benefited by bypass surgery is severe disease that involves all three main arteries of the heart; for the same reason, a high risk of dying.[68] However, more recent results with medical therapy have challenged the advantage of surgery for patients with extensive three vessel disease.[69,70] One more thing that should be kept in mind when considering surgery as treatment for left main coronary artery disease and severe disease of all three vessels, is that the risk of both angiography and bypass surgery is much greater the more severe the disease.[24,69]

Even though the need for surgery for severe left main coronary artery disease is almost unquestioned by physicians and the belief that three vessel disease is best treated by surgery is widely held, there is an important and recent dissenting opinion from a respected group of researchers. You need

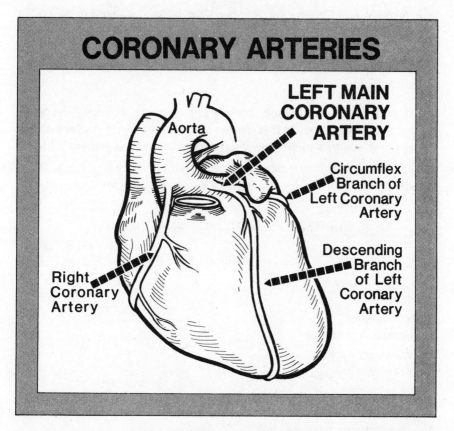

CORONARY ARTERIES

Aorta

LEFT MAIN CORONARY ARTERY

Circumflex Branch of Left Coronary Artery

Descending Branch of Left Coronary Artery

Right Coronary Artery

There are three large coronary arteries that supply the surface of the heart. The left main coronary artery provides the greater share of blood to the heart muscle; therefore a blockage of this artery can be highly lethal.

to be aware of this opposing opinion based on scientific study when deciding on your course of treatment along with your doctor's advice. Evidence from researchers from the Cardiovascular Laboratories, Harvard School of Public Health has shown that, even with severe coronary artery disease, good medical care along with changes in diet and lifestyle will give equal or better results than surgery.[67] Their series included some patients with left main coronary artery closure of 50 to 80 percent, and many with severe disease of all three vessels. As I've mentioned, many physicians would consider these situations as absolute indications for bypass surgery. But these patients postponed surgery. With an annual death rate of only 1.4 percent among their patients, these investigators challenged the need for bypass surgery in even some of the most serious cases of coronary atherosclerosis.[67] Criteria for the need for bypass surgery is based on symptoms of coronary artery disease which interfere with the patient's life and are unrelieved by medication-dietary-lifestyle changes, rather than results of the treadmill and findings of the condition of the coronary arteries on an angiogram.[15,67]

After all is said and done, how long I'm going to live is the most important thing to me. Is there some agreement among doctors about those situations in which bypass surgery will save the patient's life?

The following table presents the general feeling among physicians about the survival benefits of bypass surgery as a treatment for most patients with heart disease:[71,72]

SURGERY VS. MEDICAL MANAGEMENT

CIRCUMSTANCE	PROLONGS LIFE	FAILS TO PROLONG LIFE
One and two arteries diseased		X
All three arteries diseased extensively	?	
Left main coronary artery diseased	X	
Unstable angina		X
Variant (Printzmetal) angina		X
After a heart attack (acute myocardial infarction)		X
Cardiogenic shock		X
Arrhythmias		X
Congestive heart failure		X

Will this surgery stop my chest pain?

The most common reason why patients are sent to bypass surgery these days is chest pain that is not relieved by medical therapy. As may be expected, the primary benefit bypass surgeons claim for their efforts is the great job that the operation does in relieving chest pains, since they would have difficulty in claiming that lives have been saved. However, even the claim for pain relief is under considerable attack for several reasons. The 90 percent improvement or complete relief of chest pains that is reported one year after surgery decreases with the passage of time. Long-term follow-up of patients who have been operated on show that in five years the proportion without symptoms has fallen below 70 percent, and after ten years less than half the survivors are without symptoms.[73]

Several important reasons can be found for the relief of chest pain after the operation that cannot be credited to this surgery.

Pain relief can simply be a placebo effect; in other words, it is not the result of any physical change or improvement in the patient but is entirely psychological in origin. This placebo effect was dramatically demonstrated by observations reported in a study published in 1960.[74] In the 1950's a popular operation for angina was tying off the internal mammary artery located just under the breastbone. The theory supporting this approach maintained that it would divert more blood to the heart arteries and thereby relieve the chest pain. In order to evaluate the effectiveness of this procedure, an experiment was performed on eighteen patients, each of whom had a classic history of angina pectoris and a distinctly abnormal treadmill stress test or EKG. Five of the eighteen patients were given a sham operation; nothing more than a incision in the skin was made and then sewn up. The thirteen other patients had the internal mammary artery tied off according to the usual procedure. All patients reported improvement in their chest pains, some to the complete relief of angina, and also an improved ability to work. Yet they showed little improvement in their treadmill stress tests. The five who received the sham operation did as well as those in whom the internal mammary artery had been tied off during surgery. The conclusion is that there is a psychological benefit from simply being cut.

Another reason for pain relief is a heart attack in the part of the heart that was the source of the pain before the attack occurred. A heart attack results in the death of the portion of the heart muscle that was supplied with blood by the diseased artery. Dead tissues no longer hurt. Heart attacks have been reported to occur during or soon after operation in 5 to 50 percent of patients.[75-78] However, with improved surgical techniques the number of serious heart attacks may be lowered to as few as 5 to 6 percent of the bypass surgeries.[48] Obviously, this is not the preferred way to stop chest pains!

Relief of chest pains is also believed to be the result of severing the nerves around the heart during surgery. The combination of the placebo effect, heart attacks, and nerve damage from surgery will account for many of the patients who gain relief of chest pain from bypass surgery. Yet, in such patients who have no symptoms to warn them that something may be wrong, a dangerously compromised supply of blood to the heart muscle can still be threatening them.

Relief of chest pains can also be the result of improved circulation to the heart muscle—which, of course, is the purpose of bypass surgery.[79]

However, even successful surgery does not prolong life in most cases. I argue that removal of the warning sign—the chest pain—is a disservice to the patient. This unpleasant reminder that something is wrong can serve a person better as a strong motivation to improve their diet and lifestyle—a method which, as we shall soon discuss, can bring tremendous benefits.

My job and recreation are very important to me. Will I be able to do more if I choose bypass surgery?

One large study found a sevenfold increase in retirement for patients less than fifty-five years old who had previously been able to work, and an elevenfold increase for those over fifty-five after bypass surgery.[80] Among physicians, the consensus is one of disappointment: improvement in job and recreational activities after surgery is generally not found.[31,32,81-84] In contrast, among a series of patients who did not have surgery, a cardiac research team was able to improve performances of 90 percent of patients less than sixty years of age who had had recent heart attacks simply by relying on encouragement and rehabilitation.[85]

Can't a doctor just ream out my arteries without cutting me open? Sort of how they clean out a sewer pipe?

One alternative to bypass surgery is a technique called *coronary angioplasty,* introduced in 1977.[86] This technique is an outgrowth of coronary angiography and uses a long plastic tube with a very small bladder at its tip that can be inflated and deflated by the operator. The operation begins with passing this small catheter tip into a section of blood vessel where atherosclerotic narrowing has occurred. Then the bladder is inflated with fluid, squeezing aside the plaque to enlarge the opening in the blood vessel. In most cases, this treatment allows an improved flow of blood to the heart muscle and relief of associated chest pain.

Results of coronary angioplasty are encouraging, judging by the relief of chest pain in 55 to 77 percent of cases, depending on the experience of the surgeon performing the procedure.[87] Complications are serious in about 10 percent of patients, but this method is certainly less of an ordeal and an expense for a patient than bypass surgery.[88] The major complications are heart attack in 5 percent of cases and death in 1 percent of cases.[89] Unfortunately, there is also evidence that injury to the inside lining of the artery caused by the catheter results in an accelerated progression of atherosclerosis following the procedure.[90] Angioplasty should be tried only in patients who otherwise would be sent to surgery. Also, because of the risk of complications with the procedure, immediate surgical help should be available. In 5 to 7 percent of cases, patients have to be hurried to

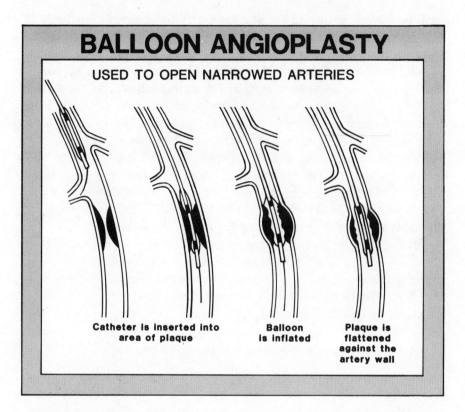

BALLOON ANGIOPLASTY

USED TO OPEN NARROWED ARTERIES

Catheter is inserted into area of plaque

Balloon is inflated

Plaque is flattened against the artery wall

bypass surgery because of failure to improve the patient's condition or a complication.[91] To date, studies have not been done to show improved survival rates for patients having angioplasty compared with those treated by medical-drug therapies or bypass surgery. However, the results are likely to be found comparable. Closing of the opened vessel accompanied by a recurrence of chest pain is the greatest problem for patients who undergo this procedure. About 30 percent of patients suffer reclosure of the vessel.[92,93] Fortunately for them, repeat angioplasty is very successful in reopening many of these arteries after an initial failure. Even with allowances for reoperations, angioplasty is estimated to offer financial savings of 40 to 50 percent over bypass surgery.[89]

Reclosure of the blood vessels is the same reason for failure after bypass surgery. Why don't these operations provide a more permanent solution?

The closure that occurs soon after either of these procedures is caused by sudden formation of blood clots. Aspirin and other blood thinning drugs have had some success in keeping the grafts and arteries open longer.[94] However, one of the most important factors that increases the tendency for clots to form is rarely changed—and this is the high content of animal fats in the American diet. Saturated or animal fats cause platelets, the blood-clotting elements, to form clumps, and they also activate clotting factors in the blood. As a result, the tendency to form blood clots is increased and the hard work of many a good surgeon is destroyed, not to mention the lives of the hopeful patients.[95-99] Decreasing the intake of animal fats in one's diet and increasing that of vegetable fats will quickly reverse this tendency toward excessive clotting. To avoid problems of obesity, blood sludging, bleeding, and possibly a higher risk of gallbladder disease and cancer, the best dietary change is simply to reduce the consumption of animal-type fats without increasing that of the vegetable fats.[100]

Health professionals and patients will make little or no progress in their campaign against heart disease until the factors that cause the disease in the first place are eliminated. The primary factors in developing atherosclerosis are, first, dietary habits, which we can control, and, second, heredity, which we can do nothing about.[101,102] Secondary factors, which are also very important and need our attention, include smoking, obesity, high blood pressure, physical inactivity, and emotional stress.

How can physicians justify doing all this surgery if it doesn't save lives?

The fact is that bypass surgery should be reserved for a last-ditch effort. The official indication for recommending bypass surgery is angina, or chest pain that is unrelieved by medical therapy.[15,31,103] In the minds of most physicians, good medical therapy consists of writing prescriptions, which, ultimately, give a patient a medicine cabinet full of antianginal drugs, including such preparations as nitroglycerin, beta blockers and calcium antagonists.[31,103] However, much more can be done for a patient with atherosclerosis and angina.

More progressive doctors are paying close attention to the nutritional and lifestyle habits of their patients and are making sincere recommendations for their patients to stop indulging in tobacco, coffee, and alcohol; to lose excess weight; to exercise moderately; and to follow a low-fat, no-cholesterol diet. Most people with heart disease and angina should not even be considered for angiography, angioplasty, or bypass surgery unless all other approaches fail—diet, lifestyle, and recommended medications.[15,31,103] Certainly, people who are faced, sooner rather than later, with the likelihood of a heart attack, extensive surgery, or sudden death, should be willing to eat better foods and adopt a lifestyle that will offer the best possible chance to resolve their problems and to recover from this potentially deadly condition. A change in diet will give the most satisfying results, and each of us has 100 percent control over the foods we eat.

Isn't it too late, now that I have the disease, to change my diet and expect any benefit? Why do you believe diet has such a great influence on heart disease and angina?

Atherosclerotic diseases of the blood vessels occur almost exclusively in parts of the world where the diet is rich in fat and cholesterol, based on meats, dairy products, eggs, and refined and processed foods.[101,102,104] Factors that cause disease also promote further disease. Studies have shown that the progression of arterial disease can be slowed or stopped with a decrease in blood cholesterol reached by proper diet and/or medications.[105-107] If enough corrective measures can be made towards lowering the cholesterol level in the blood, then the atherosclerotic disease is actually reversible.[107]

Is using diet a new treatment for heart disease and angina?

Not at all. Scientific studies relating to the dietary treatment of atherosclerotic heart disease and its accompanying chest pains date back to 1955. This long history may make you wonder why all the heroics of bypass surgery ever became popular, when such an effective and simple treatment was already available. Investigators from the Cleveland Clinic in the 1950's treated their heart patients with a low-fat diet and obtained excellent relief of angina in a few days.[108-110]

One important experiment demonstrated that a high-fat diet fed to heart patients brought on chest pains very quickly.[109] Fourteen patients were fed a single high-fat meal and the result was fourteen attacks of angina in six of those patients in the next four hours. EKG changes confirmed that the pain was from the heart. No attacks of angina occurred when those same heart patients were later fed a low-fat diet having comparable volume and calorie content. Measurements of the oxygen content of the blood (PO_2) in other patients fed a high-fat diet have shown a fall of 20 percent soon after that single meal.[110] This lower oxygen content, combined with the sluggish flow of blood through the arteries narrowed by atherosclerotic disease, were the two factors that brought on pain.

A third factor that reduces blood flow to the heart muscle is the sludging of the blood cells that occurs when the fat from a meal enters the bloodstream. At the University of South Carolina Medical School, investigators observed this sludging in the blood vessels in the whites of patients' eyes after a high-fat meal.[111] This sludging effect was associated with the onset of chest pains in those patients soon after they ate the meal. The effects of this burden of fats on the heart were confirmed by changes in the patients' EKGs.

Recently, a study at the Baylor College of Medicine combined a low-fat vegetarian diet with a relaxing environment. The results of observations of twenty-three heart patients were published in 1983 in an issue of *The Journal of the American Medical Association.*[112] The investigators found a 91 percent reduction in frequency of angina attacks and a 55 percent increase in work capacity after only twenty-four days of this cost-free, pain-free kind of treatment. Cholesterol levels also decreased by 20 percent, on the average, during this three-week alternative diet. It's nice to know that there are no complications to this treatment, as well as a 40 percent reduction in food bills.

Further investigations into the benefits of a low-fat diet on the metabolism of the heart have recently been published.[113] Patients with angina were treated with a low-fat diet for three months. After the dietary treatment, these patients could walk for a longer time before chest pains began. Definite improvements in the energy metabolism of the heart muscle were observed as a result of a low-fat diet. Cholesterol levels, incidentally, dropped by an average of 28 percent.

The effectiveness of a low-fat diet and exercise in the management of coronary artery disease was recently tested at Brigham and Woman's Hospital, Boston.[114] Results of thirty-two patients who participated in a diet and exercise program for ten to sixteen weeks showed a reduction in body weight, blood cholesterol and triglycerides. There was a significant improvement in work capacity and reduction in systolic blood pressure. Patients had almost 22 percent less angina occurring during exercise stress testing than before the program. The diet, not the exercise or the drug therapy, was believed to be the determining factor in the angina improvement.

Other investigators have shown benefits for heart patients suffering from angina who changed their diets and lifestyles.[115,116] More studies everyday are appearing in the medical journals that confirm the essential part played by diet and lifestyle changes in the rehabilitation of a victim of heart disease. In fact, state-of-the-art health care is not being provided for the patient if these changes are not emphasized as first line therapy in medical care and postoperative care of bypass and angioplasty patients.

Would a proper dietary change also improve the survival of medically treated patients if this change was commonly prescribed by doctors?

Many studies have been performed during the last forty years to determine whether or not survival of heart patients can be improved by a change to a low animal-fat diet and a subsequent reduction in blood cholesterol levels.[49,101,102,117-121] The results have been very encouraging, but until very recently they were not convincing enough for most physicians. In January 1984 "The Lipids Research Clinics Coronary Primary Prevention Trial Results" were released by the National Heart, Lung, and Blood Institute.[120,121] This study showed a definite decrease in numbers of deaths from heart disease when subjects achieved a drop in blood cholesterol levels. Evidence was also provided that suggested a decrease in the need for bypass surgery in the treated group and a reversal of atherosclerosis. The scientific literature is reporting more all the time now about the benefits of changes in diet and lifestyle, and how these changes can replace medications and surgery with better results.

See if these comparisons can help you to decide which is the best choice for you:

COMPARISON OF MEDICAL-DIETARY AND SURGICAL MANAGEMENT OF HEART DISEASE

	TREATMENT		
	SURGICAL		MEDICAL-DIETARY
FACTOR	BYPASS	ANGIOPLASTY	
Operative mortality (elderly)	2% 5%	1%	zero
Operative complications	13%	10%	zero
Operative heart attacks	5%	5%	zero
Blood transfusions likely	yes	no	no
Operative brain injury from heart-lung machine	100%	zero	zero
Persistent brain dysfunction from heart-lung machine	15+%	zero	zero
Cost of operation	$25,000+	$10,000+	zero
Closure of grafts (early)	20%	30%	zero
Operative pain and suffering	100%	100%	zero
Stress on family from surgery	100%	100%	zero

	TREATMENT		
	SURGICAL		MEDICAL-DIETARY
FACTOR	BYPASS	ANGIOPLASTY	
Survival time (five-year results with no diet change)	90%*	unknown (probably 86-90%)	86%*
Initial relief of angina	excellent	excellent	excellent
Diet and lifestyle change necessary	yes	yes	yes
acceleration of atherosclerosis caused by procedure	yes	yes	no
atherosclerosis slowed, stopped, and/or reversed	no	no	yes
future studies likely to demonstrate even more benefit	no	possibly	yes

*The survival values of 86 percent and 90 percent are essentially the same and should not imply that surgery offers an advantage over medical treatment. This small difference can be purely the result of experimental design, and as time goes on the surgical results get worse. The addition of dietary change and lowering the cholesterol level will also make a further improvement in survival rates in medically over surgically treated patients when the studies are done—unless, of course, more surgeons become farsighted enough to change the diets of their patients after surgery. Then both groups will benefit equally.

I would eat cardboard to keep myself away from the surgeon's knife. I'm certainly glad you've given me a scientifically backed alternative to rushing off to surgery.

If there were an ideal therapy that gave consistent excellent results without risks or adverse effects, then there would be no room for discussion or decision. Unfortunately, this ideal is unlikely to be achieved. Studies comparing results of medical and surgical treatments have shown not only that medical treatment is as good for most patients but also that surgery can be put off safely until later, if not forever, and that the more conservative, less painful, less expensive approaches should be tried first. Surgery, rather than medical-dietary therapy, should be employed only if the advantages of the operation justify the risks, costs, and psychological stress to the patient. In most cases they don't!

℞

● Prevention of heart disease with a low-fat, no-cholesterol, high-fiber diet, moderate exercise, and a health-promoting lifestyle should be everyone's goal.

● If you develop chest pains, go to your doctor in order to find their cause. An internist or a cardiologist would be the best physician to consult. If you are very ill, you may need to be hospitalized. Demand low-fat, no-cholesterol foods while you're in the hospital. No sense in allowing the hospital's dietary department to impair your heart's circulation any further. Besides, at no other time is your level of motivation likely to be any higher; you might as well begin immediately with this sensible changeover.

● From your history and EKG your doctor should have a good idea whether or not the pain is from coronary artery disease.

● If your doctor suspects that you do have coronary artery disease, then your primary goal should be to stop the pain so that no further testing or surgery will be necessary, at least for the present. This relief of chest pain is best accomplished by an immediate change to a low-fat, no-cholesterol, low-salt, high-fiber, high-complex-carbo-hydrate diet.

● When you are feeling better, start a program of moderate exercise. Increase your activity as you feel stronger. Exercise just short of the point where pain develops.

● If the angina persists, take antianginal medication. Nitroglycerin pills are easy to use and effective. With them, you take the medication only when you need it instead of routinely, as is necessary with other medicines. The next set of drugs to try for relief of pain are the beta blockers and the calcium antagonists. If you do take these long acting medications and your pain is relieved, do not be lead into believing your disease is healed. The medication does not stop the relentless progress of atherosclerosis.

● Somewhere in the evaluation of your chest pain and the likelihood of disease of your coronary arteries, you should have a treadmill stress test to evaluate the severity of your condition and determine the need for further testing and treatment.

● If the treadmill stress test is normal, or shows only minor changes, then you have little reason to rush into angiography or surgery. If the angina continues with a normal treadmill stress tests, you along with your doctor should persist with the diet and drug therapy.

● If the treadmill stress test is very abnormal, suggesting serious coronary artery disease, then you will need further testing to determine the severity of the disease. The next test recommended is a radionuclide heart scan.

• A negative teadmill stress test and exercising nuclide scan virtually exclude serious coronary artery disease. However, if these tests are positive then the next step is angiography.

• Both a positive treadmill stress test and a positive radionuclide scan are required before making a diagnosis of coronary artery disease or performing a coronary angiography in someone with an atypical history of chest pain or in someone with no pain at all.

• Angiography is performed as a precondition to bypass or angioplasty surgery in cases of known coronary artery disease already selected on the basis of continued symptoms or evidence of involvement of a large area of the heart muscle based on severely diseased vessels as determined by treadmill stress tests and/or radionuclide scan.

• Severe artery disease, determined by angiography, that involves the left main coronary artery or all three of the major coronary arteries, is believed by most physicians to be best treated with surgery. Also if a portion of the heart muscle, called the ventricle, functions poorly, then surgery is believed to give better results than medical therapy. Remember, that some highly respected investigators still feel that surgery is not always the best treatment for everyone, even for left main coronary artery disease and extensive three-vessel atherosclerosis. The decision for surgical intervention with bypass or angioplasty should be weighted by chest pain and other symptoms of coronary artery disease unrelieved by medical therapy, not on the basis of the disease seen in the heart arteries on angiography.

This is your decision to make, and you have the most to gain or lose from the treatment you select. But take the time to have your cardiologist explain the risks versus the benefits to you, clearly and carefully.

• If you can't find relief from the chest pains, severe enough to interfere with your life, by a diet-lifestyle-drug approach, then angiography followed by angioplasty or bypass surgery may be your last, and best, and only choice. Angioplasty, if applicable, is a better choice than bypass surgery.

• If you have already had bypass surgery, you should be eating a low-fat, no-cholesterol diet. You should also exercise and give up unhealthy habits; otherwise, you are likely to get into trouble again.

• You most likely will need to reduce the dosage and/or discontinue medications after you change your diet and lifestyle. This should be done under you doctor's supervision.

• Whenever you have chest pain that is severe and long-lasting, go for emergency treatment. This may be the beginning of a heart attack.

REFERENCES

[1]Kannel W. Incidence and prognosis of unrecognized myocardial infarction. An update on the Framingham Study. *N Engl J Med* 311:1144, 1984.

[2]Zukel W. Survival following first diagnosis of coronary heart disease. *Am Heart J* 78:159, 1969.

[3]Kannel W. Natural history of angina pectoris in the Framingham Study: Prognosis and survival. *Am J Cardiol* 29:154, 1972.

[4]Harris P. Outcome in medically treated coronary artery disease. Ischemic events: nonfatal infarction and death. *Circulation* 62:718, 1980.

[5]Cohn P. Silent myocardial ischemia in patients with a defective anginal warning system. *Am J Cardiol* 45:697, 1980.

[6]Jaffe M. Warm-up phenomenon in angina pectoris. *Lancet* 2:934, 1980.

[7]Thompson P. Incidence of death during jogging in Rhode Island from 1975 through 1980. *JAMA* 247:2535, 1982.

[8]Thompson P. Death during jogging or running: a study of 18 cases. *JAMA* 242:1265, 1979.

[9]Morris J. Vigorous exercise in leisure-time: protection against coronary heart disease. *Lancet* 2:1207, 1980.

[10]Mohr R. Treatment of nocturnal angina with 10 degrees reverse Trendelenburg bed position. *Lancet* 1:1325, 1982.

[11]Kennedy H. Frequent or complex ventricular ectopy in apparently healthy subjects: a clinical study of 25 cases. *Am J* Cardiol 38:141, 1976.

[12]Weiner D. Exercise stress testing: correlations among history of angina, ST-segment response and prevalence of coronary-artery disease in the Coronary Artery Surgery Study CASS. *N Engl J Med* 301:230, 1979.

[13]Epstein S. Value and limitations of the electrocardiographic response to exercise in the assessment of patients with coronary artery disease: controversies in cardiology II. *Am J Cardiol* 42:667, 1978.

[14]Bruce R. Value of maximal exercise tests in risk assessments of primary coronary heart disease events in healthy men: five year's experience of the Seattle Heart Watch Study. *Am J Cardiol* 46:371, 1980.

[15]Campbell R. Strategy for detection and management of coronary artery disease. "Physiology before anatomy." editorial essay. *Chest* 88:287, 1985.

[16]Gibson R. Should exercise electrocardiographic testing be replaced by radioisotope methods? In: Rahimtoola S, ed. *Controversies in Coronary Artery Disease*. Philadelphia: F.A. Davis, 1983, pp 1-31.

[17]Coronary artery bypass surgery: a consensus. *Lancet* 2:1288, 1984.

[18]Weisburst M. Significance of the negative exercise test in evaluation of patients with chest pain. *Clin Cardiol* 2:7, 1979.

[19]Editorial: Coronary artery disease: what is a reasonable diagnostic strategy? *Ann Intern Med* 95:385, 1981.

[20]Roberts W. The Coronary Artery Surgery Study (CASS): do the results apply to your patients? *Am J Cardiol* 54:440, 1984.

[21]Webster J. Natural history of severe proximal coronary artery disease as documented by coronary cineangiography. *Am J Cardiol* 33:195, 1974.

[22]Burggraf G. Prognosis in coronary artery disease: angiographic, hemodynamic, and clinical factors. *Circulation* 51:146, 1975.

[23]Gersh B. Coronary arteriography and coronary artery bypass surgery: morbidity and mortality in patients ages 65 years or older. A report from the Coronary Artery Surgery Study. *Circulation* 67:483, 1983.

[24]Fisher M. Editorial: Coronary angiography: safety in numbers? *Am J Cardiol* 52:898, 1983.

[25]Welch C. Cinecoronary arteriography in young men. *Circulation* 42: 647, 1970.

[26]Page I. Prediction of coronary heart disease based on clinical suspicion, age, total cholesterol, and triglyceride. *Circulation* 42: 625, 1970.

[27]Favaloro R. Saphenous vein graft in the surgical treatment of coronary artery disease: operative technique. *J Thorac Cardiovasc Surg* 58:178, 1969.

[28]Editorial: Coronary bypass with the internal mammary. *Lancet* 2:1253, 1984.

[29]Preston T. Marketing an operation. *Atlantic* December 1984 p- 32.

[30]Hollier L. The case against prophylactic coronary bypass. *Surgery* 96:78, 1984.

[31]Braunwald E. Editorial retrospective. Effects of coronary-artery bypass grafting on survival: implications of the randomized Coronary-Artery Surgery Study. *N Engl J Med* 309:1181, 1983.

[32]McIntosh H. The first decade of aortocoronary bypass grafting, 1967-1977: a review. *Circulation* 57:405, 1978.

[33]Kuan P. Coronary artery bypass surgery morbidity. *J Am Coll Cardiol* 3:1391, 1984.

[34]Orenstein J. Microemboli observed in deaths following cardiopulmonary bypass surgery: Silicone antifoam agents and polyvinyl chloride tubing as sources of emboli. *Hum Path* 13:1082, 1982.

[35]Hill J. Neuropathological manifestations of cardiac surgery. *Ann Thorac Surg* 7:409, 1969.

[36]Editorial: Brain damage after open-heart surgery. *Lancet* 1:1161, 1982.

[37]Henriksen L. Evidence suggestive of diffuse brain damage following cardiac operations. *Lancet* 1:816, 1984.

[38]Aberg T. Release of adenylate kinase into cerebrospinal fluid during open-heart surgery and its relation to postoperative intellectual function. *Lancet* 1:1139, 1982.

[39]Henriksen L. Brain hyperfusion during cardiac operations: Cerebral blood flow measured in man by intra-arterial injection of xenon 133: Evidence suggestive of intraoperative microembolism. *J Thorac Cardiovasc Surg* 86:202, 1983.

[40]Taylor K. Editorial: Brain damage during open-heart surgery. *Thorax* 37:873, 1982.

[41]Savageau J. Neuropsychological dysfunction following elective cardiac operation. 1. Early assessment. *J Thorac Cardiovasc Surg* 84:585, 1982.

[42]Kornfeld D. Delirium after coronary artery bypass surgery. *J Thorac Cardiovasc Surg* 76:93, 1978.

[43]Barash P. Cardiopulmonary bypass and postoperative neurologic dysfunction. *Am Heart J* 99:675, 1980.

[44]Orr W. Sleep disturbances after open heart surgery. *Am J Cardiol* 39:196, 1977.

[45]Hampton J. Coronary artery bypass grafting for the reduction of mortality: an analysis of the trials. *Br Med J* 289:1166, 1984.

[46]Grondin C. Late results of coronary artery grafting: is there a flag on the field? *J Thorac Cardiovasc Surg* 87:161, 1984.

[47]Kolata G. Consensus on bypass surgery: in most cases, the operation has not been shown to save lives, but patients do say they feel better after surgery. *Science* 211:42, 1981.

[48]Rahimtoola S. Coronary bypass surgery for unstable angina. *Circulation* 69:842, 1984.

[49]Goldman L. The decline in ischemic heart disease mortality rates. An analysis of the comparative effects of medical interventions and changes in lifestyle. *Ann Intern Med* 101:825, 1984.

[50]The Veterans Administration Coronary Artery Bypass Surgery Cooperative Study Group. Eleven-year survival in the Veterans Administration randomized trial of coronary bypass surgery for stable angina. *N Engl J Med* 311:1333, 1984.

[51]Buccino R. Aortocoronary bypass grafting in the management of patients with coronary artery disease. *Am J Med* 66:651, 1979.

[52]Rahimtoola S. Coronary bypass surgery for chronic angina-1981. A perspective. *Circulation* 65:225, 1982.

[53]Campeau L. The relation of risk factors to the development of atherosclerosis in saphenous-vein bypass grafts and the progression of disease in the native circulation. A study 10 years after aortocoronary bypass surgery. *N Engl J Med* 311:1329, 1984.

[54]Palac R. Risk factors related to progressive narrowing in aortocoronary vein grafts studied 1 and 5 years after surgery. *Circulation* 66 (suppl I): I-40, 1982.

[55]Cashin W. Accelerated progression of atherosclerosis in coronary vessels with minimal lesions that are bypassed. *N Engl J Med* 311:824, 1984.

[56]Campeau L. Loss of the improvement of angina betweeen 1 and 7 years after aortocoronary bypass surgery. Correlations with changes in vein grafts and in coronary arteries. *Circulation* 60 (suppl I):I-1, 1979.

[57]McNeer J. Complete and incomplete revascularization at aortocoronary bypass surgery: experience with 392 consecutive patients. *Am Heart J* 88:176, 1974.

[58]Valdes M. "Sham operation" revisited: a comparison of complete vs. unsuccessful coronary artery bypass. *Am J Cardiol* 43:382, 1979.

[59]Block T. Improvement in exercise performance after unsuccessful myocardial revascularization. *Am J Cardiol* 40:673, 1977.

[60]Bartel A. Exercise stress testing in evaluation of aortocoronary bypass surgery. Report of 123 patients. *Circulation* 48:141, 1973.

[61]Stanton B. Hospital readmissions among survivors six months after myocardial revascularization. *JAMA* 253:3568, 1985.

[62]Foster E. Comparison of operative mortality and morbidity for initial and repeat coronary artery bypass grafting: the Coronary Artery Surgery Study (CASS); registry experience. *Ann Thorac Surg* 38:563, 1984.

[63]Champeau L. Left main coronary artery stenosis. The influence of aortocoronary bypass surgery on survival. *Circulation* 57:1111, 1978.

[64]Takaro T. The VA cooperative randomized study of surgery for coronary arterial occlusive disease. II. Subgroup with significant left main lesions. *Circulation* 54 (suppl III):III-107, 1976.

[65]Battock D. Left main coronary artery disease—is surgery always indicated? *Am J Cardiol* 33:125, 1974.

[66]Sung R. Left main coronary artery obstruction. Follow-up of thirty patients with and without surgery. *Circulation* 51 & 52 (suppl I):I-112, 1975.

[67]Podrid P. Prognosis of medically treated patients with coronary-artery disease with profound ST-segment depression during exercise testing. *N Engl J Med* 305:1111, 1981.

[68]Prospective randomised study of coronary artery bypass surgery in stable angina pectoris. Second interm report by the European Coronary Surgery Study Group. *Lancet* 2:491, 1980.

[69]Kennedy J. Clinical and angiographic predictors of operative mortality from the Collaborative Study in Coronary Artery Surgery (CASS). *Circulation 63:793, 1981.*

[70]Braunwald E. Coronary artery bypass grafting *N Engl J Med* 310:1263, 1984.

[71]Editorial: Coronary artery bypass surgery—indications and limitations. *Lancet* 2:511, 1980.

[72]Freeman Z. Coronary by-pass surgery: a reappraisal. *Aust N.Z. J Med* 12:309, 1982.

[73]Lawrie G. Clinical results of coronary bypass in 500 patients at least 10 years after operation. *Circulation* 66:suppl II-1, 1982.

[74]Dimond E. Comparison of internal mammary artery ligation and sham operation for angina pectoris. *Am J Cardiol* 5:483, 1960.

[75]Brewer D. Myocardial infarction as a complication of coronary bypass surgery. *Circulation 45 & 46 (suppl II):II-69, 1972.*

[76]Hultgren H. Ischemic myocardial injury during coronary artery surgery. *Am Heart J* 82:624, 1971.

[77]Kansal S. Acute myocardial injury following aortocoronary bypass surgery. *Am J Cardiol* 31:140, 1973.

[78]Williams D. Myocardial infarction during coronary artery bypass surgery. *Am J Cardiol* 31:164, 1973.

[79]Ribeiro P. Different mechanisms for the relief of angina after coronary bypass surgery: physiological versus anatomical assessment. *Br Heart J* 52: 502, 1984.

[80]Rimm A. Changes in occupation after aortocoronary vein-bypass operation. *JAMA* 236:361, 1976.

[81]Barnes G. Changes in working status of patients following coronary bypass surgery. *JAMA* 238:1259, 1977.

[82]Symmes J. Influence of aortocoronary bypass on employment. *Can Med Assoc J* 118:268, 1978.

[83]Anderson A. Retention or resumption of employment after aortocoronary bypass operations. *JAMA.* 243:543, 1980.

[84]Hammermeister K. Effect of surgical versus medical therapy on return to work in patients with coronary artery disease. *Am J Cardiol* 44:105, 1979.

[85]Mulcahy R. Natural history of postinfarction angina pectoris. *Br Heart J* 38:873, 1976.

[86]Gruntzig A. Transluminal dilatation of coronary-artery stenosis. *Lancet* 1:263, 1978.

[87]Kelsey S. Effect of investigator experience on percutaneous transluminal coronary angioplasty. *Am J Cardiol* 53:56C, 1984.

[88]Dorros G. National Heart, Lung and Blood Institute registry report of complications of percutaneous transluminal coronary angioplasty. *Am J Cardiol* 47:396, 1981.

[89]Editorial: The expanding scope of coronary angioplasty. *Lancet* 1:1307, 1985.

[90]Pope C. Detection of platelet deposition at the site of peripheral balloon angioplasty using Indium-111 platelet scintigraphy. *Am J Cardiol* 55:495, 1985.

[91]Cowley M. Emergency coronary bypass surgery after coronary angioplasty: the National, Heart, Lung, and Blood Institute's percutaneous transluminal coronary angioplasty registry experience. *Am J Cardiol* 53:22C, 1984.

[92]Meier B. Repeat coronary angioplasty. *J Am Coll Cardiol* 4:463, 1984.

[93]Jones E. Comparison of coronary artery bypass surgery and percutaneous transluminal coronary angioplasty including surgery for failed angioplasty. *Am Heart J 107:830, 1984.*

[94]Lorenz R. Improved aortocoronary bypass patency by low-dose aspirin (100 mg daily): Effects on platelet aggregation and thromboxane formation. *Lancet* 1:1261, 1984.

[95]Greig H. Inhibition of fibrinolysis by alimentary lipaemia. *Lancet* 2:16, 1956.

[96]Mustard J. Effect of different dietary fats on blood coagulation, platelet economy, and blood lipids. *Br Med J* 2:1651, 1962.

[97]Hornstra G. Influence of dietary fat on platelet function in men. *Lancet* 1:1155, 1973.

[98]O'Brien J. Acute platelet changes after large meals of saturated and unsaturated fats. *Lancet* 1:878, 1976.

[99]Simpson H. Hypertriglyceridaemia and hypercoagulability. *Lancet* 1:786, 1983.

[100]McDougall J. *The McDougall Plan*. Piscataway: New Century, 1983.

[101]Connor W. The key role of nutritional factors in the prevention of coronary heart disease. *Prev Med* 1:49, 1972.

[102]Stamler J. Lifestyles, major risk factors, proof and public policy. *Circulation* 58:3, 1978.

[103]Editorial: Complementary roles of surgical and medical therapy for angina pectoris. *Ann Intern Med* 102:848, 1985.

[104]Editorial: Diet and ischaemic heart disease-agreement or not? *Lancet* 2:317, 1983.

[105]Duffield R. Treatment of hyperlipidemia retards progression of symptomatic femerol atherosclerosis. *Lancet* 2:639, 1983.

[106]Nikkila E. Prevention of progression of coronary atherosclerosis by treatment of hyper-lipidaemia: a seven year prospective angiographic study. *Br Med J* 289:220, 1984.

[107]Barndt R. Regression and progression of early femerol atherosclerosis in treated hyper-lipoproteinemic patients. *Ann Intern Med* 86:139, 1977.

[108]Kuo P. Lipemia in patients with coronary heart disease. Treatment with low-fat diet. *JADA* 33:22, 1957.

[109]Kuo P. Angina pectoris induced by fat ingestion in patients with coronary artery disease. Ballistocardiographic and electrocardiographic findings. *JAMA* 158:1008, 1955.

[110]Kuo P. The effect of lipemia upon coronary and peripheral arterial circulation in patients with essential hyperlipemia. *Am J Med* 26:68, 1959.

[111]Williams A. Increased blood cell agglutination following ingestion of fat, a factor contributing to cardiac ischemia, coronary insufficiency and anginal pain. *Angiology* 8:29, 1957

[112]Ornish D. Effects of stress management training and dietary changes in treating ischemic heart disease. *JAMA* 249:54, 1983.

[113]Thuesen L. Beneficial effect of a low-fat low-calorie diet on myocardial energy metabolism in patients with angina pectoris. *Lancet* 2:59, 1984.

[114]Ribeiro J. The effectiveness of a low lipid diet and exercise in the management of coronary artery disease. Clinical investigations. *Am Heart J* 108:1183, 1984.

[115]Ellis F. Angina and vegan diet. *Am Heart J* 93:803, 1977.

[116]Pritikin N. *Diet and exercise as a total therapeutic regimen for rehabilitation of patients with severe peripherial vascular disease.* 52nd Annual Session of the American Congress on Rehabilitation Medicine, Atlanta, 1975.

[117]Editorial: Trials of coronary heart disease prevention. *Lancet* 2:803, 1982.

[118]Gordon T. Diet and its relation to coronary heart disease and death in three populations. *Circulation* 63:500, 1981.

[119]Kallio V. Reduction in sudden deaths by a multifactorial intervention programme after acute myocardial infarction. *Lancet* 2:1091, 1979.

[120]Lipid Research Clinics Program. The Lipid Research Clinics Coronary Primary Prevention Trial results. I. Reduction in incidence of coronary heart disease. *JAMA* 251:351, 1984.

[121]Lipid Research Clinics Program. The Lipid Research Clinics Coronary Primary Prevention Trial results. II. The relationship of reduction in incidence of coronary heart disease to cholesterol lowering. *JAMA* 251:365, 1984.

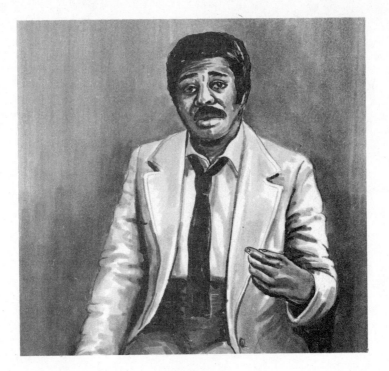

John

Maybe you'll think this is a little problem, much less important than a heart attack or a stroke. But to me it might as well be the end of my life. I can't get an erection since I started taking blood pressure pills, and I'm only thirty-five years old!— My wife says she understands, sort of.

I have never felt sick and only discovered my blood pressure was high recently when I took an insurance physical. Our family doctor started me on medication when she found my pressure was 145/95 on my first visit to her. Now my pressure is 130/80 with the pills. Another effect I've noticed from the treatment is that I am more tired now, all the time. It's even hard for me to get interested in going to work in the morning, probably because I'm feeling kind of depressed about being incurably ill.

My doctor told me that my diet has little effect on my condition. She said that information about the effects of different kinds of foods on blood pressure is not at all settled. She even said there is evidence that salt isn't important anymore, especially if I drink plenty of milk. My doctor might be a little confused about what to do, but I'm sure clear about one thing: I want off of these pills.

6

HYPERTENSION

How can a healthy young guy like me have high blood pressure?

You're not unusual. Studies of school-age children in the United States show that as many as one in eight have blood pressures that are considered to be too high and unhealthy.[1] Overall, about 23 million American adults have high blood pressure also referred to as *hypertension,* with values greater than 160/95.[2] Some estimates range as high as 50 million people in this country with hypertension—and that means one in four of us has a life-threatening illness.[3] Each year Americans make about 25 million visits to their doctors to see about high blood pressure, and drugs are prescribed in 89 percent of those cases.[4] This is the leading cause of visits to a physician's office because of illness, accounting for 9 percent of all office visits.[4] The treatment of hypertension has become the country's leading reason for prescriptions.[5] High blood pressure is definitely big business for doctors and pharmaceutical companies. And that high prevalence of hypertension and drug therapy also reveals the sorry plight of the American people.

In this country, blood pressure rises with increasing age, and so does the number of diagnoses of hypertension.[6] People who show elevated blood pressure readings early in life have a greater tendency to develop hypertension as they get older. Of the adolescents who show borderline hypertension, 56 percent progress to permanent elevated hypertension within four years.[7]

Half of the population over the age of sixty-five has hypertension with readings greater than 160/95.[2] However, in underdeveloped countries such as New Guinea and several countries in Africa, blood pressures in natives remain at the same low level of approximately 110/70 throughout life.[8] Among such fortunate people this immunity from hypertension is not inherited.

Blacks in America, whose ancestors came from African societies where hypertension is still unknown today, have adopted an affluent diet and lifestyle and now are threatened by hypertension in shocking numbers.[9] Approximately 28 percent of American black men and women have high blood pressure, whereas an estimated 16 to 18 percent of white men and women suffer from this health problem which is out of control.[2] High blood pressure "runs in families," but, as always, the question is how much of this is a genetic factor, passed on to our children, and how much is caused by the diet and lifestyle we teach them?[10] In almost every case the social influences on eating and lifestyle overwhelm inherited strengths and weaknesses. When blacks move from villages in Africa to the cities they change to a diet more typical of affluent countries and they develop both obesity and high rates of hypertension.[11]

With high blood pressure this common, it certainly sounds like most of us are doing something seriously wrong, or else nature had an off day when such a frail human body was created. Why should I worry about my blood pressure if I don't feel sick?

Hypertension is called a silent disease because most people do not feel any symptoms to warn them that their blood pressure is higher than it should be. However, if your blood pressure is high, you have increased risks over someone of comparable age with a normal blood pressure to end up with one or all of the following:[12-14]

- twice the chance of dying from anything at all.
- twice the chance of closure of the arteries in the legs.
- three times the chance of dying from heart attacks.
- four times the chance of heart failure.
- seven times the chance of having a stroke.

Generally, the more elevated the blood pressure is, the worse is the condition of the body and the greater the likelihood of future complications. This is not to say that high blood pressure alone is the only health problem you might have now that increases your chance of trouble. All these possible future diseases are basically complications of atherosclerosis, a disease of the arteries and a condition that is strongly associated with elevated cholesterol and triglyceride levels.[14,15] When considering the risks to life related to high blood pressure and the need for treatment with medications, all other factors must be considered. Other important risk factors, such as family history, use of alcohol and tobacco, amount of exercise, and obesity are important when evaluating the needs and the risks of someone like yourself who has high blood pressure.[16,17] Here is a short list of these important risk factors:

**FACTORS INCREASING YOUR RISK OF
ATHEROSCLEROTIC COMPLICATIONS**

Major factors:	**Minor factors:**
Higher systolic and diastolic blood pressure	Elevated blood levels of triglycerides and uric acid
Age (older), sex (male), and race (black)	Family history of complications of atherosclerosis
Damage already present in heart, kidney, brain, eye (retina), arteries	Obesity
Cigarette smoking	Stress and personality type
Elevated cholesterol level	Physical inactivity
Diabetes mellitus	

What should the blood pressure be for a black person my age living in America?

With growth from infant to teenager there is a rise in blood pressure, but then after the teens, in healthy people blood pressure remains about the same throughout adult life.[6] Unfortunately, because of diet and lifestyle in this country, people suffer progressive deterioration in health as the years pass, and one of the signs of this downhill course is an increase in blood pressure with age. In Third World societies, where strokes and heart attacks are virtually unknown, a person in the eighth decade of life has the same blood pressure as a teenager.[8]

All racial groups have approximately the same value for what is considered a normal blood pressure. No racial group is immune to high blood pressure. So, in this respect at least, blacks are not different from whites, browns, yellows, or reds. It is not a coincidence that the societies where blood pressure remains the same throughout adult life are the same as those where blood levels of cholesterol, triglycerides, and uric acid are also low and obesity is uncommon. All these characteristics are common to people who follow a diet based on grains, potatoes, and other starchy foods, and who also have a low intake of salt. When these people move to a country like the United States and learn to eat rich foods loaded with fats, cholesterol, salt, and calories, but deficient in fiber, they develop all of the disease conditions associated with atherosclerosis, not simply high blood pressure. Their lives are placed at risk, just like the lives of native-born Americans.

A higher pressure called the *systolic* and a lower pressure called the *diastolic* are recorded for each blood pressure reading. Normal systolic and diastolic blood pressure can mean different things to different people. For a long time, normal blood pressure has been assigned a value that is common to most Americans, and that value has been set at about 120/80. But, according to our national record on health, the average American is ill; therefore, the typical physical and laboratory values associated with this poor health are not necessarily desirable—or what is ideally considered to be normal.

Health authorities are now aware that diastolic blood pressures as low as 80 to 89 can be associated with increased risks to health.[18] For example, the chances of heart attacks are doubled at this level over those with levels below 80. This new definition of hypertension will mean that almost half of all Americans live at some increased hazard of suffering from heart attacks, strokes, kidney failure, and the eventual assault of death.

When normal blood pressure means a value associated with a long life, with little chance of heart and blood vessel diseases, then that value should be around 110/70 or less throughout the adult years. Any sustained elevation above this value is reflected in a decrease in life expectancy and an increased risk of suffering from diseases such as heart attacks and strokes.

Do you think 145/95 is all that high? I was told it was a sign of mild hypertension.

A general classification that physicians use for high blood pressure values tells them the severity of the disease and the likelihood of complications from it. These figures refer to the lower number of the blood pressure reading, the diastolic pressures measured in millimeters of mercury.

- Mild hypertension: 90 to 104 mm
- Moderate hypertension: 105 to 114 mm
- Severe hypertension: 115 mm and greater

It is difficult to say whether or not you have hypertension on the basis of elevated readings taken on only two occasions. And neither of those readings was taken under the correct circumstances. You should have been relaxed and not caught up in the anxiety-producing atmosphere of an insurance physical examination or a five-minute visit to a doctor's office. Diagnostic decisions made on the basis of too few measurements under less than ideal circumstances all too often lead to an incorrect diagnosis and unnecessary treatment for a nonexistent disease.[19-21] A more meaningful reading would have been obtained if you had been lying down quietly for fifteen minutes without internal or external stresses to affect you. Physical activity, emotional stress, and pain will naturally raise your blood pressure, but this temporary elevation in pressure caused by the excitement of the moment is not a reflection of a diseased circulatory system. Furthermore, blood pressure varies throughout the day; generally it is highest in the midmorning, falls subsequently during the day, and is at its lowest point during the first few hours of sleep.[22]

At least three elevated blood pressures on three separate occasions should be observed under proper conditions before a diagnosis should be made. More than half of the people with elevated first readings will have acceptable readings on subsequent examinations.[21]

I do feel anxious when I'm in the doctor's office. I've felt this way ever since I was a kid. Could I take my own blood pressure at home?

Blood pressure is very easy to measure, and these days stethoscopes and blood-pressure cuffs are inexpensive and available at almost any drug store. The readings you get at home when you are relaxed are much more reliable than those taken in a doctor's office.[19] Measurements recorded by patients are often lower than those observed in a doctor's office. This is especially true for people like yourself who have been diagnosed as having mild hypertension. One study found that 28 percent of so-called mild hypertensives had normal blood pressure values when they were measured at home for a week.[23] However, the first week of measuring blood pressure at home has been found to be somewhat stressful. If people with elevated pressures will continue to check their pressures over the next several weeks, after they become comfortable with using the equipment, then approximately half of these people find their blood pressure readings are normal.[24] Even for people taking medication for blood pressure, measurements recorded by themselves are helpful in evaluating treatment and detecting overtreatment.[19] Then too, you can save plenty of money on visits to the doctor if you have your own equipment at home. Sometimes you might think your pressure is up a bit because you feel tense. With your own equipment you will be able to know what your actual pressure is and not have to guess about it based on your feelings. Believe it, you can't really feel an elevated blood pressure.

What would I hear if I took my blood pressure, and what does it mean? I wouldn't know where to start.

Taking your own blood pressure or having a friend or relative do it for you is really quite easy and can be very accurate once you learn the method. A blood-pressure cuff is fastened tightly around your upper arm just above the elbow. The right arm is preferred, and the cuff should be large enough so that the rubber bladder fits all the way around the arm including its major artery. The blood pressure is measured in terms of millimeters of mercury. This measurement is related to the force required to raise a standard column of mercury by 1 millimeter. Air is pumped under pressure into the rubber bladder inside the cuff. When the air pressure in the cuff becomes greater than the highest pressure of blood being pumped by the heart through the body's arteries, the flow of blood in the major artery of the arm stops completely. At this time you will hear no sound when a stethoscope is placed over the artery near your elbow.

When, by releasing some air, the pressure in the cuff's bladder is lowered to a point that is equal to the greatest force of the blood caught in the artery, then blood is allowed to pass through the artery. Because the blood spurts intermittently through the narrowed opening under this higher external cuff pressure, it slaps against the inside of the blood vessel and makes a sharp sound. The beginning of this sound is taken to represent the moment of the highest pressure of the blood flow. This is called the *systolic* pressure and is the force achieved during the strongest contraction of the heart. This is recorded as the higher number in a blood pressure reading.

The slapping sound continues as the air pressure in the cuff is reduced until the lowest pressure in the circulatory system is reached. This occurs at the moment the heart is not forcefully contracting, at a time when the heart muscle is at rest. The slapping sound stops because below this cuff pressure the blood vessel in the arm is filled continuously with blood. Sometimes a muffled whisper is heard before the complete disappearance of all sound. There is some argument about whether the pressure at the time of the muffled sound or at the complete disappearance of the sound is the better one to record. The moment of complete disappearance is probably the pressure you should record.[19]

Most authorities consider the lower value, called the *diastolic* pressure, to be the best indicator of the health of your circulatory system. It is recorded as the lower number in the blood pressure reading. When this number is low, the blood is flowing easily through the body's blood vessels. The higher number, indicating systolic blood pressure, is also a reliable predictor of future complications involving the heart and blood vessels.

What causes high blood pressure? I've never been a tense person, and no one in my family has high blood pressure.

Elevated blood pressure is an indication that something is wrong with the circulatory system—that is, with the heart and all the blood vessels. Actually, high blood pressure can be a sign of several different problems. This is similar to the way in which a fever can be caused for several different reasons : an infected toe, for example, or pneumonia or a common cold.

To help you understand the changes that take place in your body at any level of blood pressure, you might compare the heart to a mechanical pump and the blood vessels to an elastic hose with many branches of all sizes. This illustration is an oversimplification of the way the system works, but will give you some idea of the reasons why the blood pressure rises or falls and how treatments can lower blood pressure. Consider three possible changes in the functions of this pumping system that can raise the pressure inside the hose.

Think of the heart as a pump that can be turned up to do more work. The first mechanism that can raise the blood pressure is an increase in the contractions of the heart muscle. If the rate or force of the pump is increased, then the pressure in the system rises. In the case of the heart muscle, this can be caused by a surge in the amount of adrenalin released into the bloodstream. This happens when we become emotionally excited or increase our physical activity. This temporary blood response in pressure is necessary for proper functioning of the body and is in no way harmful. When the stimulating activity ceases, the blood pressure returns to lower levels; to normal in people who are healthy.

The second way to raise the pressure is by putting extra fluid into the system. The hose expands against the contracting elastic forces of the walls when more fluid is forced through it. The fuller the hose becomes, the higher will be the pressure within it. In a similar manner, an increase in the amount of fluid forces the elastic blood vessels in the body to expand. One way the amount of fluid increases is affected by the amount of table salt you eat.[25-27] The sodium from the salt draws water into the blood vessels. This causes the blood pressure to rise, and it stays elevated for several days until the salt and extra fluid are eliminated through sweat and kidneys. If salt is eaten daily, even in relatively small amounts in some people, the pressure remains elevated.

PUMP

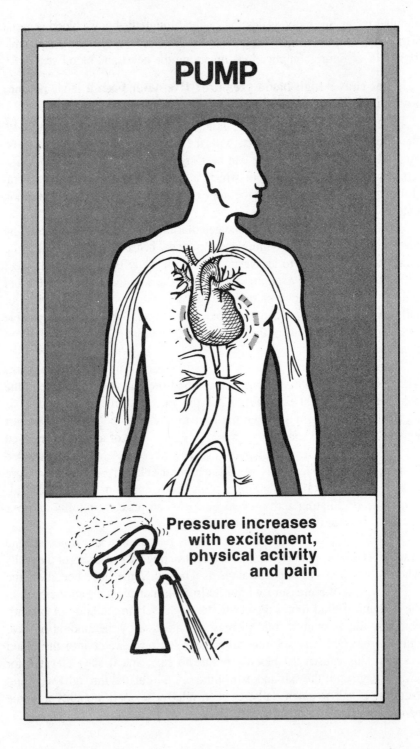

Pressure increases with excitement, physical activity and pain

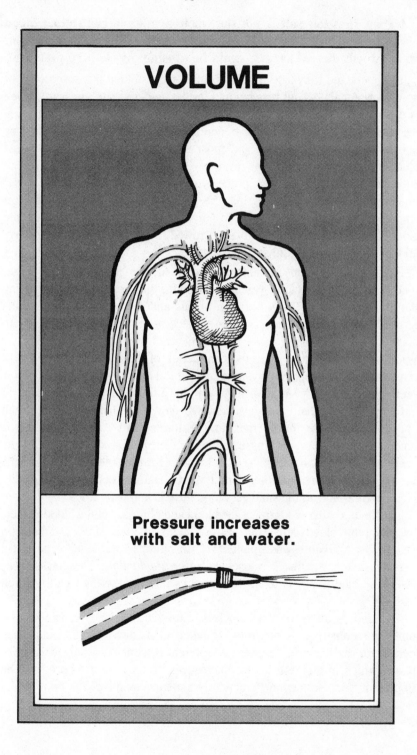

VOLUME

Pressure increases
with salt and water.

I know that low salt is not the whole answer to controlling blood pressure; otherwise, my problem would have been solved when I went on a low-salt diet. What else could be causing my elevated pressure?

To understand the most important influence on blood pressure, think of how the water shoots out stronger and farther, under greater pressure, when you place your finger over the end of a garden hose. By partly blocking the opening of the hose, you have increased the resistance against the easy flow of the water. The third and most important mechanism that raises blood pressure in Americans who eat foods high in fats and high in cholesterol is similar to this process of squeezing the end of the hose, except that the blood vessels may be squeezed at any place along their lengths and in their branchings. To gain this kind of rise in pressure, the blood vessels can be squeezed or narrowed, and their resistance to easy flow of blood increased in several ways.[28-30]

First of all, plaques of atherosclerosis fill the insides of the large, medium, and small blood vessels, narrowing their caliber and impeding the flow of blood.[30] The infiltration of fats and cholesterol into the walls of all the blood vessels causes them to become less elastic and thereby to accommodate less blood at any one moment. Failure of the diseased blood vessels to expand easily with the contraction of the heart is reflected by a rise of pressure, especially systolic pressure. This systolic hypertension is seen most frequently in the elderly, who have the most atherosclerosis.[31]

Other changes that cause resistance to flow take place soon after each and every meal for most Americans. Saturated fats eaten in dangerous amounts cause blood clotting elements, called *platelets,* and also all the various kinds of blood cells, to stick together forming clumps that slow the flow of blood in medium and small vessels and on occasion completely block normal flow in the smallest blood vessels and capillaries.[30,32-34] Even vegetable fats cause sludging of the blood and plugging of the blood vessels by clumping blood cells, but do not seem to have similar effects on platelets.[33,34] Finally, when platelets form clumps, they release powerful blood-vessel-constricting hormones called *prostaglandins.* These substances cause the blood vessels to go into spasms and narrow their caliber even further.[35]

The end result of all this blocked, clumped, sludged, spasmed, and otherwise constricted circulation is called in medical terms, "increased peripheral resistance." To you, the different detrimental changes that take place, which in their effects are like squeezing the end of a hose, will be important because they are practically announcements of the poor health

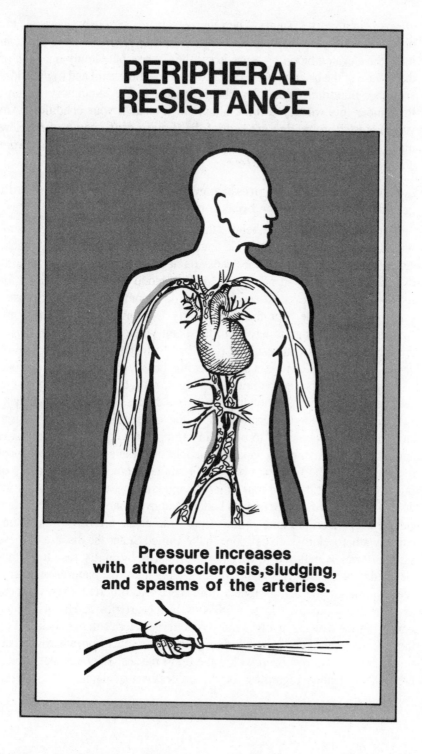

PERIPHERAL RESISTANCE

Pressure increases with atherosclerosis, sludging, and spasms of the arteries.

of your circulatory system. When the vessels are seriously diseased, the blood inside them cannot circulate easily and the pressure rises. Thus, in itself the elevated blood pressure is not the disease but is only one sign of the disease of the blood vessels. Elevated levels of cholesterol and triglycerides are other important signs of probable trouble in the circulatory system. Remember this when you think about ways to treat your condition. Are you interested in treating the sign of the disease or the cause of it? How much help does an aspirin tablet give when you have a general fever from an infection in your little toe?

Shouldn't I watch my pressure every day to make sure it doesn't get any higher and maybe break a blood vessel?

Many people mistakenly believe that even a slight elevation of pressure will burst their blood vessels wide open and cause a stroke or heart attack. Actually, elevated pressure does cause damage, but only over long periods of time and not only in one place. A high blood pressure, sustained for many years, is believed to accelerate the development of atherosclerosis, especially in people over the age of forty.[36] Eventually, the arteries are weakened by the atherosclerosis to the point where they will burst under any pressure. This can result in brain hemorrhages that are one type of stroke. When the arteries get so filled with cholesterol and fat that a stroke or heart attack is on the verge of happening, a slight elevation in pressure will have little or no additional effect to hasten the onset of the tragedy.

The elevated blood pressure that is the consequence of eating large amounts of salt is believed to be the most important cause of hypertension and atherosclerosis among Japanese people, and therefore the factor most responsible for the high rate of strokes among them. In certain areas of Japan, people eat three to four times the amounts of salt each day that we do in the United States. Scientists believe that over many years the constant elevation of blood pressure injures the inside of the arteries to the brain, causing atherosclerosis to develop. In the United States the disease of these same arteries is believed to be caused primarily by injury resulting from elevated cholesterol levels in the blood. Interestingly, the patterns of atherosclerosis inside the blood vessels from these two different causes appear as two distinct distributions of plaques in the arteries.[37] The American version of the disease involves mostly the large arteries in the neck and on the outer surfaces of the brain, whereas the Japanese suffer from atherosclerosis in the smaller arteries deep within the brain tissues. However, the strokes are just as deadly, regardless of the processes that damage the arterial walls.

Healthy blood vessels are capable of sustaining very high elevations in pressure that occur intermittently. When you exercise, your pressure increases a great deal and the arteries respond with better health.

Aren't the drugs I've been given going to solve the problem?

The drugs will lower your blood pressure by only a few millimeters of mercury and possibly will decrease slightly the acceleration of the atherosclerosis from the continuing elevated pressure. But the drugs lead to other problems that cancel out any such slight benefit. In your case, and in the cases of the other 25 million people with mild hypertension in this country, you will fare as well, if not better, without the medication. [16,37-43] Again, I'll turn to an oversimplification to help you understand how drugs lower blood pressure. Let's talk once again about the mechanical pump and the elastic hose. Drugs work on the heart and blood vessels in a variety of ways in an attempt to counteract one of the three mechanisms that can cause pressure to rise. These drugs directly oppose normal tissue functions and reactions.

One group of drugs decreases the strength of the pump. These are classed as beta receptor blockers, or simply *beta blockers*. Both the rate and the force of contraction of the heart are reduced by blocking the natural effect of the stimulant adrenalin on the beta receptors of the heart muscle.

Naturally, we pay a price for using drugs to lower blood pressure. The side effects of these drugs are considered to be mild by many doctors who prescribe them. However, many patients can't feel the lowered blood pressure, and notice only fatigue all day long, especially while they exercise.[44] The reason for this fatigue, in part, is a blunted response of the heart caused by the medication; the heart rate increases very little in response to exercise, and as a result, the circulatory system can not keep up with the physical demands made by the activity.[44] It has been claimed that at least 30 percent of patients on full doses of beta blocker medication complain of weakness of the leg muscles and inability to hurry on hills or stairs.[45] Occasionally, the weakening effect on the heart muscle from these drugs can be so severe that heart failure occurs in persons who have heart disease; the blood backs up into the lungs, and the patient drowns in his or her own body fluids.

Beta blockers also have side effects that worsen asthma and raise blood sugar levels when they are used in combination with diuretics.[46] These medications can also have the counterproductive effects of increasing the risk factors for atherosclerosis by raising blood triglyceride levels and lowering the levels of so-called ''good'' HDL-cholesterol.[47,48]

Those side effects of beta blockers would be serious for me because I like sports. What other drugs are available?

The pressure in the system can also be lowered by decreasing the amount of fluid in it. A second group of drugs slows down the normal mineral-conserving mechanisms of the kidneys. This causes the loss of sodium ions and water and thereby decreases the volume of fluids in the circulatory system. The American consumer has a great appetite for both the hidden and the obvious salt found in almost all of those enticing processed and packaged foods that are displayed on market shelves and also in the salt shaker at home. Drugs classified as diuretics are prescribed in an attempt to make a partial compensation for a high salt intake.

What kinds of side effects can I expect with these diuretics?

Recent statistics indicate that diuretics, including hydrochlorothiazide and chlorthalidone, appear to increase a patient's chance of dying from a heart attack.[49-53] Studies indicate that there is a 2 times greater incidence of sudden death, and deaths due to heart failure are more likely in treated than in untreated hypertensive patients with similar disease severity.[51-53] One reason for this is that these drugs raise the blood cholesterol, triglycerides, sugar, and uric acid levels, all of which are known risk factors for people who have developed the complications of atherosclerosis.[54-57] Another reason for the increase in death from heart disease may be arrhythmias that are common consequences of mineral imbalances, especially low potassium levels, caused by diuretics.[58] The increased chances of dying among people taking diuretics are especially high when these patients have definite diseases of the heart arteries as shown by EKGs or angiograms.[49-53] Unfortunately, in the age groups of people likely to be treated for high blood pressure with diuretics, most do have disease of the heart arteries.

I certainly don't want any medications that will increase my risk of having a heart attack and dying. After all, isn't this what I'm trying to avoid by taking medication? Aren't there any other drugs to try?

The last group of drugs that are employed will dilate the blood vessels and thereby reduce the effects of squeezing the end of the hose. These include a wide variety of medications that work by equally diverse mechanisms. Generally, these chemicals are more powerful than the others we've talked about and have more side effects. By working on the nervous system and the vessels directly, these drugs inhibit contraction of the muscles in the walls of the blood vessels. Segments that are still elastic will dilate to accommodate more blood. Of course, segments that are stiffened by atherosclerosis will not dilate because they are made rigid by the hard fibrous plaques in and on them.

These all sound like powerful drugs with lots of side effects. How can my body tolerate such medications?

The side effects of many of this last group of drugs, the *blood vessel dilators,* can be especially strong. Blood pressure that is too low can be a complication resulting from any kind of medication for treating high blood pressure, but some of the drugs that dilate blood vessels are notorious for their profound effects on blood pressure.

Long-term surveillance of the adverse effects of all blood pressure medications reveals that nearly 10 percent of people have definite or probable side effects severe enough to stop the medication. In addition, nearly 25 percent more stop treatment for suspected side effects.[59] The likelihood of side effects varies with the type of medication, the concurrent use of other medications, the dosage, and the individual. Common side effects include low blood pressure, low blood potassium, upset stomach, joint pains, heart arrhythmias, heart failure, skin rash, nasal stuffiness, muscle cramps, dehydration, nightmares, headache, depression, drowsiness, weakness, and dizziness. Some medications can hamper physical performance, prolong reaction time, and increase the errors during driving.[60] Adverse effects on intellectual performance have also been suspected with certain medications.[60] Failing memory is noted. Impotence is the most frequently reported side effect for all of these drugs, and a decrease in sexual interest is the next most common complaint.[59]

Simply labeling someone as hypertensive causes a rise of 80 percent in the number of days he or she stays home from work.[61] Diagnosing an individual as having high blood pressure has been found to impair marital adjustments and to lower the sense of well being.[62-64] People actually become hostile and depressed and feel unwell when faced with the incurable illness of hypertension.[62-64]

Since the list of possible side effects is so long, when you are taking a medication you should become familiar with the possible adverse reactions. Sources for this information are found in bookstores and libraries. One of the best books is the *Physicians Desk Reference,* which presents information supplied by drug companies. Also, your physician should tell you, clearly and specifically, what you should look for in the way of adverse reactions.

With all of these side effects, I guess the benefits for health must be great. Is that why drug treatment is so popular?

Many studies have attempted to show that drugs that lower blood pressure will improve survival rates and reduce risks of stroke and heart attacks. And indeed some benefits are noted for some groups of patients. A small minority of patients suffer from moderate to severe hypertension, with a diastolic level above 104. Those people with severe disease have been shown to benefit with a decrease in risk for strokes when their blood pressure is lowered with medication.[38]

However, the results from treatment of the large majority of people with elevated blood pressure, those with mild hypertension like yourself, with a diastolic level below 105 millimeters, have been disappointing. Five of the six large studies performed during the last two decades show no significant reduction in deaths from cardiovascular disease, and only one of the six shows any protection from heart attacks with drug therapy in cases of mild hypertension.[16,38-43] Even in this one study the benefit derived was an absolute reduction in the number of deaths by only 1.3 percent. This means that for every 100 patients treated, 1 derived some benefit and the other 99 did not.[39] Here a basic question must be asked: Should we subject a large number of people to long-term treatment with potentially harmful medications having unpleasant side effects when the chances of any one person deriving benefit from the treatment is so small?[39] Since the benefits are questionable and side effects and the costs are definite, the latter become the dominant issue.

Even though the evidence from the studies on drug treatment of mild hypertension show the beneficial effects are seriously in doubt, this fact has been ineffectively communicated to practicing doctors.[43] In 1977 the Joint National Committee on Detection, Evaluation, and Treatment of High Blood Pressure recommended that persons with diastolic pressures of 90 to 104 millimeters, mild hypertension, receive individual approaches with consideration to be given to weight control and salt intake. They recommended that virtually all patients with blood pressures greater than 105 millimeters be treated with medication. In 1978 the New York Heart Association conducted a survey of doctors to assess the impact of the Committee recommendations. Of the doctors responding, 92 percent answered that they routinely prescribed medication for people with mild hypertension, 90 to 104 millimeters.

Enthusiasm runs high for proving the benefits of drug therapy for mild hypertension because a study showing such good effects can mean millions of dollars in profits for people in the drug-prescribing and drug-producing businesses. Once a patient is put on blood pressure medicine, he or she is given the message that this treatment is going to be for life. This means that the physician will be able to charge the patient for monthly office visits to "keep an eye on the pressure." There will also be a steady business from treating the side effects of the medications prescribed. The drug companies have a guaranteed future market because of the prevailing attitude instilled in physicians and patients about the treatment of this disease; the view that hypertension is incurable.

One of the reasons why the medications to control hypertension fail is that these drugs have little or no positive effects, and sometimes exert one or more adverse effects, on the processes that cause the diseased blood vessels. They do little to change the progress of the atherosclerosis and the eventual time of disability and death. A national reorientation of treatment goals toward preventing the *causes* of cardiovascular disease and hypertension, rather than the present concentration upon the treatment of *signs*, will be slow because of the financial incentives involved in caring for sick people. A pharmaceutical company might easily spend $25 million to $50 million on developing and testing one new drug for treating hypertension. Compare this enormous budget to the total amount of money that has been spent on studying the effects of sodium and potassium, which are suspected of being involved in the dietary causes of high blood pressure. One estimate for this budget guesses that throughout the years it has probably been less than $100,000![65]

Should the top number, the systolic blood pressure, be treated?

Sustained elevations of systolic blood pressure without similar elevations of diastolic pressure are most often seen in elderly people. This is definitely associated with an increased risk of complications such as heart attacks and strokes.[66,67] However, there is little evidence that lowering systolic blood pressure with drug therapy benefits these patients.[67] And there is some evidence that harm can be done.[68] Future studies may lead to other opinions. Elderly people are especially sensitive to the side effects of medications and with them even more caution is required.[69]

I've decided that I don't want to take any medicine at all. Let's talk about the habits I can change.

Elevation of blood pressure is a sign of disease, and regardless of how common this health-problem has become, it is not a normal condition. We need to look at its causes to find clues for its cure. When the factors that cause disease are corrected, the body heals unless the disease process has gone too far. Fortunately, when they first gain a doctor's attention, most people have not passed their ability to recover full function and the chance for an active, healthy, long life.

People in some countries of the world maintain the same low blood pressure throughout life.[8,11,70] These people have certain lifestyle and dietary characteristics in common. Their diet is low in sodium, fats, and animal products, and it is high in potassium and fiber. Their foods are primarily starches, vegetables, and fruits, they are physically active, and obesity is uncommon. Studies of people in our society with a comparable diet and lifestyle, and with low blood pressure as well, confirm the value of these safeguards to health.

Other practices in diet and lifestyle that are associated with elevated blood pressure are eating meat, drinking caffeine, drinking alcohol, and smoking cigarettes.[71-75] Polyunsaturated vegetable fats tend to lower blood pressure, and saturated animal fats will raise it.[76] The reason for this difference is related to the synthesis of a group of blood-vessel-relaxing hormones called prostaglandins that increase with intake of vegetable oils.[76] Certain of these hormones cause the dilation of the blood vessels, a resulting decrease in resistance of the wall of the peripheral vein and arteries, and a lowering of blood pressure. Prostaglandins also may increase the excretion of salt from the body. There are many kinds of prostaglandin hormones that have a wide variety of actions in the body.

Moderate daily exercise and loss of weight will help to lower blood pressure.[77-80] Some evidence indicates that certain methods of relaxation also help to lower elevated blood pressure.[80]

I've been told to drink milk and eat cheese if I want to lower my blood pressure. What is the reason for this?

It is interesting to note how some so-called discoveries in health make their way to the public's attention so easily by way of the national media. When some scientific "fact" or "finding" supports the sales of a product for a big industry, it is publicized immediately and widely. Better yet, if this information allows us to eat with a guilt-free conscience the foods we have learned to love, then the information quickly gains acceptance as a reliable fact.

Recently a study showed that blood pressure was lower in people who for some reason or other had greater amounts of calcium in their diets.[81] The investigators also found that salt had no adverse effect on high blood pressure in the people being studied.[81] This work gained national attention overnight. Some readers instantly forgot or ignored the simple truth that this announcement contradicted nearly sixty years of scientific investigations made by hundreds of other investigators, all of which showed that the amount of salt eaten in the diet was very important.[8,25-27,65,82,83] Instead, the conclusions of this new study were hailed with joy by millions of people who had found that a low-salt diet was unpalatable and by millions more who craved milk and cheese, regardless of the harm they did. At least part of the credit for the research showing the beneficial effects of calcium on high blood pressure must be given to the the the National Dairy Council. With great foresight and admirable generosity, they provided some of the financial support for these investigators.[84,85]

Several mechanisms for lowering blood pressure with the aid of calcium have been proposed.[85,86] More calcium taken into the body through the diet causes the kidneys to excrete more sodium, the primary ingredient in table salt that raises blood pressure. Calcium will also dilate the blood vessels and lower the resistance in the peripheral blood system, thus lowering blood pressure.

We're told that dairy products are excellent sources of calcium. It seems to me like a healthy way to lower my blood pressure would be by drinking more milk and eating more cheese, and maybe a little ice cream on the side. What's wrong with that?

Some studies fail to support this association of calcium intake and lower blood pressure, but let's assume that the findings of this research are at least partly correct.[87,88] Even so, the advice to increase the amount of dairy products that you eat can be very dangerous to your health.

We want to lower blood pressure because we want to reduce the risk of dying from heart attacks and strokes. These tragedies occur because the blood vessels are diseased, having the condition known as atherosclerosis. The consumption of dairy products is believed to be a leading cause not only of atherosclerosis, but also of complications—heart attacks and strokes.[89-91] Worldwide, the highest incidence of death from heart disease occurs in Finland.[92] The people in Finland are also among the very highest consumers of dairy products in the world.[93] Compared to the United States population, the Finnish have approximately one and a half times the mortality from heart disease and consume one and a half times as much cow's milk products.[92,93] The saturated fats and cholesterol present in large amounts in those tasty dairy foods are the culprits. Therefore, any slight benefit in lowering blood pressure that may be gained from the calcium in milk and cheese will be offset many times over by the relative quantities of athero-sclerosis-producing cholesterol and saturated fats in those same double-crossing foods.

Couldn't I eat low-fat dairy products or take calcium pills to get the extra calcium to lower my pressure?

This approach may provide minimal benefit. However, this is not necessarily going to make you any healthier or reduce your risk of developing atherosclerosis and reaching an early death unless you make other serious modifications in your diet. Eating and drinking low fat dairy products can create other problems for some people. Often the milk proteins are causes of allergies; and in many people the milk sugar, lactose, can cause stomach cramps, diarrhea, and excessive gas. If you are not bothered by such allergies, problems with digestion, and other adverse reactions some people have from low-fat milk, then your plan is OK as far as it goes.

Calcium pills may offer a slight benefit, but taking them as your only medication is an unsuitable way to treat high blood pressure. The actual amount by which calcium does lower the pressure is quite small. Remember, as with blood pressure pills, anything else, like calcium tablets, that disguises the tell-tale sign of an elevated blood pressure, does not necessarily reduce the risk of dying from complications of atherosclerosis. This is so often the case with treatments that deal with signs and symptoms of any disease while they ignore the causes of it.

Let us consider one final thought that focuses on the inappropriateness of us using calcium in an effort to correct high blood pressure: We should all agree that hypertension is not a disease due to "cow's milk deficiency" or "calcium pill deficiency"!

Is it true that limiting salt is no longer considered important for preventing or lowering high blood pressure?

Most people do not appear to be harmed by the amount of table salt they use each day. However, health authorities estimate that about 20 percent of the American population will suffer some kind of distress from the amount of salt they eat. The average daily salt intake is approximately two teaspoons, about 10 grams of sodium chloride a day. The more salt a person eats, the more likely he or she is to be troubled by it. But we must realize that salt alone is not the only cause of our present frightening outbreak of hypertension.

Studies on vegetarians have focused attention on the fact that other components of diet are also very important.[94-97] Certain groups of strict vegetarians follow principles of macrobiotics, emphasizing brown rice and vegetables in their diets. These people also include generous amounts of salt, but their blood pressures are not elevated by it.[95,96] Other aspects of their diets apparently compensate for the high salt intake. Their foods are high in potassium and fiber and practically devoid of any kind of meat. These components have an overriding influence, and the level of table salt is tolerated reasonably well.

Potassium plays an important role in high blood pressure, acting in counterbalance with sodium. In studies of volunteers with and without hypertension, their blood pressures fell when their diets were supplemented with potassium.[65,98,99] This does not mean that you should take potassium salts or pills to treat your problem. Instead, you should emphasize high-potassium foods, which are vegetables and fruits.

Just like taking an aspirin to relieve a fever doesn't cure a cold any sooner, blood pressure pills, dairy products, and calcium and potassium pills aren't going to solve my problem. OK, I'm ready for the message. What is it?

To improve the health of your circulatory system, you need to change your diet, get some exercise, stop drinking caffeine and alcohol, and quit smoking. A health-supporting diet centered around starches, with plenty of vegetables and fruits and practically no salt, will give the best results for lowering your blood pressure and improving your health in general.[80,100-109] I strongly advise that you give up feasting on rich foods, at least until you are better. By that I mean when your blood pressure is down and you are off all medication. After about three weeks on this health-supporting diet most people can stop taking medication, and most attain a reasonable blood pressure.

How will I know when I am better? After all, I feel fine now except for the side effects of the medications.

A lower blood pressure will tell you when your condition has been improved. Your goal is 110/70 or lower when you are at rest and no longer taking medication. Also, you can check the other indicators of a healthier circulatory system. Blood tests for cholesterol, triglycerides, blood sugar, and uric acid will reflect the changes you have made in your diet. Of these risk factors for disease, your cholesterol level is most important, and your goal is to reduce that to 160 milligram percent or less.

I want to remind you that this is not an all-or-nothing choice. The more changes in lifestyle and diet you make, the more you will gain in health. Even if you don't follow my advice, for whatever reason, you should realize that with your mild degree of high blood pressure you will be better off without any medication. However, you will still be at a considerably increased risk of dying earlier than a man of your age should, unless you correct the disease that is progressing in your body.

How do I go about getting off the medication that my other doctor put me on?

Under a doctor's supervision, you will need to decrease slowly, day by day, the dosage you're taking now and at the same time monitor your blood pressure. In general, you should begin by reducing or stopping the strongest one first, the one that causes the worst side effects. Usually, the strongest medications are the ones a doctor adds last. Here is a list showing an order in which medications can be dealt with; those in step 1 are the most powerful.

STEP-DOWN ON MEDICATIONS
step 1. Minoxidil, guanethidine,
step 2. Hydralazine, captopril, clonidine, prazosin, methyldopa, reserpine
step 3. Beta blockers (propanolol, metoprolol, nadolol, atenolol); Reduce dosage slowly, usually cut in half every three days
step 4. Diuretics (furosemide, hydrochlorothiazide, other thiazides, ethacrynic acid, spironolactone, triamterene, amiloride)
step 5. Off all medications

Proceed under your doctor's supervision, while monitoring your blood pressure in the doctor's office and at home. Begin with the most powerful drugs in step 1 and work through to step 5.

When the dosage is large, cutting the amount of one type of medication by a third or half may be the first step. Wait about three days before beginning the next decrease in dosage of this medication. When you have gained the smallest dosage in which the medication is packaged, then the next step is to stop it altogether. If, with the dietary change, blood pressure falls to levels that are too low, such as 110/70 or lower, or if a person becomes dizzy, then the dosages should be lowered more rapidly. When adjusting medications in this manner, try to keep the blood pressure below 160/100. Don't worry if the pressure is this high for a few days. This elevation for a short time does not place you in any extra danger.

However, most people with high blood pressure have a very serious disease of the arteries and therefore are at a high risk of having a hazardous complication. Even so, if a stroke or heart attack did occur while an individual was making adjustments, in most cases that would simply be a coincidence. The actual cause of the climactic event would be many years of serious damage to the arteries from abuses caused by diet and lifestyle, not from the reduction in medication and the slight rise in blood pressure that sometimes may follow a lower dosage.

Actually, during this short period of adjustment the danger is greater from too much medication than from too little. Overenthusiastic treatment of blood pressure can be dangerous. The attempt to lower blood pressure to normal levels with medication in people with extensive atherosclerosis has been shown to result in a fivefold increase in heart attacks.[110]

Beta blockers should be reduced slowly, because rapid withdrawal can cause bothersome strong or rapid heartbeats. There is also some evidence that too rapid a decrease in dosage of beta blockers will cause chest pains and heart attacks in susceptible people. On the other hand with withdrawal of some medications, such as clonidine, a rapid rise in blood pressure may happen, attended by symptoms of nervousness, agitation, and headache. The medication should be reduced slowly, at intervals of three days.

Let's take you for an example. You need to stop taking only two medications; 80 milligrams of a popular beta blocker medication called Corgard and 25 milligrams of hydrochlorothiazide as a diuretic. After you start the health-supporting diet, take only 40 milligrams of Corgard and all of the diuretic. If the blood pressure readings are reasonable, say 140/90 or less for three days, then stop the Corgard altogether. If the pressure stays reasonable for another three days, then the next step is to see what your pressure does without the diuretic. If the pressure goes up and stays up, you can always start to take the medication again, in the reverse order, with no harm done. Going without the medication for many days, and probably for many weeks, will do very little, if any, harm. Remember that the effects of high blood pressure are from damaging the blood vessels over a long term. If you don't try this step-down approach, you may never know whether or not you really need all, or any, of the medication.

Your goal is to lower your blood pressure to 110/70 or less without medication. Some people will not realize this ideal pressure, even with a strict low-salt, low-fat vegetarian diet, and a clean lifestyle, because the damage to the circulatory system is already too severe. Also, a small minority of people have hypertension from causes other than years of poor diet and lifestyle practices, which need attention other than changes in their habits. Your doctor will need to identify these rare cases.

For those people who are unable to reach an ideal blood pressure, if readings can be maintained below 160/100 and if other risk factors are not involved, then medications are likely to do more harm than good.[16,38-42] When evaluating the need for medication in order to lower blood pressure, other factors must be considered, such as evidence of disease of the blood vessels, heart, and kidneys, and elevated levels of cholesterol, triglycerides, blood sugar, and uric acid. Also consider body weight, family history, and daily exercise. Someone affected by few of these other adverse factors will tolerate an elevation in blood pressure much better and will be less likely to benefit from medication. Think of hypertension as a disease that involves the whole body, not just something that has gone wrong only with the pressure.

People who have blood pressure readings of 160/100 or greater, and some of those with slightly lower pressures who are threatened by other risk factors, should be placed on medication. The blood pressure should be lowered by medication to a level of about 140/80. Decreasing the pressure to a level lower than this increases the risk of hypotension, which can make some people dizzy or faint. Also, too low a pressure in blood vessels that are narrowed by atherosclerosis may lead to a situation where no flow at all goes to the tissues and may lead ultimately to a stroke or heart attack.

I certainly understand and like all the things you're telling me. I really do want to be healthier. After all, I'm a successful person. I have a fine job and a wonderful family. Everything is going right for me. Why should I fail in my health, the one thing that is basic to all the rest of my life? I'm more than willing to put all the effort that's needed into remaking me.

A major problem in the treatment of any disease by any method is the patient who won't follow the doctor's directions. In the case of blood pressure, 25 to 50 percent of patients fail to follow their physicians' instructions.[111] The problem becomes even greater when people are told to change their diet and lifestyle rather than simply to swallow a pretty-colored pill every morning.

Changes in diet and lifestyle are highly effective. The doctor's first step in easing the many health problems of hypertension is to make hypertensive people aware that they have a second option; that they need not choose only drugs and enduring an "incurable" illness. Once they are told about this way out, then the real obstacle to success is getting people to make the change and to take care of themselves without the intervention of more doctors, more pills, and much more distress to mind and body. People who enjoy life and who generally like themselves and their associates find that the transition is easy to make and certainly worth all the effort required. People who don't care about their jobs, families, personal relationships, or themselves are almost beyond helping. As a doctor I receive a tremendous reward from my successes when I help a patient like you gain back something so important to you and your family—your good health.

℞

- Prevention and treatment of hypertension is based upon a diet low in salt, high in fiber, low in animal products, and generous with starchy foods, vegetables, and fruits.
- Moderate exercise and reduction in weight in cases of obesity will help lower blood pressure.
- Drinking caffeine and alcohol and smoking tobacco should be stopped as soon as possible.
- Monitor your blood pressure at home, not only in a doctor's office.
- When you change your diet and lifestyle, decrease your medication in graded stages while monitoring your blood pressure under a doctor's supervision.
- Your goal is to reach a blood pressure of 110/70 or less without medication.
- Reduce all controllable risk factors and periodically check your blood levels of cholesterol, triglycerides, and sugar.
- Take medication to lower blood pressure if it is higher than 160/100 and bring it down to about 140/80. Beta blockers are safer for most people than diuretics as a first choice for medication when necessary.[16] If you are on medications, report regularly to your doctor for follow-up. Report side effects to your doctor.
- Don't give up too soon and don't be impatient. After all, most of us spent years getting ourselves into the shape we're in.

REFERENCES

[1]Loggie J. Hypertension in the pediatric patient: a reappraisal. *J Pediatr* 94:685, 1979.

[2]Roberts J. *Blood pressure levels of persons 6-74 years, United States, 1971-1974. DHEW Pub No. (HRA) 78-1648 203,* 1977.

[3]Kaplan N (ed). *Clinical Hypertension.* Baltimore: Williams and Wilkins, 1982.

[4]Cypress B. *Medication therapy in office visits for hypertension: National Ambulatory Medical Care Survey, 1980. National Center for Health Statistics Advanced Data,* No. 80, July 22, 1982.

[5]Baum C. Drug use in the United States in 1981. *JAMA* 251:1293, 1984.

[6]Editorial: Why does blood-pressure rise with age? *Lancet* 2:289, 1981.

[7]Falkner B. Cardiovascular response to stress in adolescents, in Onesti G, Kim K (eds). *Hypertension in the young and the old.* New York: Grune & Stratton, 1981 pp 11-17.

[8]Freis E. Salt, volume and the prevention of hypertension. *Circulation* 53:589, 1976.

[9]Editorial: Hypertension in blacks and whites. *Lancet* 2:73, 1980.

[10]Biron P. Familial aggregation of blood pressure and its components. *Pediatr Clin North Am* 25:29, 1978.

[11]Sever P. Blood-pressure and its correlates in urban and tribal Africa. Lancet 2:60, 1980.

[12]Kannel W. Should all mild hypertension be treated? Yes. In: Lasagna L. (ed) *Controversies in Therapeutics* Lasagna L (eds.) Philadephia: W.B. Saunders Co, 1980. p-299.

[13]Fry J. Deaths and complications from hypertension. *J Roy Coll Gen Pract* 25:489, 1975.

[14]Evans P. Relation of longstanding blood-pressure levels to atherosclerosis. *Lancet* 1:516, 1965.

[15]Stamler J.. Lifestyles, major risk factors, proof and public policy. *Circulation* 58:3, 1978.

[16]Kaplan N. Mild hypertension: when and how to treat. *Arch Intern Med* 143:255, 1983.

[17]Madhavan S. The potential effect of blood pressure reduction on cardiovascular disease: a cautionary note. *Arch Intern Med* 141:1583, 1981.

[18]An epidemiological approach to describing risk associated with blood pressure levels. Final report of the Working Group on Risk and High Blood Pressure. *Hypertension* 7:641, 1985.

[19]O'Brien E. Blood pressure measurement: Current practice and future trends: Regular review. *Br Med J* 290:729, 1985.

[20]Armitage P. The variability of measurements of casual blood pressure I. A laboratory study. *Clin Sci* 30:325, 1966.

[21]Carey R. The Charlottesville blood-pressure survey. Value of repeated blood-pressure measurements. *JAMA* 236:847, 1976.

[22]Millar-Craig M. Circadian variation of blood-pressure. *Lancet* 1:795, 1978.

[23]Julius S. Home blood pressure determination. Value in borderline (''labile'') hypertension. *JAMA* 229:663, 1974.

[24]Traub Y. Home blood-pressure recording. *Lancet* 2:126, 1975.

[25]Meneely G. High sodium-low potassium environment and hypertension. *Am J Cardiol* 38:768, 1976.

[26]Dahl L. Salt and hypertension. *Am J Clin Nutr* 25:231, 1972.

[27]Parfrey P. Relation between arterial pressure, dietary sodium intake, and renin system in essential hypertension. *Br Med J* 283:94, 1981.

[28]Freis E. Hemodynamics of hypertension. *Physiol Rev* 40:27, 1960.

[29]Frohlich E. Re-examination of the hemodynamics of hypertension. *Am J Med Sci* 257:9, 1969.

[30]Malhotra S. Dietary factors causing hypertension in India. *Am J Clin Nutr* 23:1353, 1970.

[31]Stamler J. Hypertension screening of 1 million Americans: Community Hypertension Evaluation Clinic (CHEC) program, 1973 through 1975. *JAMA* 235:2299, 1976.

[32]Friedman M. Serum lipids and conjunctival circulation after fat ingestion in men exhibiting type-A behavior pattern. *Circulation* 29:874, 1964.

[33]Friedman M. Effect of unsaturated fats upon lipemia and conjunctival circulation. A study of coronary-prone (pattern A) men. *JAMA* 193:882, 1965.

[34]O'Brien J. Acute platelet changes after large meals of saturated and unsaturated fats. *Lancet* 1:878, 1976.

[35]Hamberg M. Thromboxanes: a new group of biologically active compounds derived from prostaglandins endoperoxides. *Proc Nat Acad Sci USA* 72:2994, 1975.

[36]McGill H. Persistent problems in the pathogenesis of atherosclerosis. *Atherosclerosis* 4:443, 1984.

[37]Kuller L. An explanation for variations in distribution of stroke and arteriosclerotic heart disease among populations and racial groups. *Am J Epidemiol* 93:1, 1971.

[38]McAlister N. Should we treat 'mild' hypertension? *JAMA* 249:379, 1983.

[39]Pickering T. Treatment of mild hypertension and the reduction of cardiovascular mortality. The 'of or by' dilemma. *JAMA* 249:399, 1983.

[40]Boyd G. The pressure to treat. *Lancet* 2:1134, 1980.

[41]Venkata C. Should mild hypertension be treated? *Ann Intern Med* 99:403, 1983.

[42]Kaplan N. Therapy for mild hypertension. Toward a more balanced view. *JAMA*. 249:365. 1983.

[43]Thomson G. High blood pressure diagnosis and treatment: Consensus recommendations vs actual practice. *Am J Public Health* 71:413, 1981.

[44]Editorial: Fatigue as an unwanted effect of drugs. *Lancet* 1:1258, 1980.

[45]Stone R. Proximal myopathy during beta-blockade. *Br Med J* 2:1583, 1979.

[46]Dornhorst A. Aggravation by propranolol of hyperglycaemic effect of hydrochlorothiazide in type II diabetics without alteration of insulin secretion. *Lancet* 1:123, 1985.

[47]Leren P. Effect of propranolol and prazosin on blood lipids: the Oslo study. *Lancet* 2:4, 1980.

[48]Editorial: Antihypertensive drugs, plasma lipids, and coronary disease. *Lancet* 2:19, 1980.

[49]Multiple Risk Factor Intervention Trial Research Group. Multiple Risk Factor Intervention Trial. Risk factor changes and mortality results. *JAMA* 248:1465, 1982.

[50]Holme I. Treatment of mild hypertension with diuretics. The importance of ECG abnormalities in the Oslo Study and in MRFIT. *JAMA* 251:1298, 1984.

[51]Kannel W. Sudden death: Lessons from subsets in population studies. Lessons from epidemiology. *J Am Coll Cardiol* 5:141B, 1985.

[52]Anti-HT therapy seems to add to sudden death risk in some. *Intern Med News* 18:60, 1985.

[53]Higher death rates in hypertensive patients treated with diuretics raise many questions. *Cardiovascular News* Oct 1984. p-12.

[54]Grimm R. Effects of thiazide diuretics on plasma lipids and lipoproteins in mildly hypertensive patients. A double-blind controlled trial. *Ann Intern Med* 94:7, 1981.

[55]Ames. R. Serum cholesterol during treatment of hypertension with diuretic drugs. *Arch Intern Med* 144:710, 1984.

[56]Editorial: Diuretics, hyperuricaemia, and tienilic acid. *Lancet* 2:681, 1980.

[57]Murphy M. Glucose intolerance in hypertensive patients treated with diuretics; a fourteen-year-follow-up. *Lancet* 2:1293, 1982.

[58]Holland O. Diuretic-induced ventricular ectopic activity. *Am J Med* 70:762, 1981.

[59]Curb J. Long-term surveillence for adverse effects of antihypertensive drugs. *JAMA* 253:3263, 1985.

[60]Editorial: Intellectual performance in hypertensive patients. *Lancet* 1:87, 1984.

[61]Haynes R. Increased absenteeism from work after detection and labeling of hypertensive patients. *N Engl J Med* 299:741, 1978.

[62]Editorial: Possible dangers of the label hypertension. *Lancet* 1:547, 1982.

[63]Editorial: Mental health and hypertension. *Lancet* 2:80, 1984.

[64]Editorial: More on hypertensive labelling. *Lancet* 1:1138, 1985.

[65]MacGregor G. Dietary sodium and potassium intake and blood pressure. *Lancet* 1:750, 1983.

[66]Kannel W. Systolic versus diastolic blood pressure and risk of coronary heart disease. The Framingham Study. *Am J Cardiol* 27:335, 1971

[67]Cressman M. Controversies in hypertension: mild hypertension, isolated systolic hypertension, and the choice of a step one drug: Brief review. *Clin Cardiol* 6:1, 1983.

[68]Traub Y. Hazards in treatment of systolic hypertension. *Am Heart J* 97:174, 1979.

[69]Editorial: Hypertension in the over-60s. *Lancet* 1:1396, 1980.

[70]Finn R. Blood pressure and salt intake: an intra-population study. *Lancet* 1:1097, 1981.

[71]Sacks F. Effect of ingestion of meat on plasma cholesterol of vegetarians. *JAMA* 246:640, 1981.

[72]Burstyn P. Effect of meat on BP. *JAMA* 248:29, 1982.

[73]Curatolo P. The health consequences of caffeine: review. *Ann Intern Med* 98:641, 1983.

[74]Freestone S. Effect of coffee and cigarette smoking on the blood pressure of untreated and diuretic-treated hypertensive patients. *Am J Med* 73:348, 1982.

[75]Potter J. Pressor effect of alcohol in hypertension. *Lancet* 1:119, 1984

[76]Iacono J. Reduction of blood pressure associated with dietary polyunsaturated fat. *Hypertension 4* (supp III): III-34, 1982.

[77]Boyer J. Exercise therapy in hypertensive men. *JAMA* 211:1668, 1970.

[78]Sims E. Obesity and hypertension. Mechanisms and implications for management. Special communications. *JAMA* 247:49, 1982.

[79]Editorial: Weight reduction in hypertension. *Lancet* 1:1251, 1985.

[80]Kaplan N. Non-drug treatment of hypertension: Review. *Ann Intern Med* 102:359, 1985.

[81]McCarron D. Blood pressure and nutrient intake in the United States. *Science* 224:1392, 1984.

[82]Dahl L. Salt intake and salt need. *N Engl J Med* 258:1152, 1958.

[83]Finn R. Salt and hypertension. *Lancet* 2:632, 1981.

[84]McCarron D. Calcium, magnesium, and phosphorus balance in human and experimental hypertension. *Hypertension* 4 (supp III):III-27, 1982.

[85]Henry H. Increasing calcium intake lowers blood pressure: the literature reviewed. *JADA* 85:182, 1985.

[86]Belizan J. Reduction of blood pressure with calcium supplementation in young adults. *JAMA* 249:1161, 1983.

[87]Johnson N. Effects on blood pressure of calcium supplementation of women. *Am J Clin Nutr* 42:12, 1985.

[88]Sowers M. The association of intakes of vitamin D and calcium with blood pressure among women. *Am J Clin Nutr* 42:135, 1985.

[89]Viikari J. Multicenter study of atherosclerosis precursors in Finnish children-pilot study of 8 year-old boys. *Ann Clin Res* 14:103, 1982.

[90]Hartroft W. The incidence of coronary artery disease in patients treated with the Sippy diet. *Am J Clin Nutr* 15:205, 1964.

[91]Oski F. Is bovine milk a health hazard? *Pediatrics 75* (suppl): 182, 1985.

[92]Truswell A. ABC of Nutrition. Reducing the risk of coronary heart disease. *Br Med J* 291:34, 1985.

[93]*Food Balance Sheets. 1979-81 Average.* Rome: FAO, 1984.

[94]Burr M. Plasma cholesterol and blood pressure in vegetarians. *J Hum Nutr* 35:437, 1981.

[95]Sacks F. Blood pressure in vegetarians. *Am J Epidemiol* 100:390, 1974.

[96]Armstrong B. Urinary sodium and blood pressure in vegetarians. *Am J Clin Nutr* 32:2472, 1979.

[97]Ophir O. Low blood pressure in vegetarians: the possible role of potassium. *Am J Clin Nutr* 37: 755, 1983.

[98]MacGregor G. Moderate potassium supplementation in essential hypertension. *Lancet* 2:567, 1982.

[99]Khaw K. Randomised double-blind cross-over trial of potassium on blood-pressure in normal subjects. *Lancet* 2:1127, 1982.

[100]Kempner W. Treatment of hypertensive vascular disease with rice diet. *Am J Med* 4:545, 1948.

[101]Parijs J. Moderate sodium restriction and diuretics in the treatment of hypertension. *Am Heart J* 85:22, 1973.

[102]Morgan T. Hypertension treated by salt restriction. *Lancet* 1:227, 1978.

[103]Stamler J. Prevention and control of hypertension by nutritional-hygienic means: long-term experience of the Chicago Coronary Prevention Evaluation Program. *JAMA* 243:1819, 1980

[104]Beard T. Randomised controlled trial of a no-added-sodium diet for mild hypertension. *Lancet* 2:455, 1982.

[105]MacGregor G. Double-blind randomised crossover trial of moderate sodium restriction in essential hypertension. *Lancet* 1:351, 1982.

[106]Editorial: Lowering blood pressure without drugs. *Lancet* 2:459, 1980.

[107]Rouse I. Blood-pressure-lowering effect of a vegetarian diet: controlled trial in normotensive subjects. *Lancet* 1:5, 1983.

[108]Gillum R. Nonpharmacologic therapy of hypertension: the independent effects of weight reduction and sodium restriction in overweight boderline hypertensive patients. *Am Heart J* 105:128, 1983.

[109]Iacono J. Effect of dietary fat on blood pressure in a rural Finnish population. *Am J Clin Nutr* 38:860, 1983.

[110]Stewart I. Relation of reduction in pressure to first myocardial infarction in patients receiving treatment for severe hypertension. *Lancet* 1:861, 1979.

[111]Sackett D. Randomised clinical trial of strategies for improving medication compliance in primary hypertension. *Lancet* 1:1205, 1975.

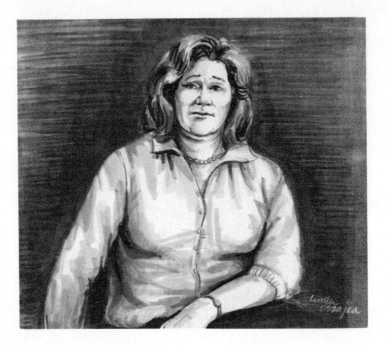

Kim

I remember how, as a little girl, I dreaded getting shots. Now I have to poke myself every morning, just to stay alive. When I was only taking pills for my diabetes I didn't really feel like I was very sick. But this year, since I was changed to insulin, I do realize that I have a serious disease. I feel pretty good except for those low blood sugar reactions I get when I don't eat on time. Then I get weak and dizzy, and one time I was so confused that I couldn't find my way home. I don't notice much difference when my sugar is too high, except that I drink a lot more water and I'm almost constantly in the bathroom passing urine.

The exchange diet leaves me cold. How can dietitians honestly believe that anyone can follow their complicated rules? Even when I tried to follow them, my blood sugar levels weren't any better. What a waste of time. And now, of all things, I've just read how eating starches can help someone with my disease.

Sometimes I do get depressed about this illness, especially when I see other people with diabetes. They don't look well. I've met some people who are blind and others who have lost their toes or their feet from complications of this disease. I really need help soon.

7

DIABETES

I'm not overreacting, am I? This is a very serious disease, isn't it?

Having to take your medications must remind you daily that you are incurably ill and that life-threatening complications from your diabetes can be expected to show up at any time. Before 1921, when insulin was first used in treatment, the lives of people with diabetes were menaced by uncontrollable levels of blood sugar, accompanied by a buildup of metabolic wastes, called *ketoacidosis,* leading to eventual coma and early death.[1] These threats to a long and active life were changed by the miracle of insulin, only to be replaced by problems of accelerated degeneration of the body caused by many years of living with diabetes. As a victim of this common illness, you face an 80 percent possibility of suffering from damage to the eyes which all too often progresses to blindness.[2] You run, at the least, twice the risk of dying prematurely from a heart attack and a chance eighteen times greater than usual of developing serious kidney damage, which probably would tie you to a kidney machine for the last few years of your life.[2-4] Statistics show that *diabetes mellitus,* to give its medical name, is the seventh leading cause of death in the United States. You're not alone: 1 in 20 people has diabetes in this country.[5]

I wouldn't unload all this pessimism on you if I didn't know about ways that could make life much better for you. An easy and effective alternative to drug therapy and complications is possible, which not only can dramatically change a diabetic patient's future, but also can decrease the number of people who will develop diabetes.

Taking pills wasn't so bad. I was told once that I had the type of diabetes that could be treated with pills. Why do I have to take insulin now? Did I develop another kind of diabetes?

That is unlikely. There are two general kinds of diabetes mellitus, but one kind rarely, if ever, turns into the other. Your doctor probably changed you to insulin simply because your disease has advanced to the point where it has become too difficult to control with the pills.

One form is called *childhood-onset* diabetes. This disease usually, but not always, starts in children or young adults. This type is also referred to as *insulin-dependent* diabetes mellitus, because it is caused by actual lack of insulin in the body and therefore requires injections of insulin for treatment.[6] Childhood-onset diabetes represents less than 5 percent of the cases of diabetes, but I consider it the more tragic kind because its victims are usually so young.[5]

The more common form of diabetes is called *maturity-onset* or *adult-onset* diabetes because usually it develops as people get older, and usually fatter. This form is also referred to as *noninsulin-dependent* diabetes mellitus, because in most cases insulin therapy is not required to maintain life or health.[6] This is the kind of diabetes you have.

What actually happens in the body to cause these two forms of diabetes and make the blood sugar level so uncontrollably high?

The fact that the blood sugar levels are elevated in both forms of the disease is a characteristic they share and the reason why both are called diabetes. However, they represent two different problems with insulin. Childhood-onset diabetes is caused by the fact that the body can produce only an insufficient amount of insulin. Adult-onset diabetes is caused by a lowered effectiveness of the insulin that the body does produce.

Insulin is a hormone made in the pancreas that regulates the amount of sugar present in the circulating blood. Insulin performs this job by helping the sugar to pass through the cell membranes, to get inside to the cell's "machinery."[5,6] Once inside a cell, the sugar is converted into compounds that eventually yield energy. If too little insulin is produced, as in the childhood-onset diabetic, or if the insulin fails to function properly, as in the adult-onset diabetic, then the cells will be starved for energy. This happens because the cells' usual food source, which is sugar, is blocked out. Since the sugar cannot enter the cells, the sugar level in the blood rises. Insulin also serves many other functions in the body, and when those are not performed normally, the failures will cause serious metabolic changes in a diabetic.

How do the cells survive if they can't get any sugar for energy?

Because the sugar cannot get into the cells to provide energy, the body switches to fats as alternative fuel sources. Body fats are broken down into fatty acids. These can pass into the cell without the aid of insulin and can provide life-sustaining energy. However, the use of this alternative metabolic pathway for yielding energy creates other problems. When a fat is "burned" for energy, it produces ketones and acids; these by-products of fat metabolism cause an acidic system, losses of cell fluids, and mineral imbalances. The fruity aroma of the ketones can be detected on a diabetic's breath. This characteristic odor is often an important clue in the diagnosis of diabetes that is out of control.

I never get that kind of odor on my breath, but I do get very thirsty. Why?

High levels of sugar in the blood spill out of the body through the kidneys into the urine. The sugar draws water out of the body, and dehydration can develop even to the point where it is life-threatening. Among the earliest signs of severe diabetes are frequency of urination and increased thirst in an attempt to replace the lost water.

The sugar lost in the urine also represents calories lost from the body. Before insulin therapy was available, most people with diabetes wasted away to bare bones skeletons. These days, many diabetics are too fat and could afford to lose a few more calories through their urine, or, better yet, to take in a few less calories.

Why do diabetics develop so many health problems? The insulin is being replaced with shots, and it seems to me that ought to take care of everything.

When insulin became available, the insulin-dependent childhood-onset diabetic was given a chance to live and does live long enough to develop other problems. But insulin seems to have done little to improve the life span and possibly the quality of life for most adult-onset diabetics, such as yourself.[6,7]

Diabetes is a disease that affects the entire body and alters the metabolism that regulates many different functions. Bodies burdened with the metabolic problems of diabetes are unable to defend themselves normally from environmental threats. When exposed to a variety of physical stresses, the diabetic individual suffers injury more easily and more severely than a healthy person. Minor bacterial infections in the toes can lead to gangrene, which means the loss of a foot or a leg and, occasionally, ends in death. The usual American diet, rich in proteins, salt, fats, and cholesterol, is much more dangerous for the weakened diabetic body. Many diseases that healthy people can avoid for longer periods are more likely to torment a person with diabetes. Among these are osteoporosis, different kinds of cancer, gout, high blood pressure, heart attacks, strokes, kidney failure, gangrene of the feet and legs, and blindness, to name just a few.[9,10] The future can be grim indeed for a diabetic. Serious complications can begin soon after the diagnosis of diabetes is established, and most people, within seventeen years of the onset of either form of this disease, have been struck by a major health catastrophe.[11]

One serious problem for the diabetic is the extra molecules of sugar that are floating around in the blood. They will attach themselves to molecules of different proteins in the body and in doing so change the shapes and surfaces of those protein molecules.[12] For those proteins to function normally,

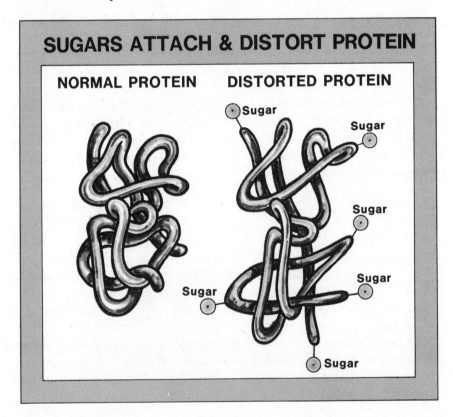

SUGARS ATTACH & DISTORT PROTEIN

NORMAL PROTEIN   **DISTORTED PROTEIN**

Sugar
Sugar
Sugar
Sugar
Sugar
Sugar

they must maintain their specified natural shapes and surfaces. The more important proteins act as hormones, as oxygen-carrying hemoglobin, as components of the immune system, and as parts in the body's structural architecture. Their functions are adversely affected by high levels of blood sugar. Some of the damage to the body that happens because of this attachment of sugar to proteins are suspected to be: alteration of the hemoglobin, causing decreased delivery of oxygen to all tissues; distortion of nerve and kidney proteins, causing the failures that are so commonly seen in diabetes; making the lens of the eye opaque, thus causing cataracts; and alteration of the cholesterol-triglyceride-protein packets called *lipoproteins,* thereby speeding up atherosclerosis.[13-17] Notoriously, diabetics have earlier and more severe complications from atherosclerosis, which lead to kidney failure, heart attacks, and strokes.[2-4,18]

I'm scared! There must be something reasonable I can do to prevent or slow down some of these complications.

Some clues about preventing these complications can be found by observing how diabetes affects people who follow different diets and lifestyles. For instance, Asians who have diabetes and who live in their native countries and follow a rice-centered diet with foods low in fats and cholesterol have few complications.[19,20] In contrast, diabetics from these same Asian ethnic groups who live in Hawaii and eat the typical high-fat American foods have marked increases in blood levels of cholesterol and triglycerides and severe complications of atherosclerosis.[20]

In all diabetics the physical stresses that cause damage must be avoided as much as possible. Cholesterol, salt, fats, and refined foods are the culprits that cause degenerative diseases even in people who do not have diabetes. These harmful foods are considerably more damaging for diabetics. A diet that supports health—one that is low in fats and salt, reasonable in content of proteins, high in fiber and complex carbohydrates, and with no cholesterol at all—is easy to plan around starches, vegetables, and fruits. Furthermore, it is enjoyable.

This kind of health-supporting diet, when it is eaten by diabetics, has been shown to decrease the risk factors that are associated with atherosclerosis and the complications of this disease, including heart attacks, strokes, interference with circulation to the feet and legs, and kidney failure.[21-23] The level of cholesterol in the blood is the most reliable predictor of future complications from atherosclerosis. This level can be lowered substantially, by as much as 32 percent in diabetics who adopt the recommended diet.[21] Contrary to the belief of many health professionals, the triglyceride levels are also lowered by a diet high in complex carbohydrates that is also high in natural plant fiber.[21] Without the fiber however, the triglycerides tend to rise with higher carbohydrate diets.[21] Fruits, with their high contents of simple sugars, must be restricted also when triglyceride levels need to be lowered.

A diet that is higher in complex carbohydrates and lower in fats, along with better control of the blood sugar levels with frequent insulin injections, has been found to slow the development of two common diabetic problems.[24] Both nerve and kidney function have been better preserved in patients maintained on this combined diet and insulin program, as compared with patients who are less carefully controlled.[24]

Damage to the eyes is one of the most common disabling complications for a diabetic who is dependent on insulin. An estimated 15 to 30 percent of childhood-onset diabetics lose vision later in life.[25] More than twenty-five years ago two independent groups of researchers showed that a low-fat diet would dramatically improve the poor condition of the retina, the light-sensitive part of the eye.[26,27] Disease of the retina, called *retinopathy*, cleared substantially in a matter of months, as the cholesterol and triglyceride levels fell after the change to the low-fat, low-cholesterol diet. Benefits for the eyes were seen in most patients. From these observations you can draw more than just a bit of hope for prevention of complications from diabetes, and even for the improvement of some existing conditions.

You mentioned that drugs to keep the blood sugar under better control may reduce my risk of having those complications. Can you tell me a little more about the reasons for making a choice between insulin and pills?

Long-term therapy for almost all childhood-onset diabetics requires daily injections of insulin because their bodies fail to produce enough of it. Failure to take a sufficient amount of insulin each day can lead to coma, ketoacidosis, and death. Both insulin injections and pills are prescribed by doctors for people with adult-onset diabetes in an attempt to normalize their blood sugar levels. Many people with adult-onset diabetes are treated with a class of pills called *sulfonylureas;* these stimulate the pancreas to release more insulin than usual and seem to cause other changes in the body that lower the blood sugar level.[28] Although the exact mechanism of action is poorly understood, the changes in the body caused by these pills are supposed to compensate for the diminished activity of the insulin the pancreas is secreting.[28]

In some cases the blood sugar levels are reduced toward normal with diabetic pills alone. On the other hand, many people receive little or no improvement in blood sugar control from pills only.[28] Since you were recently changed from pills to insulin, I suspect you are one of those people.

Keeping blood sugar levels as close to normal as possible has been considered important for preventing complications. Most investigators are encouraged by their efforts toward this end.[29-32] Others are not convinced, however, and feel that the control of blood sugar has little, if any, benefit in reducing complications.[7,8] Regardless of the debate, all agree that diabetic pills and daily injections of insulin cannot control blood sugar levels as well as a normal pancreas can. As a result, medical science strives toward improving control over blood sugar levels with the means that are available while trying to discover new and better methods.

Better control can be attained by using shorter-acting insulin which is given more frequently, often four times a day at regular intervals. Of course, for most people the frequent injections are uncomfortable and bothersome.

A new insulin delivery system, called an insulin pump, is worn all the time. A pump is expensive, costing between $1000 and $2500.[33] This system introduces short-acting insulin continuously into the body, and frequent adjustments in the amount of insulin delivered to the body can be made to keep the blood sugar level as close to normal as possible. With this device the control of sugar levels is much improved, and many of the metabolic defects that are common in diabetics can be corrected.

The insulin pump sounds great. Are there any hazards from this treatment that I should know about?

Helpful as this pump is, it is still not even close to being as good as a healthy pancreas. The pump can fail to inject insulin, and when it does so, the blood sugar can rise quickly to a very high level, causing ketoacidosis and coma in a person with childhood-onset diabetes.[34] Also an opposite kind of failure of the pump could inject too much insulin into the body and cause a life-threatening reduction in blood sugar.[34] Furthermore, infections are common at the needle site, occurring in almost 30 percent of patients.[34]

Many physicians consider the insulin pump to be a breakthrough in therapy because they hope that better control of blood sugar levels will decrease the complications from diabetes. Unfortunately, in some ways this stricter form of insulin therapy has been disappointing. Even though a slowing of deterioration in body functions is likely to happen in most patients who are equipped with a pump, no reversal of complications has been gained.[33] In fact, too rigid control of blood sugar with the insulin pump has resulted in worsening of eye disease after the pump has been in use for only three to six months.[35] This deterioration is believed to be caused by frequent episodes of hypoglycemia which injure the sensitive nerve cells in the retina at the back of the eye.[35] Tight control of blood sugar level with multiple daily injections results in a similar deterioration of the retinas. Return to less rigid control improves the retinopathy caused by stricter control for many, but not for all, patients in about a year.[35]

You said I was an adult-onset, noninsulin-dependent diabetic. That means I don't have to take insulin, right? Does the one shot of insulin each morning do me any good?

Insulin injections will lower the blood sugar level during part of the day, when the hormone has maximum activity. However, at other times of the day sugar levels are usually quite high. The primary role of insulin therapy for an adult-onset diabetic is to control symptoms caused by the disease. Insulin can help to correct problems of excessive weight loss, frequent urination, and thirst. Although as yet the evidence is far from convincing, insulin is also supposed to decrease the probability of complications later in life.[7,8]

I had some side effects when I was taking the diabetes pills. How safe are they?

Sulphonylureas, as they are called, have been used since 1956 to treat adult-onset diabetes.[28] The most frequent complication is an overdose of medication or insufficient food intake, either of which results in serious low blood sugar reactions, called *hypoglycemia*. A partial list of other serious reactions to diabetic pills includes jaundice, skin rashes, anemia, and, rarely, death.

One important finding is that adult-onset diabetics who take these pills more than double their risk of death from heart attacks, as compared with diabetics who receive no medicine at all or those who take injected insulin. This disturbing conclusion was reported in 1970 by investigators in a large study involving several medical centers at major universities.[36-38] Release of this information to the medical profession resulted in a sharp drop in sales of the sulfonylureas. The reaction to this study stimulated a great debate during the next decade, and there was criticism of the report by some medical investigators.[39] Many practicing physicians now believe that the university study has been discredited, and they have started again to prescribe diabetic pills, feeling confident that they are safe. To the delight of the pharmaceutical companies, the sales of these highly profitable medications are much better these days. However, the increased risk from complications of atherosclerosis are known to the drug manufacturer. The fact that the product information that accompanies their medical journal advertisements states, in very small print, a "special warning on increased risk of cardiovascular mortality," is evidence enough that the pharmaceutical companies are aware of the potential health hazards from their little pills.

SPECIAL WARNING ON INCREASED RISK OF CARDIOVASCULAR MORTALITY

The administration of oral hypoglycemic drugs has been reported to be associated with increased cardiovascular mortality as compared to treatment with diet alone or diet plus insulin. This warning is based on the study conducted by the University Group Diabetes Program (UGDP), a long-term prospective clinical trial designed to evaluate the effectiveness of glucose-lowering drugs in preventing or delaying vascular complications in patients with non-insulin-dependent diabetes. The study involved 823 patients who were randomly assigned to one of four treatment groups (Diabetes, 19 [Suppl 2]: 747-830, 1970).

UGDP reported that patients treated for 5 to 8 years with diet plus a fixed dose of tolbutamide (1.5 grams per day) had a rate of cardiovascular mortality approximately 2-1/2 times that of patients treated with diet alone. A significant increase in total mortality was not observed, but the use of tolbutamide was discontinued based on the increased in cardiovascular mortality, thus limiting the opportunity for the study to show an increase in overall mortality. Despite controversy regarding the interpretation of these results, the findings of the UGDP study provide an adequate basis for this warning. The patient should be informed of the potential risks and advantages of TOLINASE and of alternative modes of therapy.

Although only one drug in the sulfonylurea class (tolbutamide) was included in this study, it is prudent from a safety standpoint to consider that this warning may apply to other oral hypoglycemic drugs in this class, in view of their close similarities in mode of action and chemical structure.

Because nowadays the primary purpose in care of diabetics is to reduce the complications from the disease, prescribing a medication that may more than double the risk of death from heart disease makes no sense. Therefore, if an adult-onset diabetic needs therapy in order to lower blood sugar, and few people actually do need it, then insulin is the only defensible choice.

I hear some people get used to their daily injections after awhile. That hasn't happened for me. I wish my body made enough insulin so I didn't have to take any drugs at all.

Your body makes all the insulin you'll ever need. An important and surprising discovery about people with adult-onset diabetes is that their pancreases produce as much natural insulin as, and frequently more than, people who don't have diabetes.[40] The difference between the two groups is that the insulin from adult-onset diabetics fails to function as efficiently as it should. Therapy with pills and insulin shots is directed at increasing the quantity of functioning insulin in the blood in an attempt to overcome the inefficiency of the insulin. Diabetic pills also change the way the body's cells respond to insulin.

I don't understand how I might help my body's insulin work better. I was told I was incurable and that diabetes is inherited.

You think you are incurable only because of what you don't know about diabetes. Even though in some families the tendency is passed on genetically, making some people more susceptible than others to adult-onset diabetes, heredity isn't the primary cause. The kind of diabetes you have is really caused by the foods your parents taught you to eat. If you had been raised on a healthier diet, it is highly likely that you would not have become a diabetic.

Diabetes is rare among Africans, Asians, and Polynesians who eat foods that are primarily starches, vegetables, and fruits.[19,20,41,42] However, when these people learn to eat the things offered by the rich Western diet, diabetes and complications of atherosclerosis flourish in all of them.[19,20,41,42]

Recently, a tragic effect upon general health caused by foolish eating habits has evolved on the small island of Nauru in Micronesia.[42] Before World War II, Nauruans lived in isolation, eating the traditional Polynesian foods of taro, breadfruit, coconuts, some vegetables, and fresh fish. They enjoyed excellent health and a very low incidence of diabetes. After the war their only natural resource, phosphates, from bird dung deposited on the island during many centuries, proved to be a valuable commodity in the modern world. As a result of this demand, Nauruans became the richest people in the world. Their diet changed with mounting wealth, and they began importing new and rich foods from the Western world. Their fat intake increased and fiber consumption decreased with the introduction of canned and frozen meats, fish, oils, white rice, and soft drinks. It is not unusual for Nauruans to have two or three different meats and fish at the same meal. During the last decade, diabetes has appeared in 34.4 percent of the population over the age of fifteen. Not only does one-third of the population have diabetes, but obesity and the complications of atherosclerosis are also common now among these modern-day Polynesians.

What in their diet can cause healthy individuals to get diabetes so easily?

Three harmful components in the rich American diet cause adult-onset diabetes. First, the fats and the oils, which account for 40 to 50 percent of the calorie content of our diet, act by interfering with insulin activity.[43-47] The cells of the body become unable to respond to the natural insulin produced by the pancreas and also to insulin injected by means of a syringe. This effect of fats and oils has been known for more than fifty years.[43]

In 1927, Dr. S. Sweeney fed young, healthy, medical students for two days on a diet very high in fats, consisting of olive oil, butter, mayonnaise made with egg yolks, and 20 percent cream.[44] Then he gave them a glucose tolerance test. All of his students showed blood sugar levels high enough to classify them as diabetic. Some were severely diabetic.[44]

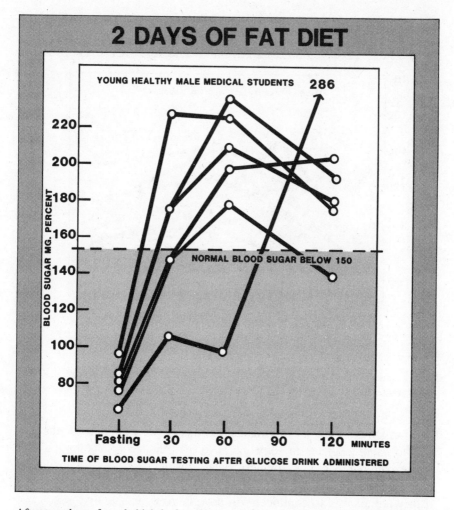

After two days of meals high in fat, glucose tolerance tests in otherwise healthy people become markedly abnormal.[44] These test results would be interpreted as pre-diabetic and as clearly diabetic responses.

In another experiment employing the same students, before running glucose tolerance tests, Dr. Sweeney fed them simple and complex carbohydrates consisting of sugar, candy, pastry, white bread, baked potatoes, syrup, bananas, rice, and oatmeal.[44] After this high-starch and high-sugar diet, maintained for two days, glucose tolerance tests showed that all of them were normal, without evidence of diabetes.

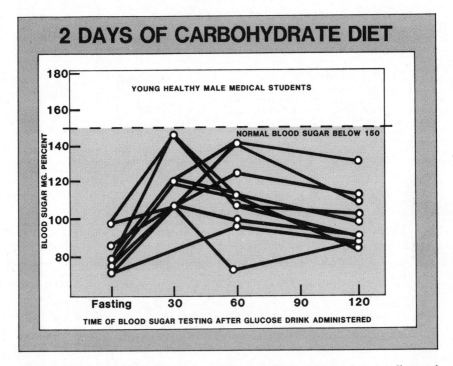

2 DAYS OF CARBOHYDRATE DIET

YOUNG HEALTHY MALE MEDICAL STUDENTS

NORMAL BLOOD SUGAR BELOW 150

BLOOD SUGAR MG. PERCENT

Fasting   30   60   90   120

TIME OF BLOOD SUGAR TESTING AFTER GLUCOSE DRINK ADMINISTERED

After two days of meals high in sugar and starch the glucose tolerance tests are all normal in otherwise healthy people.[44]

From Dr. Sweeney's experiments and others, we can conclude that one way to cause diabetes in someone is to feed them lots of fats and oils. These ingredients are the greatest dietary insults to the body, causing not only diabetes but all sorts of other interferences with normal functions that, if they are allowed to continue, will provoke recognizable diseases.

As surprising as this may sound, carbohydrates, both simple and complex, have effects opposite to those of fats. Carbohydrates can actually increase the power of insulin. Even sugar fed to a diabetic does not make control of the blood sugar more difficult but actually makes it a little easier. When subjects with mild diabetes were changed from a diet containing 45 percent simple sugar to one providing 85 percent sugar, fasting blood sugar levels fell and results of the glucose tolerance test improved.[48] The conclusion is clear: a high-carbohydrate diet, even one loaded with simple sugars, will increase the sensitivity of body tissues to the action of the insulin it is producing.

These experiments, and others, show that diabetics and non-diabetics can safely eat both simple and complex carbohydrates.[49] However, we must not overlook the fact that foods high in simple carbohydrates, with the exception of fruits, can be unhealthy when used in excess because they are mostly "empty calories," providing little real sustenance for the body's needs.

From these studies we can also conclude that the lack of adequate amounts and kinds of carbohydrates contributes to the development of diabetes. Foods containing these carbohydrates make up too small a portion of the American diet. Red meat, poultry, fish, milk, and cheese are practically devoid of these essential nutrients. What little carbohydrates may be present in cow's milk are poorly digested by most adults. On the other hand, the carbohydrate content of most starches, vegetables, and fruits ranges from 60 to 90 percent of the calories contained.

The third characteristic of the American diet that encourages the diabetic condition is the lack of fiber. All animal products lack fiber entirely. Most processed foods, such as white rice and white bread, have had much of their fiber removed. Fiber is made up of long chains of sugar molecules that are connected by linkages that are relatively resistant to the digestive processes. In nature, fiber is mixed with the digestible complex and simple carbohydrates that are present in starchy foods, fruits, and vegetables. Fiber, by several mechanisms, slows the absorption into the bloodstream of the products of digestion of simple and complex carbohydrates found in the foods.[50-54] This gradual release of sugars into the bloodstream is believed to be better synchronized with the action of the body's insulin-secreting cells.[50-54] Simply adding more fiber to a diet without changing its content of fats and carbohydrates improves the blood sugar levels in diabetics.[51]

Indirectly, the obesity that is so prevalent in people who eat high-fat, low-carbohydrate, low-fiber foods also contributes to development of diabetes.[55] In an obese person, the tissue cells are less sensitive to the varied actions of insulin, and the blood sugar can rise to abnormally high levels.

Another complementary quality of a starch-centered diet is that it aids, almost effortlessly, weight reduction in obese persons until they reach a healthy, trim body weight. Thus, the obese diabetic will gain one additional advantage when he or she chooses the right foods. Trim diabetics may actually gain a little weight as their health improves, but rarely do they lose weight to a harmful extent when they start eating these high-carbohydrate foods.

You shouldn't think that all the beneficial characteristics of a good diet are found in starches, vegetables, and fruits simply by coincidence, or the opposite, that harmful characteristics of an unhealthy diet are characteristics of dairy products, red meats, poultry, and fish only by chance. There are foods intended for human nutrition that support health and there are delicacies that are consumed for other reasons than improved health. The important thing is that you know the difference. By nature's plan the human body—with or without diabetes—was designed to live on a starch-based diet supplemented by a plentiful variety of fruits and vegetables.

Should I add extra fiber—maybe some miller's bran—to my diet? Or are there any vitamins and minerals I should take, like chromium? I've heard that was good for diabetes.

The fibers that are most helpful for someone with diabetes are the ones that are naturally present in foods.[50,52-54] Adding extra wheat fiber from miller's bran will do little more than generate extra bowel gas and possibly some painful bowel cramps. There are two large general classes of fibers, and they affect the blood sugar and also the cholesterol levels differently. Fibers that are poorly soluble in water act as roughage and are found in high concentrations in wheat, certain other grains, and most vegetables. Fibers readily soluble in water are plentiful in oats, beans, and some fruits. These soluble fibers have a greater effect on lowering blood sugar levels and cholesterol than do the insoluble ones.[53] Do not become overly concerned with the types of fibers in your diet. Fortunately, both kinds are present in all plant foods and will lead to the improvement in diabetes that you want.[53]

Edible plants provide enough vitamins and minerals, and adding more of these in the form of supplements is not likely to improve your health.[56] However, much attention has been given lately to the mineral chromium as a supplement to treat diabetes and possibly to retard atherosclerosis. Some experiments on animals and humans support evidence for this benefit. Yet a recent well-designed study failed to demonstrate any improvement in blood sugar or cholesterol levels in adult-onset diabetics receiving 200 milligrams of chromium daily.[57] Even though further studies may be necessary to resolve the question of chromium supplements, diabetics who eat a starch-based diet will be receiving plenty of this mineral and should not look to mineral tablets for further improvement in their condition.

I've read someplace that diabetics should avoid carrots and potatoes because they make blood sugar levels rise fast. Is that true?

Researchers have recently measured the absorption rates of different carbohydrates into the body. The results have been surprising and confusing for many people.[58,59] For example, table sugar is actually more slowly and less completely absorbed than carrots and potatoes.[59] The kinds of carbohydrates, as well as other properties of vegetable foods, seem to override the influence of the fibers to slow absorption through the intestinal wall. The importance of this response of blood sugar to various foods is unknown at the present.[60,61] However, the rate and the completeness of absorption of a specific carbohydrate appear to be minor factors in the development and treatment of diabetes. Besides, the purpose of the sugar in foods is to enter the body as rapidly, completely, and as safely as possible to be used for life-sustaining energy. Rest assured, nature made no mistakes with the design of the foods or the human intestinal absorption mechanisms.

Possibly the best example of the confusion created by this new finding comes from a study of the effects of eating ice cream on childhood-onset diabetics. Because only a modest change in blood sugar levels occurred after eating this dessert, the authors of a recent study concluded that ice cream could be included in the diet of a diabetic.[62] Clearly, choice of foods should be based on their nutritive value, not on their appeal to the taste buds or to the eyes. We should not make the mistake of thinking that "empty calorie" foods such as sugar or high-fat foods like ice cream are healthy for our bodies. On the contrary, starches, vegetables, and fruits, regardless of their rates of absorption, are best, with their generous content of proteins, carbohydrates, fibers, vitamins, and minerals, and their lack of harmful ingredients.

Does the way I prepare my foods make any difference?

Cooking foods will increase the digestibility of the carbohydrates by breaking them down into the simpler sugars, and therefore the blood sugar will rise faster to a slightly higher level.[63,64] Also, simply grinding a food will change the blood sugar response, as when brown rice is ground into rice flour; an equal amount of flour will cause a greater increase in the blood sugar response than the whole rice kernel when eaten.[65] Even disrupting the fibers by using a kitchen blender will change the blood sugar and insulin response.[66] Therefore, to take fullest advantage of a food, it should be consumed raw in its natural state. However, the actual overall advantages to eating all foods in that way are small at most and inconvenient, to say the least. For almost every diabetic, simple cooking or grinding of the food, without removing the fiber has no serious nutritional consequence to their condition and makes the foods a lot more palatable.

Is the childhood-onset type of diabetes also caused by eating the wrong food?

The childhood-onset form is the result of serious injury to the pancreas, causing destruction of the insulin-producing cells. At present, viruses, particularly those of the Coxsackie B group, are thought to be the ones that damage the pancreas and cause diabetes.[67,68] However, children who are properly nourished and in good health would be more likely to resist viral infections and other injurious agents from their environment, thus decreasing the chances of suffering a serious loss of the pancreas' insulin production. In this sense, then, good and proper foods are better safeguards than junk foods or those provided in the rich American diet.

I've heard there are diabetics who are resistant to insulin therapy. Is that also because of the wrong diet?

Many diabetics of both types who take daily injections are considered to be *insulin resistant*. They may have to take three or four or more times the usual dose of insulin. Sometimes this is necessary because of their high-fat, low-carbohydrate, low-fiber diet. Fats and their derivatives circulate in the bloodstream in the form of triglycerides. High levels of triglycerides cause insulin to be less effective, and that is when insulin resistance develops.[43-47] A change to the more health-supporting diet can reduce insulin needs dramatically.

When I faithfully followed a diabetic exchange diet, it didn't seem to make me any better. Did I do something wrong?

The exchange diet is the official word preached by many health professionals. The exchange diet portions foods from the basic four foods groups, allowing the patient to plan a meal by exchanging foods of similar carbohydrate content. The aim of the diabetic exchange diets has been to restrict the carbohydrate intake while meeting requirements for protein and calories. However, this dietary plan offers a person with diabetes far less than an ideal chance of improving his or her health and little hope of stopping daily medications. The diabetic exchange diet is similar to the rich American diet that made you ill in the first place. Even worse, the various diets that have been recommended for diabetics during the past fifty-five years have actually favored the development of some dreaded complications. These diets have provided damaging concentrations of fats, cholesterol, and proteins and insufficient quantities of beneficial fibers and complex carbohydrates.

All those damaging ingredients are suspected of contributing to conditions that lead to blindness, heart attacks, kidney failure, and osteoporosis.

In recent years, some improvements have been made in the exchange diet recommended for diabetics.[69] However, even today the best official dietary advice is to take 50 to 60 percent of your calories as carbohydrates, 20 to 38 percent as fats, and 12 to 20 percent as proteins, with way too much cholesterol and far too little fiber.[70] Diabetics deserve a much better chance to regain their health. They should be taught the kind of diet that will best support their health and give them a better chance to stop taking daily medications. This weak compromise is not the answer to their needs.

Can the insulin needs of adult-onset and childhood-onset diabetics be reduced with such a diet change? Do you think I could ever be cured?

There is more hope for victims of diabetes than most people realize. Like you, many adult-onset diabetics are overweight. Losing weight makes the body's cells more responsive to the insulin that the pancreas is producing, and this change alone will "cure" many diabetics.[55] Regular exercise will promote weight loss, and has the further advantage of making the body's natural insulin more potent by increasing the sensitivity of the body cells.[71] However, the most effective approach to improving diabetes is a sensible change in the body's intake of its basic sources of energy.

Instead of the diet high in fats, proteins, and refined foods that is devoured by most Americans, you need to switch to a low-fat diet offering much more carbohydrates and fiber. The proportions for this ideal diet are 80 to 90 percent carbohydrates, 5 to 12 percent proteins, 5 to 10 percent fats, with no cholesterol at all, and a high content of fiber. This kind of diet will reduce the blood sugar levels of most diabetics, and thereby reduce or eliminate the need for insulin and diabetic pills for most adult-onset diabetics.[72-78] Foods that make up this kind of meal plan are starches, vegetables and fruits.

Please note that this is the same sensible diet that cuts down on the amounts of those harmful components that contribute to the development of complications in diabetes, such as atherosclerosis, heart attacks, kidney failure, and blindness.

Will I be able to stop taking my insulin if I eat this way?

Chances are good that you will. As many as 75 percent of adult-onset diabetics who take insulin can stop all medication soon after making this diet change.[76-78] Many people who have been taking insulin injections for years are cured of their disease with this simple change in diet. Unfortunately, this is not true for insulin-dependent childhood-onset diabetics.

Under your doctor's supervision, medications should be lowered quickly after you make the diet change; your need for insulin and diabetic pills can decrease in a matter of hours. The safest initial reduction in medication after changing your diet is to cut that day's insulin dose in half of the amount previously taken. The urine sugar levels should be tested four times a day, every day, before meals and at bedtime, and used as guides to changing future insulin dosages. If all urine sugar tests are negative for two days, then the next day's dose should be dropped by five to ten units. Similarly, for every two days that all urine tests are negative throughout both days, the dosage is dropped by five to ten more units. If the urine tests are strongly positive for two days, then an upward adjustment of five to ten units every two days may be necessary. If hypoglycemic reactions occur, treat them as usual with simple sugars in fruit juice, white sugar, or hard candy; then reduce the next day's insulin dose by 50 percent or more. Your goal is to have most of the urine tests weakly positive after taking any particular dosage. When urine sugar tests are weakly positive, you may have to wait for a few days before they become negative and you make further adjustments. As the body's condition improves, you will find the urine clearing of sugar and your insulin needs decreasing. Most people are off all insulin within one to six weeks after the diet change. The danger of overtreating with too much insulin is far greater than that of underdosing.

While you are taking insulin, you should eat your meals so that food will be in the intestinal tract at the time the insulin is having its greatest effects. For the intermediate-acting insulins, this is usually about four to six hours after injection; for short-acting insulin, the time is one to four hours. During the time when you are adjusting insulin dosages, often the easiest way to eat is three to four meals a day at regular intervals. You should eat as much as you want of the starchy foods and the vegetables. Fruits should be limited to two or three a day in order to keep the triglycerides under control. Only rarely will someone have to pay attention to their total calorie intake while trying to lose weight. The switch in food is usually enough to ensure a two- to three-pound weight loss each week in obese persons.

Will this diet work as well for people on diabetes pills?

On this diet almost all diabetics taking pills can be freed of that daily medication.[72,77,78] The safest way to make the change is to stop taking the pills as soon as the diet is started. After all, by definition, patients on pills are not dependent on insulin and have plenty of their own insulin. For this reason, there is little chance that they will go into a diabetic coma, even if they stayed on a high-fat diet. Fortunately, with the diet change their health will improve rapidly. The blood sugar level should come down close to normal, if not in a few days, then in just a few weeks.

Adjusting medication dosages may seem simple to experienced diabetics. However, if you plan to change your diet and lifestyle and you are on medication, then you should do so *only under the supervision of your physician.* As an extra check on progress, fasting blood sugar levels in the morning should be checked by the doctor once or twice a week while the insulin dosage is being decreased or after the pills are stopped. A normal blood sugar level ranges from 60 to 115 milligram percent. While you are still taking insulin and changing your diet, the fasting blood sugar levels should be kept over 150 milligram percent to avoid hypoglycemic reactions. Low blood sugar reactions are much more harmful to you than high sugar levels. Levels below 350 milligram percent without medication are acceptable, but not ideal. If you show signs of excessive weight loss, urination or thirst, then a decision may be made to treat with insulin in order to relieve those symptoms. Levels of 150 to 300 milligram percent are often the best and safest that can be obtained, even with standard insulin treatment. If an adult-onset diabetic does require medication, insulin is preferred over pills because it introduces less risk for complications of atherosclerosis.

Can people with insulin-dependent childhood-onset diabetes also be cured if they change to this diet?

Childhood-onset diabetics can rarely eliminate their need for insulin, but frequently they can lower their daily dosage with this recommended diet and a little exercise. Furthermore, with a healthier diet, their wide and uncomfortable swings in blood sugar levels are calmed down; in medical terms, they are "less brittle." One consistent result I have seen is that people with diabetes feel better almost immediately after changing to the healthier diet. This is a most welcome relief for someone who feels poorly much of the time.

A safe first step for a person with childhood-onset diabetes is to lower the usual dosage for insulin by 30 percent on the day the new diet is started. This reduction will help to prevent hypoglycemia from too much insulin. Further adjustments in dosage are made, up or down, based on urine and blood tests.

This reduction in daily insulin dosage is only a minor benefit for a person with childhood-onset diabetes. The decreased risk from complications is the real gain. No one deserves the benefits of a low-fat, high-fiber, no-cholesterol diet more than a young victim of diabetes. This helpful diet will offer such a person, faced otherwise with a very bleak future, the best possibility for enjoying a long life with all of his or her body's parts functioning properly in later years. During World War II in occupied

European countries, the death rate from diabetes decreased dramatically when the consumption of rich foods high in fat and cholesterol were replaced by more whole grains and vegetables.[79]

Why aren't more victims of diabetes aware of the improvements in health that they can gain for themselves by changing their diet and getting a little exercise?

Research and education take money. Recommending simple foods and exercise is advice that makes profits for no one—not the drug companies, not even the doctor who gives it. The health care profession finds little incentive for spreading this information among the diabetic population or even among physicians who treat those unfortunate people.

Using a high-carbohydrate diet to treat diabetes is not a new idea. In 1930, long before diabetic pills were available, Dr. I. M. Rabinowitch reported that "a potential diabetic can be transformed into a completely diabetic individual by administration of the time-honored carbohydrate-free diet of meat and fat."[80] Fifty-five years ago, before most people who have diabetes today were even born, Dr. Rabinowitch successfully treated his diabetic patients with a high-carbohydrate, low-fat diet. For many of them the need for insulin was ended, and for others the dosage of insulin was reduced. Dr. Rabinowitch reported that his patients preferred the diet over taking daily insulin injections.

In 1928, Dr. E. P. Joslin, founder of the famous Joslin Diabetic Center in Boston, suspected that the high-fat, high-cholesterol diet might favor the acceleration of atherosclerosis in diabetics.[81] He wrote: "Can it be that the prevalence of arteriosclerosis in diabetes is to be attributed to the high-fat diets we have prescribed and more especially to these diets having been rich in cholesterol? I suspect this may be the case. At any rate it is reasonable to maintain the cholesterol in the blood of our patients at a normal level and that I shall strive to do. This may result in the limitation of eggs, each one of which is .38 gm. of cholesterol...This therapeutic procedure is adaptable for experimental investigation and should not require long for solution."

More than fifty-five years have passed since these two pioneers in the treatment of diabetes clearly identified effective approaches to the disease and the prevention of complications. How many diabetics have suffered needlessly because their physicians have failed to give them this information? How many physicians have stood by helplessly, watching their diabetic patients become blind and disabled, and finally die early because they knew of no effective treatments to prevent the course of those expected events? How needless the suffering, the waste, the despair. The time for better treatment is now.

Rx
- A high-complex-carbohydrate, high-fiber, low-fat, moderate-protein, no-cholesterol diet is the key to the prevention and treatment of adult-onset diabetes and of the complications seen with both forms of diabetes.
- All damaging factors in the environment will have greater impact on a victim of diabetes than on someone in good health. A health-supporting diet and lifestyle are especially important for reducing the injury those elements can cause. Avoid all cholesterol, excess salt, excess proteins, excess fats, and environmental contaminants. Also avoid alcohol, caffeine, and tobacco.
- Exercise daily, in moderation.
- Make adjustments in your diet and medications only under the supervision of a qualified physician.
- Reductions in medication after a change in diet depend upon the case:

  For adult-onset diabetics:
  Cut dose of insulin in half on day of dietary change; reduce by five to ten units every two days thereafter, based upon negative urine sugar tests or improved blood sugar readings.
  Stop taking diabetic pills on day of change, check response with urine sugar and blood sugar tests.
  Patients still requiring medication should be
  treated with insulin rather than pills.

  For childhood-onset diabetics:
  Reduce dose of insulin by 30 percent on day of dietary change.
  Adjust insulin needs according to tests for sugar in the urine and blood.

- Treat hypoglycemic reactions as usual with simple sugars.
- Check cholesterol and triglyceride levels initially and once a month while adjusting to the new diet and medication dosages.
- Your goals are:
  To live long and function fully by avoiding complications of diabetes
  To take little or no medication for adult-onset diabetics.
  To improve control over blood sugar levels
  To avoid hypoglycemia
    To lower levels of cholesterol and triglycerides
  To lose excess body weight
  To feel well every day

REFERENCES

[1]Allan F. Diabetes before and after insulin. *Med Hist* 16:266, 1973.

[2]Winegrad A. Editorial: The complications of diabetes mellitus. *N Engl J Med* 298:1250, 1978.

[3]Kannel W. Diabetes and cardiovascular risk factors: the Framingham study. *Circulation* 59:8, 1979.

[4]National Commission on Diabetes "The long-range plan to combat diabetes." Vol 1 DHEW Publication No (NIH) 76-1018, 1975.

[5]National Institutes of Health. "Diabetes Mellitus. Trans-NIH Research." NIH Pub No. 84-1982, May 1984.

[6]Kaplan S. Diabetes mellitus. *Ann Intern Med* 96:635, 1982.

[7]Ashikaga T. Multiple daily insulin injections in the treatment of diabetic retinopathy: the Job study revisited. *Diabetes* 27:592, 1978.

[8]The University Group Diabetes Program. Effects of hypoglycemic agents on vascular complications in patients with adult-onset diabetes. VIII. Evaluation of insulin therapy: Final report. *Diabetes* 31:(Suppl 5);1, 1982.

[9]Marble A. *Joslin's Diabetes Mellitus.* (11th ed) Philadelphia: Lea & Febiger, 1971.

[10]Weintroub S. Is diabetic osteoporosis due to microangiopathy? *Lancet* 2:983, 1980.

[11]Report of the National Commission on Diabetes to Congress of the United States. Vol III, part 2, DHEW pub. no. (NIH) 76-1022, 1975.

[12]Editorial: Glycosylation and disease. *Lancet* 2:19, 1984.

[13]McDonald M. Functional properties of the glycosylated minor components of human adult hemoglobin. *J Biol Chem* 254:702, 1979.

[14]Vlassara H. Excessive nonenzymatic glycosylation of peripheral and central nervous system myelin components in diabetic rats. *Diabetes* 32:670, 1983.

[15]Lubec G. Enzymatic reversibility of nonenzymatic glycosylation of the glomerular basement membrane. Is the diabetic glomerulopathy principally reversible? *Nephron* 33:26, 1983.

[16]Stevens V. Diabetic cataract formation: potential role of glycosylation of lens crystallins. *Proc Natl Acad Sci USA* 75:2918, 1978.

[17]Witzum J. Nonenzymatic glucosylation of low-density lipoprotein alters its biologic activity. *Diabetes* 31:283, 1982.

[18]Cohen A. Myocardial infarction and carbohydrate metabolism. *Geriatrics* 23:158, 1968.

[19]West K. *Epidemiology of diabetes and its vascular lesions.* New York: Elsevier, p. 353-402, 1978.

[20]Kawate R. Diabetes mellitus and its vascular complications in Japanese migrants on the island of Hawaii. *Diabetes Care* 2:161, 1979.

[21]Anderson J. Hypolipidemic effects of high-carbohydrate, high-fiber diets. *Metabolism* 29:551, 1980.

[22]Andersen E. Effects of a rice-rich versus a potato-rich diet on glucose, lipoprotein, and cholesterol metabolism in noninsulin-dependent diabetics. *Am J Clin Nutr* 39:598, 1984.

[23]Blanc M. Improvement of lipid status in diabetic boys: The 1971 and 1979 Joslin Camp lipid levels. *Diabetes Care* 6:64, 1983.

[24]Holman R. Prevention of deterioration of renal and sensory-nerve function by more intensive management of insulin-dependent diabetic patients. A two year randomised prospective study. *Lancet* 1:204, 1983.

[25]Deckert T. The prognosis of insulin dependent diabetes mellitus and the importance of supervision. *Acta Med Scand* Suppl 624:48, 1979.

[26]Kempner W. Effect of rice diet on diabetes mellitus associated with vascular disease. *Postgrad Med* 24:359, 1958.

[27]Van Eck W. The effect of a low fat diet on the serum lipids in diabetes and its significance in diabetic retinopathy. *Am J Med* 27:196, 1959.

[28]Asmal A. Oral hypoglycaemic agents: an update: review article. *Drugs* 28:62, 1984.

[29]Tchobroutsky G. Relation of diabetic control to development of microvascular complications. *Diabetologia* 15:143, 1978.

[30]Dornan T. Factors protective against retinopathy in insulin-dependent diabetics free of retinopathy for 30 years. *Br Med J* 285:1073, 1982.

[31]Steno Study Group. Effect of 6 months of strict metabolic control on eye and kidney function in insulin-dependent diabetics with background retinopathy. *Lancet* 1:121, 1982.

[32]Eschwege E. Delayed progression of diabetic retinopathy by divided insulin administration: a further follow up. *Diabetologia* 16:13, 1979.

[33]Rosenstock J. Insulin pump therapy: a realistic appraisal. *Clin Diabetes* 3:25, 1985.

[34]Editorial: Acute mishaps during insulin pump treatment. *Lancet* 1:911, 1985.

[35]Dahl-Jorgensen K. Rapid tightening of blood glucose control leads to transient deterioration of retinopathy in insulin dependent diabetes mellitus: the Oslo study. *Br Med J* 290:811, 1985.

[36]A study of the effects of hypoglycemic agents on vascular complications in patients with adult-onset diabetes: Design, methods, and baseline results. University Group Diabetes Program. *Diabetes* 19, (Suppl 2) :747, 1970.

[37]A study of the effects of hypoglycemic agents on vascular complications in patients with adult-onset diabetes: II Mortality results. University Group Diabetes Program. *Diabetes* 19 (Suppl 2):787, 1970.

[38]Knatterud G. Effects of hypoglycemic agents on vascular complications in patients with adult-onset diabetes: VII. Mortality and selected nonfatal events with insulin treatment. *JAMA* 240:37, 1978.

[39]Kilo C. The Achilles heel of the University Group Diabetes Program. Special communication. *JAMA* 243:450, 1980.

[40]Kipnis D. Insulin secretion in normal and diabetic individuals. *Adv Intern Med* 16:103, 1970.

[41]Trowell H. Dietary-fiber hypothesis of the etiology of diabetes mellitus. *Diabetes* 24:762, 1975.

[42]Ringrose H. Nutrient intakes in an urbanized Micronesian population with a high diabetes prevalence. *Am J Clin Nutr* 32:1334, 1979.

[43]Himsworth H. The physiological activation of insulin. *Clin Sci* 1:1, 1933.

[44]Sweeney J. Dietary factors that influence the dextrose tolerance test: a preliminary study. *Arch Intern Med* 40:818, 1927.

[45]Olefsky J. Reappraisal of the role of insulin in hypertriglyceridemia. *Am J Med* 57:551, 1974.

[46]Farquhar J. Glucose, insulin, and triglyceride responses to high and low carbohydrate diets in man. *J Clin Invest* 45:1648, 1966.

[47]Davidson P. Insulin resistance in hyperglyceridemia. *Metabolism* 14:1059, 1965.

[48]Brunzell J. Improved glucose tolerance with high carbohydrate feeding in mild diabetes. *N Engl J Med* 283:521, 1971

[49]Hollenbeck C. The effects of variations in percent of naturally occurring complex and simple carbohydrates on plasma glucose and insulin response in individuals with non-insulin-dependent diabetes mellitus. *Diabetes* 34:151, 1985

[50]Anderson J. Plant fiber. Carbohydrate and lipid metabolism. *Am J Clin Nutr* 32:346, 1979.

[51]Miranda P. High-fiber diets in the treatment of diabetes mellitus. *Ann Intern Med* 88:482, 1978.

[52]Rivellese A. Effect of dietary fibre on glucose control and serum lipoproteins in diabetic patients. *Lancet* 2:447, 1980.

[53]Anderson J. Health implications of wheat fiber. *Am J Clin Nutr* 41:1103, 1985.

[54]Jenkins D. Dietary fibres, fibre analogues, and glucose tolerance: importance of viscosity. *Br Med J* 1:1392, 1978.

[55]Bar R. Fluctuations in the affinity and concentration of insulin receptors on circulating monocytes of obese patients: effects of starvation, refeeding and dieting. *J Clin Invest* 58:1123, 1976.

[56]Ovesen L. Vitamin therapy in the absence of obvious deficiency. What is the evidence? *Drugs* 27:148, 1984.

[57]Uusitupa M. Effect of inorganic chromium supplementation on glucose tolerance, insulin response, and serum lipids in noninsulin-dependent diabetics. *Am J Clin Nutr* 38:404, 1983.

[58]Crapo P. Comparison of serum glucose, insulin and glucagon responses to different types of complex carbohydrate in noninsulin-dependent diabetic patients. *Am J Clin Nutr* 34:184, 1981.

[59]Jenkins D. The diabetic diet, dietary carbohydrate and differences in digestibility. *Diabetologia* 23:477, 1982.

[60]Coulston A. Utility of studies measuring glucose and insulin responses to various carbohydrate-containing foods. *Am J Clin Nutr* 39:163, 1984.

[61]Jenkins D. Dietary carbohydrates and their glycemic responses. *JAMA* 251:2829, 1984.

[62]Nathan D. Ice cream in the diet of insulin-dependent diabetic patients. *JAMA* 251:2825, 1984.

[63]Collings P. Effects of cooking on serum glucose and insulin responses to starch. *Br Med J* 282:1032, 1981.

[64]Douglass J. Raw diet and insulin requirements. *Ann Intern Med* 82:61, 1975.

[65]Collier G. Effect of physical form of carbohydrate on the postprandial glucose, insulin, and gastric inhibitory polypeptide responses in type 2 diabetes. *Am J Clin Nutr* 36:10, 1982.

[66]Haber G. Depletion and disruption of dietary fibre. Effects on satiety, plasma-glucose, and serum-insulin. *Lancet* 2:679, 1977.

[67]Gamble D. Coxsackie viruses and diabetes mellitus. *Br Med J* 4:260, 1973.

[68]Yoon J. Virus-induced diabetes mellitus: Isolation of a virus from the pancreas of a child with diabetic ketoacidosis. *N Engl J Med* 300:1173, 1979.

[69]Bierman E. Diet and diabetes. *Am J Clin Nutr* 41:1113, 1985.

[70]American Diabetes Association. Principles of nutrition and dietary recommendations for individuals with diabetes mellitus: 1979. *Diabetes* 28:1027, 1979.

[71]Soman V. Increased insulin sensitivity and insulin binding to monocytes after physical training. *N Engl J Med* 301:1200, 1979.

[72]Kiehm T. Beneficial effects of a high carbohydrate, high fiber diet on hyperglycemic diabetic men. *Am J Clin Nutr* 29:895, 1976.

[73]Simpson H. A high carbohydrate leguminous fibre diet improves all aspects of diabetic control. *Lancet* 1:1, 1981.

[74]Anderson J. High-carbohydrate, high-fiber diets for insulin-treated men with diabetes mellitus. *Am J Clin Nutr* 32:2312, 1979

[75]Simpson R. Improved glucose control in maturity-onset diabetes treated with high-carbohydrate-modified fat diet. *Br Med J* 1:1753, 1979.

[76]Singh I. Low-fat diet and therapeutic doses of insulin in diabetes mellitus. *Lancet* 1:422, 1955.

[77]Barnard R. Response of non-insulin-dependent diabetic patients to an intensive program of diet and exercise. *Diabetes Care* 5:370, 1982.

[78]Anderson J. Update on HCF diet results. *HCF Diabetes Research Foundation Newsletter* Number 4, June 1982.

[79]Himsworth H. Diet in the aetiology of human diabetes. *Proc Roy Soc Med* 42:323, 1949.

[80]Rabinowitch I. Experiences with a high carbohydrate-low calorie diet for the treatment of diabetes mellitus. *Can Med Assoc J* 23:489, 1930.

[80]Joslin E. *The Treatment of Diabetes Mellitus*. Fourth Edition. Philadelphia: Lea and Febiger, 1928.

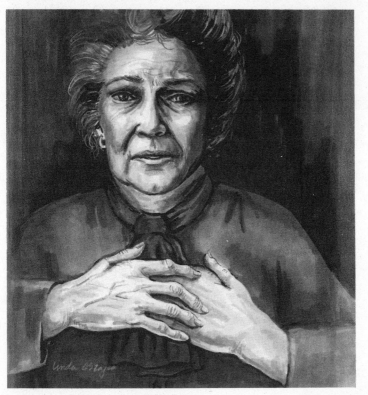

Adele

The mornings are especially hard for me because then my joints are very stiff and painful. Getting dressed each day is misery, but once the aspirin takes effect I can finally button my blouse. My fingers are starting to look ugly, twisted at all angles, and with swelling and hard lumps at the joints. I've been to see many specialists. They frighten me by the way they prescribe so freely a number of drugs that can do everything from making me blind to killing me with liver and kidney disease. But all those pills haven't done me a bit of good. I've gone the other route too. I've tried vitamins, healing herbs, and all kinds of natural concoctions, and I got no help from them either. Every time I mention trying a special diet for easing my arthritis, my doctor gets angry. So now I keep quiet and try to follow his advice to eat what he calls a ''well-balanced diet.''

8

ARTHRITIS

I have terrible pains in the joints of my fingers. It makes me feel old, crippled, and useless. What exactly is arthritis?

Arthritis is actually a general term that refers to signs and symptoms of inflammation in any joint in the body. Pain, swelling, redness, and stiffness are often present during flare-ups of disease activity in any part of the body. After years of continuous inflammation, the joints become permanently deformed and crippled. In many people the disease that is causing the arthritis affects the entire body. Involvement of joints is only one aspect of the bigger problem. In these cases many different tissues and organs can also be inflamed and prevented from functioning normally.

Tendons and bursas consist of tissues similar to those in the joints and frequently are troubled with inflammation. When they are inflamed and painful, the disorder is called *tendonitis* or *bursitis*.

I don't see any reason why I should have this problem. I am getting along in years, but most of my friends have much less trouble with their hands than I do. What causes arthritis?

There are many different causes of inflammation of the joints. A simple type of arthritis to understand is caused by a physical injury to a joint, such as twisting your ankle. In a few days or weeks the swelling and pain will go away, as long as you don't injure it again. Infections with bacteria or viruses can cause a sudden onset of arthritis that is relieved in time by healing or by treating the infection, when appropriate, with surgery and antibiotics. *Gout* is a type of arthritis caused, at least in part, by eating rich foods containing large amounts of substances called purines. Chronic and debilitating varieties of arthritis also occur, such as *rheumatoid arthritis, lupus erythematosus, psoriasis-associated arthritis* and *ankylosing spondylitis.* These conditions have more obscure origins, all of which are not fully understood. *Osteoarthritis* is said to be a natural consequence of getting old, and by the age of fifty-five years nearly everyone in the United States suffers with some degree of this joint deterioration.[1]

Why is my doctor so sure that my diet has nothing to do with my arthritis?

That is what most doctors have been taught. *The Truth About Diet & Arthritis* is published and distributed nationally by the Arthritis Foundation. It declares in bold print, ''There is NO special diet for arthritis. No specific food has anything to do with causing it. And no specific diet will cure it.''

This is a very strong position statement on diet and arthritis released by a respected national health organization. Why should anybody look any further for information on the subject? Because of this brochure and related statements, you and your doctor would reasonably assume that all needed research has been done, all the results have been analyzed, and there's no point in worrying over the possibility that what you're eating each day might affect the course of your disease.

Didn't the Arthritis Foundation investigate the effect of diet on arthritis thoroughly before taking such a position?

You may be surprised to learn that their statement is not actually founded on scientific research. In fact, the medical literature to support their dogma is practically nonexistent.[2] Most arthritis research dollars are spent on testing high-profit drug therapies. Unfortunately, only a few studies have been done on the ''nonprofit'' approach of using a health-promoting diet to treat the different types of arthritis.

The few studies that have been done on the relationship between diet and arthritis do clearly show that for many people certain foods can be very important factors in the cause, prevention, and treatment of arthritic diseases. For this reason, as well as the fact that proper foods can cause no harm, changing the diet should be considered the first-choice therapy for everyone suffering from a chronic form of arthritis for which another specific cause has not been identified and an effective treatment is not yet available.

The truth about

Diet & Arthritis

Published by

ARTHRITIS
FOUNDATION

The truth about Diet & Arthritis

may surprise you. It is simply this: There is NO special diet for arthritis. No specific food has anything to do with causing it. And no specific diet will cure it.

Gout

Gout is a special kind of arthritis, caused by an inherited defect in body chemistry, not by "high living." However, overeating and overindulgence in alcohol can trigger attacks in some patients who already have gout. Doctors recommend not drinking beer and not eating such foods as kidney, liver and sweetbreads. With new drugs, gout can be well controlled today.

The truth about Diet & Arthritis

may surprise you. It is simply this: There is NO special diet for arthritis. No specific food has anything to do with causing it. And no specific diet will cure it.

Well-meaning friends may tell you otherwise. Food fanatics and peddlers of "health and nature" foods and self-styled "experts" who write books praising their miracle "discoveries" about food and arthritis are more interested in their personal profit than they are in your health. Don't let them convince you.

The fact is, there is no valid scientific evidence that any dietary factor either causes or can help control arthritis. The only exceptions are in gout and when adjustments in a normal diet need to be made for an arthritis patient with an individual problem, such as overweight. These are explained below.

The proper diet for an arthritis patient

is a normal, well-balanced nourishing diet. Good nutrition is essential for good health whether you have arthritis or not; and it is even more important that you eat well-rounded, adequate meals regularly when your body must resist and fight off the ravages of a disease like arthritis.

There are many sources of reliable information on good nutrition. If in doubt, call upon your local chapter of the Arthritis Foundation.

Weight

Overweight. People with arthritis tend not to move around very much and may become overweight. This can put a burden on arthritic joints, increasing the inflammation and the pain. If you need a reducing diet, your doctor can advise you.

Underweight. Arthritis sometimes can make you rundown and underweight, leading to fatigue and lowered resistance. You may need extra nourishment, more high calorie foods. Let your doctor tell you what to do.

Gout

Gout is a special kind of arthritis, caused by an inherited defect in body chemistry, not by "high living." However, overeating and overindulgence in alcohol can trigger attacks in some patients who already have gout. Doctors recommend not drinking beer and not eating such foods as kidney, liver and sweetbreads. With new drugs, gout can be well controlled today.

Nutrition nonsense

A great deal that you hear and see advertised about special food products for arthritis is outright quackery. It is fantastically profitable for the sellers. For you, the arthritis sufferer, it leads to false hope and wasting of your money. So don't be lured into treating yourself. Arthritis experts do have an answer for you.

Arthritis pain now can be controlled and crippli prevented by prompt and proper treatment. See qualified physician.

How can the food we eat be important in all these different kinds of arthritis? This sounds a little like snake-oil medicine to me.

Foods provide nourishment for bones and joints and also the building materials for these tissues. Carbohydrates, fats, proteins, calcium, phosphorus, other trace elements, and vitamins are all required for the growth and maintenance of healthy bones and joints. Fortunately, nature is so generous in providing for our needs that virtually every diet followed by people around the world supplies adequate amounts of these basic raw materials.

However, most of the diseases that bother people in affluent societies are not caused by nutritional deficiencies.[3] Instead, they are due to excessive amounts of different components of the diet.[3] Arthritis appears to be no exception to this general observation.

You mentioned that gout was caused by a diet high in purines, so they must be some of the excessive amounts you are talking about. What are purines, and how do I avoid them?

Purines are some of the essential building blocks of DNA and RNA, which direct the processes by which the cells in the body reproduce and many of the chemical compounds in the body are synthesized. Foods which are plentiful in tissue cells rich in proteins, such as shellfish, fish, poultry, red meat, and legumes, are also rich in purines. DNA and RNA break down into purines, and these are degraded by the liver into uric acid, which is supposed to be excreted by the kidneys. In addition to the fact that foods high in protein are generally high in purines, the amount of protein in the diet independently affects the amount of uric acid that is produced. The more protein that is consumed, the more efficient becomes the conversion of purines to uric acid.[4] Other dietary factors, such as alcohol, also seem to influence the metabolism of uric acid and the risk of developing gout.[5]

Uric acid causes little trouble while in solution in the bloodstream. However, this substance can precipitate out of solution and form minute crystals. When these needle-like crystals are deposited inside a joint, they are very irritating. They cause sudden and severe pain, redness, and swelling, even localized fever—all the classical signs of inflammation.

When a patient consults a doctor for help with such an inflamed joint, a blood test usually is ordered to determine the level of uric acid. The results of this examination may provide some important information on the likelihood of this arthritis being an attack of gout; a high blood level of uric acid strongly suggests gout.[6] However, the diagnosis is made by sticking a needle into the exquisitely painful joint and examining a specimen of the joint fluid under a microscope. The presence of uric acid crystals in the joint fluid confirms the diagnosis.

I certainly have had my share of high-protein foods in my lifetime. Could I have gout?

That is unlikely because this disease usually begins suddenly, and the pain, redness, and swelling are intense. In most cases, only a single joint is involved at a time. The big toe is a common site for this type of arthritis. The attack subsides in a few days, with or without medication. However, medicines can bring welcome relief. Generally little, if any, permanent damage is done, although in some rare cases more severe, persistent, and deforming effects have been observed.

Do most doctors believe that gout is caused by the foods people eat?

Although in the past doctors specializing in arthritis have generally held to the belief that diet has nothing to do with the cause and cure of arthritis, these days most will admit that gout is one of the few exceptions to this rule. Since the eighteenth century, as a matter of fact, common knowledge has blamed rich foods as being the cause of gout. However, some physicians still resist the idea that foods are of great importance in causing this affliction. Instead, some doctors emphasize heredity as the primary, if not the sole, cause.

Heredity, in a way, does play a role. Metabolic rates differ among individuals, even those in the same family. Some people convert purines to uric acid faster and eliminate uric acid from their bodies through the kidneys more slowly than others do, and thereby they accumulate this arthritis-producing substance. Slower excretion is more common in certain ethnic groups, such as Filipinos.[7] Some health professionals use this basic biological difference as a reason for claiming that gout is inherited.

However, high blood levels of uric acid and gout do not occur in people who eat low-protein, low-purine foods found in healthful portions of a starch-centered diet.[7,8] Filipinos maintain low levels of uric acid when they follow their native diet which is generous with rice and vegetables.[7] But after they switch to the high-protein, high-purine diets preferred in more affluent societies such as ours, their levels of uric acid quickly rise.[7] This happens because their intake of purines and the conversion of these substances to uric acid exceeds the capacity of their metabolism to excrete this waste product. But this doesn't mean that a large proportion of the Filipino population is genetically defective.

Gout is no more an inherited disease than is a heart attack. Coronary heart disease does run in some families in the United States, but in countries where people follow a low-cholesterol, low-fat diet no one gets heart disease; therefore, this "genetic weakness," if it exists, is never expressed.[9] However, when these same people change to a diet high in cholesterol that exceeds their metabolic abilities to excrete the cholesterol they ingest, many of them do develop atherosclerosis and coronary heart disease. Similarly, if people were not overloaded with purines from their meaty diets, their ability to metabolize this waste product would not be exceeded, and they would never feel the twinges of gout.[7,8]

The Arthritis Foundation in its brochure states that "gout is a special kind of arthritis, caused by an inherited defect in body chemistry, not by high living." National health organizations often focus on uncontrollable factors like heredity in their attempts to improve health, but that approach doesn't help us very much. Even when a disease is shown to be caused by a "family tendency" passed along in our genetic material, none of us has the power to change this element. The public is poorly served when heredity is blamed and the actual culprits are simply overlooked—or hidden away. To gain improvements in personal and public health, the emphasis should be on the controllable factors of diet and lifestyle.

You're right. I can't change my heredity. So what does a person do who has this kind of arthritis? Will a change in diet cure gout?

Yes. Gout is easily stopped if you eat foods that are low in purines and as well as low in proteins.[7,8,10,11] In European countries where rich foods high in purines and proteins were rationed severely during World War II, gout was rarely, if ever, seen.[11] Just feed your body with an amount of purines that it has the ability to metabolize.

Note, however, that sometimes an unexpected attack will occur after someone changes his or her diet and begins to lose weight.[12] With weight loss from any diet, uric acid that has been stored in the body begins to move out of the tissues. This can lead to the appearance of uric acid crystals in the joints, and an unmistakable attack of gout, even after a low-purine diet is started. However, attacks of gout from weight loss are rare and occur only in people who are cursed with a very great tendency toward gout. A medication, 0.5 milligrams of colchicine taken daily, can be used for the first six months after changing to a low-purine diet to prevent an attack during the period of weight loss.[12] But this should be taken only when risk of an attack must be kept to an absolute minimum. For most people no medication is recommended or needed.

People with a history of gout or kidney stones containing uric acid can be treated routinely with any one of a variety of medications that will lower the level of uric acid in the body.[13] This preventive approach has been shown to decrease the risk of future attacks. However, with a change in diet the uric acid level will decrease, and so will the tendency to develop gout and kidney stones. In most instances, medications can be discontinued soon after the change to a low-protein, low-purine diet. Usually, the medication can be stopped abruptly. However, a few patients with a history of very serious disease may be better advised to take the medication for a time after the diet has been started, and then slowly to discontinue the medication while the blood uric acid levels are checked periodically to see if they remain low. In any case, tests of the blood uric acid level should be obtained monthly, at least initially. After the levels have fallen and have been stabilized at the lower level, blood uric acid levels need to be checked only annually. If the uric acid increases, (usually because of too many feasts), then medication should be resumed for those people who have had gout and/or uric acid stones in the past.

A person, who on routine examination, without a history of gout or kidney stones, is discovered to have high levels of uric acid presents another problem in drug therapy. In these cases, evaluation of risks against benefits shows that people are better off not taking medications because the side effects of the drugs prescribed can be serious.[14] Furthermore, present kinds of therapy for attacks of gout, if they should occur, work rapidly and effectively. Failure to treat patients is unlikely to cause any serious injury to the few who do develop an attack of gout.[14]

But, best of all, a simple change in your diet has no side effects, so don't hesitate to get started.

If you don't think I have gout, then what do I have? Once I was told that I have osteoarthritis. How about that for a diagnosis?

Osteoarthritis is a much more likely explanation for your symptoms. After all, osteoarthritis is the most common of all types of arthritis.[1,15] This form of arthritis can be identified in 35 percent of the knees of people as early as age thirty. At least 85 percent of persons aged seventy to seventy-nine have diagnosable osteoarthritis, which much of the time will compromise the quality of a person's life. This can be a very serious problem for some people. An estimated 180,000 people in the United States are bed or wheelchair invalids because of this common disease.

Osteoarthritis is seen most frequently in the joints that are most used and abused. In his later years a carpenter may find his wrists, elbows, and shoulders becoming painful and stiff. A tailor eventually develops swollen, stiff joints in the hands and fingers deformed by unsightly nodules. The obese person will show increased wear on his or her weight-bearing joints—the ankles, knees, hips, and vertebrae.

I know that the right kind of exercise is important for keeping bones and joints healthy. Are you suggesting that some people might overdo it and cause osteoarthritis? What would you consider proper exercise?

Exercise is often too severe, and injury is done to the joints, bones, and surrounding muscles and tendons. Football players, basketball players, and joggers are notable for injuries to their knees and ankles. Tennis players can have recurrent pain in their shoulders, elbows, and wrists. Later in life osteoarthritis may plague many health-conscious people who have done their best to keep fit with exercise while they were younger.

Another instance of excessive wear occurs when a bone is broken and, in setting it, the nearest joint is poorly aligned. Such a joint soon shows signs of osteoarthritis, because of the excessive wear and tear caused by that improper alignment.

No blood vessels connect directly with the joint surfaces. Oxygen and essential nutrients from the nearest blood vessels are supplied indirectly to these surfaces through the joint fluids, which are secreted by the surrounding tissues. Motion of the joints circulates these fluids. Exercise is helpful because it ensures plenty of motion of the fluids about the joints.

Beneficial exercise provides motion to all the body's parts, especially the joints, and avoids injury to any of them. For your condition, I suggest that you try walking, bicycling, dancing, or swimming. Find something you enjoy so you will keep on doing it. Exercise only to a point where the pain is not made worse; if on the next day you are more crippled, then the amount of exercise was not beneficial.

I can see how injury could lead to deterioration and arthritis of my joints, but I never injured my fingers outside of normal work. Why should my joints wear out before the rest of my body does?

That's a fair question. Our body parts were certainly designed to last a lifetime. Our bones and joints are no exception to that rule. Osteoarthritis is not an inevitable part of growing old because we can see that this affliction is rare in certain parts of the world.[16] Even in their advanced years, hard-working people in Africa are essentially free of osteoarthritis.[16,17] These people carry heavy loads and do physical work every day, from sunrise to sunset. Approximately 10 percent of the population is over the age of sixty, when this type of arthritis would be expected.[18] One of the most important differences between people of affluent countries and those of underdeveloped countries is in their diets. I suspect that the foods eaten by people in underdeveloped countries keep their bones and joints freer of disease.

The diet of those hardy Africans is low in fats, cholesterol, and proteins. Animal products are eaten in small amounts, if at all. Another bone disease common in the United States, osteoporosis, is also very rare among people of underdeveloped countries.[19] The lower animal protein content of their diet is believed to be the primary reason for the bone strength that persists into the later years of life. The excessive amounts of proteins that are consumed by most people in affluent nations weaken their bones, through many years of calcium loss from the body. The connection between osteoarthritis and osteoporosis may be that weaker bones, including their joint surfaces, are more easily injured.

When joints afflicted with osteoarthritis are examined, tiny fractures of the cartilage surface are visible under a microscope.[20] The body attempts to heal these microfractures by producing new bone. The healing is imperfect in most cases because of continued injury to weakened joint surfaces, and the end result is degeneration of the cartilage which is described as osteoarthritis. Another possible cause of weaker joint surfaces susceptible to microfractures may be poor circulation of blood to the bone underlying the cartilage surfaces.[20] This poor circulation would likely be the result of damage to the small blood vessels and sludging of blood flow caused by the large amounts of cholesterol and fat in the American diet. However, evidence that explains the relationship between the foods we eat and our susceptibility to osteoarthritis is far from clear. Other theories may be proposed as we learn more about this common disease of affluent populations consuming rich diets.

One very important recent realization in medicine has been that osteoarthritis can in some cases be arrested and even reversed.[20] This idea would have been regarded as heresy only a few years ago, because this form of arthritis was believed to be caused by progressive, unrelenting wear and tear. To improve the condition of the joints, repeated injury must be stopped. Considering the evidence of the importance of diet to the health of the bones and circulation, as well as the rest of the body, a change to a low-protein, low-fat, no-cholesterol diet would be expected to provide the best circumstances for the bones and joint surfaces to regain their strength.

Does diet have anything to do with the cause of other serious forms of arthritis? I have two friends with rheumatoid arthritis.

People with dietary customs and lifestyles different from those of Americans also offer important clues to answering this question. These diseases are rare in societies where animal products are seldom eaten and the diet is starch-centered, such as in Africa, Japan, and China.[18,21,22] In contrast, in the United States, 1 to 4 percent of the population suffers from rheumatoid arthritis. The few cases of rheumatoid arthritis that are found among people from developing cultures, who eat according to starch-based diets, are much more mild, with little or no disability.[18] In our society the disease is often crippling and sometimes fatal. When blacks in Africa move from their villages to the big cities, and adopt a rich Western diet, rheumatoid arthritis becomes as common among them as it is in America, and also as severe.[18]

What in the Western diet could cause rheumatoid arthritis?

Several theories suggest ways in which diet can be involved in the cause and aggravation of serious forms of arthritis, like rheumatoid arthritis. This form of arthritis belongs to a group of ailments called *antigen-antibody diseases* or *immune complex diseases*. Antigen-antibody complexes are formed when the immune system makes antibodies to fight invading substances. The invaders, such as bacteria, viruses, food proteins, and other "foreign" proteins are called *antigens*. These complexes, made up of antigens from outside and specific antibodies synthesized by the body, have been identified in blood specimens from patients very early in the course of rheumatoid arthritis.[23,24]

In most people these complexes are engulfed and eliminated by scavenger cells lining the blood vessels and cells in the spleen. However, in a few individuals the complexes of antibodies and antigens are not cleared from the bloodstream. Instead, they become lodged in various tissues, where they cause inflammation, much as a sliver of wood does when it is caught under the skin.[25,26] When the complexes are deposited in the joints themselves, pain, swelling, redness, and stiffness occur. Destruction of the joints and permanent deformity happen eventually as the inflammation continues.

The reasons why some people fail to clear these complexes from their systems is still unknown.[26,27] However, fats and cholesterol are known to impair the functions of the immune system, and may inhibit the efficiency of the "clearing system."[28,29] Also, the intestinal linings of some people may allow more large food proteins to enter into the body than usual.[30-32] These food proteins and the antibody complexes present in circulating blood can be measured soon after a meal.[31,32] The more "foreign" antigen substances that get into the interior of the body, the more likely it is that a problem with persistent antigen-antibody complexes will develop.

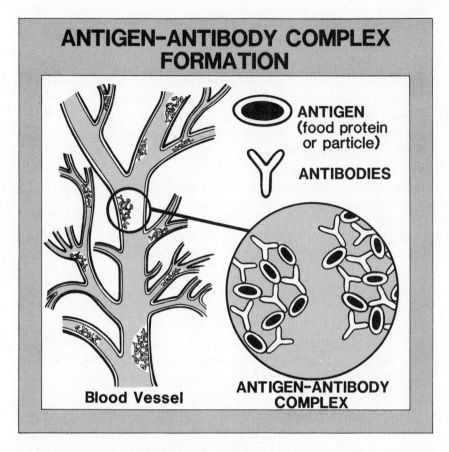

Antigen-antibody complexes are formed in many people when food proteins and other food particles pass through the intestinal wall into the bloodstream.[25,26] When these complexes persist they can lodge in the blood vessel walls and cause injury with resulting inflammation.

This explanation blames antigen-antibody complexes that float in the blood and eventually deposit in the joint tissues for the arthritis. However, another explanation for the antigen-antibody complexes found in the joint tissues is that they are formed as a result of injury that is caused by a inadequate supply of oxygen to the joint tissues.[33] This theory blames the high-fat, high-cholesterol components in the American diet for the arthritis.

How could fats and cholesterol in the diet deprive the joints of oxygen and cause rheumatoid arthritis?

Normal circulation is a vital factor in the health of all tissues, because it provides oxygen, nutrition, and a method for removing the waste products of cellular metabolism. The most common chronic disease in the United States is hardening of the arteries, or atherosclerosis. Over time a person's circulation almost expectedly decreases throughout his or her body. The blood vessels supplying the vital tissues are not simply narrowed by deposits of fats and cholesterol, but they also suffer damage from these two substances. Even in young people without evidence of extensive large vessel atherosclerosis, the microscopic and biochemical changes caused by the effects of cholesterol and fats on the blood vessels may prevent the normal transfer of oxygen from the blood to the joint tissues.[33] Joint tissues deprived of oxygen become inflamed. The inflammation causes the production of antigen-antibody complexes; the tissues swell and become painful. The clinical picture is that of rheumatoid arthritis.[33]

Another effect of diet is the disturbance of normal circulation to the joint tissues after each and every meal. Immediately after eating a single meal that is high in fats and oils, sludging of the blood cells can occur, with a dramatic reduction in the flow of blood and nutrients to the tissues. The circulation slows as blood cells stick together in clumps, and such a slowdown may last for hours especially in smaller blood vessels.[34,35] Measurement of the oxygen content in the blood has shown a drop of 20 percent (PO_2) after a person has eaten a high-fat meal, of the sort that many Americans eat three and more times a day.[36] Both animal fats and vegetable fats will decrease the amount of oxygen that reaches the tissues.[34,35]

Even though vegetable fats and animal fats will decrease effective circulation to the joints, recent evidence indicates that one type of fat may have a beneficial effect upon patients with rheumatoid arthritis.

Adding fats to my food every day sounds a lot easier than changing my entire diet. What kind of fat has been found to benefit patients with rheumatoid arthritis?

An unusual kind of polyunsaturated fat is synthesized by marine algae and plankton, which serve as food for smaller fishes. It is called *eicosapentaenoic acid*, or *EPA*. This is not the same kind of fat that is found in such vegetable oils as those expressed from sunflower seeds or corn kernels.[37] High concentrations of EPA are stored in the bodies of certain marine fish, such as mackerel. When eicosapentaenoic acid is fed to human patients, it has a drug like effect in that it suppresses inflammation. It does this by decreasing the production of prostaglandin hormones, and by inhibiting the activity of the white blood cells that take part in the inflammation processes.[38,39]

EPA, then, is a medication to reduce inflammation. But this approach does nothing to remove the cause of the arthritis. Eighteen capsules daily in divided doses have been administered with some success. Taking concentrated fish oil as a therapy for arthritis has some drawbacks, however. Eighteen capsules of fish-oil represents an extra 162 calories per day, which can add to a problem of obesity. There is evidence that oil of any type, but especially polyunsaturated varieties, may increase the risk of gallbladder disease and certain types of cancer.[40]

Inflammation has also been suppressed in experimental animals by restricting calorie intake, eating a low-fat diet, and losing weight, each independently; although these three circumstances are often present together in a starch-based meal plan.[41-44] Thus, several more possibilities can be explored as treatments for people with rheumatoid arthritis and similar conditions.

Has a dietary change actually been shown to help someone with rheumatoid arthritis?

In some people the positive effects of a dietary change are impressive. During a preliminary study, investigators at Wayne State University Medical School fed a fat-free diet to six patients suffering from rheumatoid arthritis.[45] Complete remissions of the disease were obtained in all six patients within seven weeks. The symptoms recurred within seventy-two hours when either vegetable oil or animal fats were introduced into their diets. Chicken, beef, cheese, coconut oil, and safflower oil all caused severe arthritis in these patients. The investigators concluded that "dietary fats in the amounts normally eaten in the American diet cause inflammatory joint changes seen in rheumatoid arthritis."[45]

The positive effects on the circulation by eliminating the animal and vegetable fats may have been the reason for improvement in these patients. However, the fat-free diet used by the investigators also eliminated many of the foods, such as cheese and meat, that are common sources of the antigens in the antigen-antibody complexes. Therefore, the fact that fewer reactive food antigens were present in the experimental diet may also have benefited the patients.

What sort of foods contain these potentially harmful antigens?

Many different ingredients in almost any of the foods we eat can serve as antigens in antigen-antibody complex diseases.[46] The antigens responsible for one person's troubles may be different from those that afflict another. Dairy foods are the most frequent source of the dietary antigens that cause a great variety of food allergies. Eggs run a close second. In addition to dairy and egg products, beef, wheat, corn, and many other foods and a whole host of food additives can provide the antigens that provoke arthritic symptoms, as well as many kinds of allergic manifestations.[46-48]

Is there evidence that eliminating certain foods is an effective treatment for rheumatoid arthritis?

Evidence for this approach has been sought by many doctors who are interested in allergic reactions as a cause of rheumatoid arthritis.[46] *The British Medical Journal* recently reported a dramatic improvement in arthritis achieved by the elimination of all dairy products from a patient's diet.[47] A thirty-eight-year-old woman had an eleven-year history of progressive destructive rheumatoid arthritis. She began to feel better about three weeks after eliminating from her diet all products containing cow's milk. After four months her arthritic symptoms had completely disappeared. She remained well until she agreed to accept an experimental challenge with cheese and milk. Within twenty-four hours her joints swelled, pain and stiffness set in, and she lost strength. The protein molecules from dairy products can readily pass through the intestinal wall.[30,49,50] In this patient the challenge with milk and cheese produced a slight alteration in the antigen-antibody complexes and a serious impairment in the clearing mechanisms for removing antigen-antibody complexes.[47] The investigators suspected that antigen-antibody complexes may have been the reason for this patient's destructive rheumatoid arthritis. Fortunately, she recovered her well-being a second time after returning to the milk-free diet.

In another important study, seven patients with rheumatoid arthritis were challenged with a variety of foods. Three responded to egg, two to wheat, and one each to beef and potato— the response being a notable worsening of their arthritis. Within one to four hours of eating these foods they all showed objective signs of inflammation, including measurable swelling of the joints, loss of strength, and pain. The reactions lasted up to eighteen hours. Generally, the hands were most affected, but in two patients the knees were most involved.[51]

There seem to be so many different dietary antigens. I almost feel like I should stop eating altogether.

A definite benefit is obtained when dietary antigens derived from foods are removed completely by fasting. When patients with rheumatoid arthritis are made to fast for seven to ten days, being allowed only water, joint pains are reduced and stiffness decreases.[52,53] However, when these same patients ate lacto-ovo-vegetarian foods, their problems returned and they became ill. This should not be surprising; dairy products and eggs are leading sources of antigens in food allergies. Fasting also reduced the inflammation by altering activities attributed to the white blood cells and other components of the immune system.[53]

Fasting seems so drastic. Isn't there something a victim of serious arthritis can do that is less difficult?

Not only is fasting difficult, but the results are only temporary. The reason is saddening: most patients know no alternative and hurry to return to their harmful diets, eating the foods that made them sick in the first place. All benefits gained during the days without food are lost. There are more sensible approaches to allergy and arthritis problems than fasting.

There are other reactions with the environment and the immune system besides antigen-antibody complex formation that are believed to cause arthritis. All of these reactions are generally classified as *allergies* and the substances that provoke the allergic reactions are called *allergens*. Allergy clinics investigate the sources of allergens for patients by eliminating foods, perfumes, pollens, atmospheric pollutants, and anything else that is suspect from the person's surroundings.[46,54] Some programs go so far in their attempts to discover the cause of the arthritis that they place a patient in a completely controlled, "sterile" environment. For the first week, only distilled water is allowed. After the initial week, foods and other components of the environment are introduced in a controlled manner, and the patient's reactions are observed. Scientific though it may be, this environmental laboratory approach is too expensive and impractical for most people.

What other alternative is there for the person who suspects that food is affecting his or her arthritis? I'd be interested in some cheap approach that I could try at home.

A simpler, cost-free and effective approach uses an elimination diet which can provide vital information about food sensitivities and, with luck, actual relief for many arthritis victims. The diet I recommend, in addition to being low in allergens, is also low in fats, cholesterol, and food additives. Your food bill probably will be cut in half with this diet, and you won't have to buy anything special.

The *Elimination Diet* begins by eating the foods to which most people are least likely to be allergic. It is observed strictly for at least one week. Occasionally a person may need to stay with this phase of the diet for two or three weeks in order to get a positive indication. Sometimes, too, because of an unusual sensitivity to many foods, a person may need to limit the recommended test foods to only two or three at the beginning. Starches form the center of this meal plan, and those least likely to cause allergy are sweet potatoes, brown rice, winter squashes, such as acorn, pumpkin, Hubbard, and butternut varieties, and taro or poi. Add to these basic starches your favorite cooked green and yellow vegetables and cooked non-citrus fruits. If your arthritic pains and stiffness decrease during the first one to three weeks of the test, then you have gained good evidence that some item or items in your regular diet was causing your arthritis.

Now your detective work begins in earnest. The problem is to identify which food or foods is playing the part of villain in your life. Every two days, add only one new food at a time to your basic test diet. If no reaction occurs, then you can consider it safe to eat. During each of these two-day test periods, eat a lot of the food you're considering for its effects upon your health. This use of the Elimination Diet is a highly effective way to resolve most other conditions that are caused by food allergies. Allergic reactions may be the cause of some other ailments, such as headache, muscle pains, or complaints of fatigue that accompanies arthritis. Some people will find the Elimination Diet too difficult, at least for an initial attempt at improving their arthritis. These people will benefit from the simple elimination of all animal products, especially dairy and egg products. (See the appendix for further details of the Elimination Diet.)

How little fat and protein should I eat, if I want to help my bones and joints get well?

Eating no more than 5 to 10 percent of your calories in the form of fats and 5 to 10 percent as proteins would be ideal. These figures apply to the health of your whole body, not only to your arthritis. To obtain an adequate number of calories from available foods and still keep the fat and protein levels safely low, your choices must be made from starches, vegetables, and fruits. Even among these foods, some restraint should be placed on high-protein legumes, which include beans, peas, and lentils, and on high-fat plant foods, such as nuts, seeds, avocados, olives, soybean products, and vegetable oils.

A diet low in fats and proteins sounds safe and sensible. Will a change in diet help any other types of arthritis?

Another serious disease attributed to antigen-antibody complexes is *lupus erythematosus*. It affects women mostly.[55] Arthritis is one of the principle manifestations of this disease, because antigen-antibody complexes lodge in the joint tissues and cause inflammation. These complexes are also found in the skin, lungs, brain, and kidneys, where they cause similar kinds of damage. Lupus is less common in Chinese people who live in China as compared with Chinese people who have moved to Hawaii and adopted the rich American diet, which is also rich in food antigens, fats, proteins, and calories.[56,57]

The available evidence suggests that a healthier diet will benefit patients with this disease. A form of lupus induced in experimental animals improved dramatically and consistently when they were given foods low in fats, proteins, and calories.[58,59] Furthermore, the life span of comparable experimental animals was decreased when they were fed a high-fat ration.[44]

Proteins from beef and from dairy products can form potentially harmful antigen-antibody complexes which have been found in the blood of patients with lupus, and these complexes are suspected of causing this disease in some people.[60] Higher levels of antibodies to beef proteins are found in the majority of patients who suffer from lupus, making the likelihood of antigen-antibody complex formation greater than it is with the lower levels found in people who do not have lupus.[60] Other kinds of foods, including alfalfa sprouts, have been suspected of causing a few cases of lupus.[61] Therefore, a person with lupus, who is attempting to improve his or her health should first try a low-fat, no-cholesterol, health-supporting diet, without animal products, of course. If clear improvement is not gained after a month, then the Elimination Diet should be tried to search for a specific food that may be aggravating the disease.

The possibility of benefit from a proper diet for patients with lupus has been raised recently by two groups of authors in articles published in two of the world's most respected medical journals.[55,62] They recommended a dietary approach, low in fats and meat protein. As one group wrote, "a trial of the low-fat diet should be easy to organize, particularly since overall calorie reduction is not required. This seems a useful lead to follow."[55]. The patient with lupus should understand that there is no need to wait for the professional evaluations, the long intervals while benefits of studies are being appraised, the time it takes for the information to trickle down through the medical hierarchy to the practicing doctor—who more than likely isn't interested in a dietary approach anyway.

From my clinical experience I can say that people with lupus improve considerably when they follow a low-fat, animal-product-free diet. We can hope that studies will soon be performed that support my observations.

Ankylosing spondylitis has many characteristics that are similar to those of rheumatoid arthritis. However, in this condition the arthritis is located mostly in the backbone and the hips. The disease is much less common in countries where people eat according to a starch-based diet, than where a high-fat diet is followed.[18] Because this disease is rather uncommon, even in the United States, few investigations have been made into its cause or treatment.

Psoriasis is primarily a skin disease, but many victims also suffer with severe joint pains and consequent deformation. Recently, fasting was tried in the treatment of ten patients who had psoriatic arthritis.[63] Eight reported improvement. After the fasting period they were fed a high-fat (42 percent of the total calories), pure-vegetarian diet. Their joints became worse. However, some of the patients continued to show improvement in their skin lesions, even when they stayed on this oily vegetarian diet. The improvement in arthritis and skin condition gained from fasting might be expected to be maintained on a *low-fat,* starch-based, pure-vegetarian diet. And this I have observed.

Should I take any medication for my arthritis?

Medications can be taken to relieve inflammation and reduce pain and swelling.[64] The usual treatment for the patient who does not have a severe form of the disease consists of aspirin, nonsteroidal antiinflammatory drugs, and antimalarial drugs. All of these medications act by suppressing the inflammatory responses of the body. For more resistant case of arthritis, more powerful drugs that inhibit the immune system are used, such as gold-shots, D-penicillamine, corticosteroids, and cancer chemotherapy agents. Drug therapy at this level of toxicity is far from ideal because of serious side effects and little or no improvement in the progress of the disease.[65] Medication for arthritis, as for most kinds of disease, is given to control the symptoms. The medication you choose with the help of your doctor should be the least toxic, and the least expensive, and, at the same time, the most effective. In general, drugs should be reserved for those cases that fail to respond to changes in diet.

I certainly don't like taking medications. I avoid them whenever I can. Proper food and proper exercise sound like first-choice treatments for me.

The important fact is that foods have profound effects on health and should be the first things that anyone with arthritis should investigate. The treatment I recommend is without any adverse effects and will cut your food bill considerably. Furthermore, the proper foods will benefit the arthritic patient with an improvement in general health and a helpful loss in weight for those who are overweight. Fortunately, the diet that is most likely to help in preventing and treating arthritis is also the most effective and safest way to lose those extra burdensome pounds. Weight loss in the obese arthritic patient is reason enough for a change in diet.

Other theories about the cause of arthritis have been advanced, but at the present time they offer little practical hope for the victim of arthritis. If today rheumatoid arthritis and other types of inflammatory arthritis were proved beyond a doubt to be the result of a virus infection, this discovery would do the patients no good, since we have no effective antiviral therapies. Also, believing that the several kinds of arthritis are inherited diseases does patients no good at all. How can they change their heredity? Attention toward prevention and treatment of diseases must be focused on things over which we do have control. Foremost among these are the foods we eat. At present, victims of arthritis are offered nothing in the form of a cure, considering current medical practices with drugs and surgery. The physician's prescriptions do a useful service by covering up the symptoms so that each day's pain is more endurable. But can we as doctors do more for our patients? I believe that we can help in one more very important way. We can recommend a change in diet.

The number of people whose arthritic afflictions can be cured or otherwise benefited by a dietary approach is unknown, only because so far this nonprofit kind of therapy has barely been investigated. You may be certain that many victims of arthritis will find considerable benefit and even, in some cases, an actual ''cure'' by means of this dietary approach. They have no reason to wait. I encourage anyone with arthritis to try a low-fat, no-cholesterol diet for four months, under a doctor's supervision, of course. Even stubborn cases are worth the extra effort that the Elimination Diet requires. So begin today. You deserve the chance to enjoy better health. In your predicament, nothing given up is nothing gained.

℞
• A low-fat, no-cholesterol, low-protein, low-purine, low-allergen diet is the key to prevention and treatment of the several diseases that are called arthritis.

• This health-supporting diet is centered around a variety of starches, supplemented by fresh fruits and vegetables.

• A low-protein, low-purine diet is emphasized for people suffering from gout. Try the health-supporting diet, but without the legumes, which are rich in purines. Avoid alcohol.

• A low-fat, low-allergen diet is emphasized for people who have antigen-antibody complex diseases, such as rheumatoid arthritis and lupus erythematosus. Special attention must be given to avoiding high-fat plant foods such as nuts, seeds, avocados, olives, tofu, soy beans, and all vegetable oils.

• The Elimination Diet should be tried for all cases that do not respond to the recommendations given above. (See appendix)

• The positive effects from a dietary change usually are seen within one to three weeks; however, as long as four months may be necessary in stubborn cases.

• A program of exercise should not make the joints more inflamed and painful.

• The special fish oil, EPA, should be regarded as a medication to improve symptoms by reducing inflammation, not as a cure. Eighteen capsules, in divided doses, have been used with some success. This approach should be considered after failure to obtain relief with a starch-based, health-supporting diet, and second, an elimination diet.

• Medications are to be used when needed to reduce inflammation and relieve pain and swelling. Aspirin is safest, cheapest, and most effective for patients suffering arthritis other than gout. Except for corticosteroids, most medications can be easily and safely reduced or discontinued as the condition improves. Corticosteroids must be discontinued gradually. In all cases a doctor's supervision must be obtained when strong medications are taken or discontinued.

• Attacks of gout are effectively treated with colchicine and/or a number of antiinflammatory drugs. A few people with a very strong tendency for developing gout may wish to take 0.5 milligrams of cholchicine a day for the first six months after beginning a diet that results in weight loss. Most people should not consider this as pro-phylaxis.

• Asymptomatic elevations of uric acid are not treated with drugs, but with a low-protein, low-purine diet, and avoidance of alcohol.

REFERENCES

[1]Kellgren J. Osteo-arthrosis and disk degeneration in an urban population. *Ann Rheum Dis* 17:388, 1958.

[2]Panush R. Diet therapy for rheumatoid arthritis. *Arthritis Rheum* 26:462, 1983.

[3]Connor W. Presidential address: Too little or too much: the case for preventive nutrition. *Am J Clin Nutr* 32: 1975, 1979.

[4]Bien E. The relation of dietary nitrogen consumption to the rate of uric acid synthesis in normal and gouty man. *J Clin Invest* 32:778, 1953.

[5]Gibson T. A controlled study of diet in patients with gout. *Ann Rheum Dis* 42:123, 1983.

[6]Hall A. Epidemiology of gout and hyperuricemia. A long-term population study. *Am J Med* 42:27, 1967.

[7]Healey L. Hyperuricemia in Filipinos: Interaction of heredity and environment. *Am J Hum Genet* 19:81, 1967.

[8]Zollner N. Diet and gout. *Proc. 9th Int. Congr. Nutrition,* Mexico, 1972. 1:267, 1975.

[9]Connor W. The key role of nutritional factors in prevention of coronary heart disease. *Prev Med* 1:49,1972.

[10]Elkeles R. The effect of hypolipidaemic therapy on serum uric acid concentration. *Atherosclerosis* 24:587, 1976.

[11]Emmerson B. Acquired causes of hyperuricaemia. *Aust NZ J Med* (Suppl 1) 8:149, 1978.

[12]Drenick E. Hyperuricemia, acute gout, renal insufficiency and urate nephrolithiasis due to starvation. *Arthritis Rheum* 8:988, 1965.

[13]Emmerson B. Therapeutics of hyperuricaemia and gout. *Med J Aust* 141:31, 1984.

[14]Duffy W. Management of asymptomatic hyperuricemia. *JAMA* 246:2215, 1981.

[15]Kellgren J. Rheumatic complaints in an urban population. *Ann Rheum Dis* 12:, 1953.

[16]Valkenburg H. Osteoarthritis in some developing countries. *J Rheumatol* (suppl 10) 10:20, 1983.

[17]Solomon L. Rheumatic disorders in South African Negro. Part II. Osteo-arthrosis. *S Afr Med J* 49:1737, 1975.

[18]Solomon L. Rheumatic disorders in the South African Negro. Part I. Rheumatoid arthritis and ankylosing spondylitis. *S Afr Med J* 49:1292, 1975.

[19]Walker A. The human requirement of calcium: should low intakes be supplemented? *Am J Clin Nutr* 25:518, 1972.

[20]Bland J. The reversibility of osteoarthritis: a review. *Am J Med* 74:16, 1983.

[21]Beighton P. Rheumatoid arthritis in a rural South African Negro population. *Ann Rheum Dis* 34:136, 1975.

[22]Beasley R. Low prevalence of rheumatoid arthritis in Chinese. Prevalence survey in a rural community. *J Rheumatol* (Suppl 10) 10:11, 1983.

[23]Jones V. Immune complexes in early arthritis. I. Detection of immune complexes before rheumatoid arthritis is definite. *Clin Exp Immunol* 44:512, 1981.

[24]Jones V. Immune complexes in early arthritis. II. Immune complex constituents are synthesized in the synovium before rheumatoid factors. *Clin Exp Immunol* 49:31, 1982.

[25]Theofilopoulos A. Evaluation and clinical significance of circulating immune complexes. *Ann Prog Clin Immunol* 4:63, 1980.

[26]Barnett E. Circulating immune complexes: their immunochemistry, detection, and importance. *Ann Intern Med* 91:430, 1979.

27Denman A. Nature and diagnosis of food allergy. *Proc Nutr Soc* 38:391, 1979.

28Palmblad J. Lymphomas and dietary fat. *Lancet* 1:142, 1977.

29Morrow W. Dietary fat and autoimmune disease. *Arthritis Rheum* 26:1532, 1983.

30Hemmings W. Transport of large breakdown products of dietary protein through the gut wall. *Gut* 19:715, 1978.

31Paganelli R. Immune complexes containing food proteins in normal and atopic subjects after oral challenge and effect of sodium cromoglycate on antigen absorption. *Lancet* 1:1270, 1979.

32Paganelli R. Detection of specific antigen within circulating immune complexes: validation of the assay and its application to food antigen-antibody complexes formed in healthy and food-allergic subjects. *Clin Exp Immunol* 46:44, 1981.

33Rothschild B. Pathogenesis of rheumatoid arthritis: a vascular hypothesis. *Semin Arthritis Rheum* 12:11, 1982.

34Friedman M. Serum lipids and conjunctival circulation after fat ingestion in men exhibiting type-A behavior pattern. *Circulation* 29:874, 1964.

35Friedman M. Effect of unsaturated fats upon lipemia and conjunctival circulation. A study of coronary-prone (pattern A) men. *JAMA* 193:882, 1965.

36Kuo P. The effect of lipemia upon coronary and peripheral arterial circulation in patients with essential hyperlipemia. *Am J Med* 26:68, 1959.

37Glomset J. Editorial: Fish, fatty acids, and human health. *N Engl J Med* 312:1253, 1985.

38Kremer J. Effects of manipulation of dietary fatty acids on clinical manifestations of rheumatoid arthritis. *Lancet* 1:184, 1985.

39Lee T. Effect of dietary enrichment with eicosapentaenoic and docosahexaenoic acids on in vitro neutrophil and monocyte leukotriene generation and neutrophil function. *N Engl J Med* 312:1217, 1985.

40McDougall J. *The McDougall Plan*. New Century, Piscataway, 1983.

41Fernandes G. Influence of diet on survival in mice. *Proc Nat Acad Sci USA* 73:1279, 1976.

42Fernandes G. Influence of dietary restriction on immunologic function and renal disease in (NZBxNZW) F1 mice. *Proc Natl Acad Sci USA* 75:1500, 1978.

43Gross R. Role of nutrition in immunologic function. *Physiol Rev* 60:188, 1980.

44Levy J. Dietary fat affects immune response, production of antiviral factors, and immune complex disease in NZB/NZW mice. *Proc Natl Acad Sci USA* 79:1974,1982.

45Lucas P. Dietary fat aggravates active rheumatoid arthritis. *Clin Res* 29:754A, 1981.

46Stroud R. Comprehensive environmental control and its effect on rheumatoid arthritis. *Clin Res* 28:791A, 1980.

47Parke A. Rheumatoid arthritis and food: a case study. *Br Med J* 282:2027, 1981.

48Epstein S. Hypersensitivity to sodium nitrate: a major causative factor in case of palindromic rheumatism. *Ann Allergy* 27:343: 1969.

49Cunningham-Rundles C. Milk precipitins, circulating immune complexes, and IgA deficiency. *Proc Natl Acad Sci USA* 75:3387, 1978.

50Korenblat P. Immune responses of human adults after oral and parenteral exposure to bovine serum albumin. *J Allergy* 41:226, 1968.

51Little C. Platelet serotonin release in rheumatoid arthritis: a study in food-intolerant patients. *Lancet* 2:297, 1983.

[52]Skoldstam L. Effects of fasting and lactovegetarian diet on rheumatoid arthritis. *Scand J Rheumatol* 8:249, 1979.

[53]Uden A. Neutrophil functions and clinical performance after total fasting in patients with rheumatoid arthritis. *Ann Rheum Dis* 42:45, 1983.

[54]Rea W. Food and chemical susceptibility after environmental chemical overexposure: case histories. *Ann Allergy* 41:101, 1978.

[55]Morrow W. Systemic lupus erythematosus: 25 years of treatment related to immunopathology. *Lancet* 2:206, 1983.

[56]Chang N. Rheumatic diseases in China. *J Rheumatol* (suppl 10) 10:41, 1983.

[57]Serdula M. Frequency of systemic lupus erythematosus in different ethnic groups in Hawaii. *Arthritis Rheum* 22:328, 1979.

[58]Gardner M. Type C virus expression and host response in diet-cured NZB/W mice. *Nature* 268:341, 1977.

[59]Izui S. Low-calorie diet selectively reduces expression of retroviral envelope glycoprotein gp70 in sera of NZBxNZW F1 hybrid mice. *J Exp Med* 154:1116, 1981.

[60]Carr R. Antibodies to bovine gamma globulin (BGG) and the occurrence of a BGG-like substance in systemic lupus erythematosus sera. *J Allergy Clin Immunol* 50:18, 1972.

[61]Roberts J. Exacerbation of SLE associated with alfalfa ingestion. *N Engl J Med* 308:1361, 1983.

[62]Steinberg A. Systemic lupus erythematosus: Insights from animal models. NIH Conference. *Ann Intern Med* 100:714, 1984.

[63]Lithell H. A fasting and vegetarian diet treatment trial on chronic inflammatory disorders. Effects on clinical condition and serum levels of neutrophil-derived granule proteins. *Acta Derm Venereol* (Stockh) 63:397, 1983.

[64]Pinals R. Approaches to rheumatoid arthritis and osteoarthritis: an overview. *Am J Med* 75:2, 1983.

[65]Butler R. Controversy in the treatment of rheumatoid arthritis. *Lancet* 2:278, 1984.

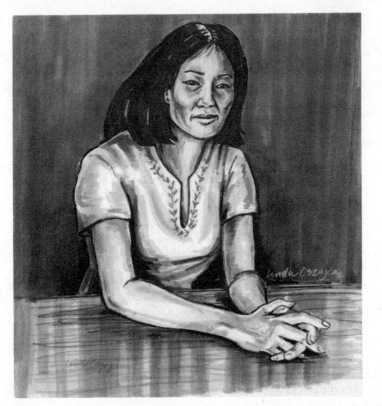

Karen

I'm told that soon I'll have a new companion, a kidney machine to spend five hours a day with, three days a week. Maybe if it makes me feel better than I do now, I'll be glad for the attachment. The nausea and the itching are enough to drive me crazy.

I don't even know what I did to get into this mess. Every month I'm becoming worse, and my doctor tells me there's no chance of stopping the deterioration of my kidneys. He calls my condition chronic glomerulonephritis. I asked if there was any special diet to follow that would help, and his reply was for me to eat, drink, and be merry. To me that's the same as telling me I'm condemned to die. After a few days he did call me on the phone and say that a low-protein diet might help. But he also went on to say that he doesn't usually recommend it to his patients because it's too hard to follow.

I've seen how people on the kidney machine spend their lives. They really don't look so great, and they waste a lot of time just lying there. I'm a busy woman with a family that needs my care. I'm determined to do something. To me following a low-protein diet seems like a small effort to make, if it will help.

9

URINARY DISEASE

I never knew anything about kidney disease until I developed it myself. How do people get into this kind of trouble?

Functional kidney tissues can be lost from a variety of diseases and injuries. For example, if a person suffers from severe shock after a serious accident or a heart attack, a sudden and long-lasting decrease in the flow of blood to the kidneys can cause some of their tissues to die. For some people, atherosclerosis can slowly narrow the large and small arteries that supply the kidneys and lead to kidney failure. Atherosclerosis is accelerated by high cholesterol levels, high blood pressure, and diabetes. In addition, both high blood pressure and diabetes have their own ways of damaging the kidneys and are notorious for causing rapid deterioration of kidney function. Chemical poisoning can destroy kidney tissues. A kidney stone can lodge in the ureter, blocking flow of the urine to the bladder, and pressure of the urine backing up to the kidney can destroy that kidney.

Medical research has made some real progress in saving kidneys or at least parts of them. In earlier times a frequent cause of kidney failure was chronic infection caused by several kinds of bacteria. Fortunately, antibiotics and surgery have been highly effective in reducing the number of cases of kidney loss from infections. Today, kidney failure more commonly occurs after years of subtle, but constantly repeated injury, causing the kind of inflammation known as *glomerulonephritis*. Unfortunately, little medical progress has been made in checking this life-threatening disease.

I still suffer from occasional bladder infections. Is there anything I can do to avoid taking all those antibiotics?

Most likely your bladder problems are not related to your kidney, even though in some people bladder infections do extend to become kidney infections. Infections of the bladder are common in women and are often associated with injury to the outlet tube of the bladder, the *urethra*. Usually this injury occurs during sexual intercourse, for which reason the infection that sometimes follows is called *honeymoon cystitis*. Obviously, injury to this delicate part of the body should be avoided. Urinating immediately after intercourse has been recommended in order to clear the urethra, but the value of this practice is questioned.

For many women the burning of the urethra on urination is caused by the soap they use in washing.[1] Women with recurrent episodes of painful urination, especially in cases when no harmful bacteria can be grown in laboratory tests, are very likely to find the cure to their distress in simply avoiding all types of soaps and using only tap water in cleaning the vaginal area.

Doctors recognize that a natural agent for treating minor bladder infections is present in cranberry juice.[2] The body converts some of this juice into an organic acid. Concentrated in the urine, this causes the bladder contents to become acidic. Most harmful bacteria cannot survive in this acid environment, and the infection subsides. To achieve adequate concentrations of the inhibiting acid, you should drink a whole quart of cranberry juice all at one time. Gulp!

The ordinary treatment of bladder infections with antibiotics calls for a ten-day course of pills taken four times a day. These days this older way may be replaced by a single dose of an antibiotic.[3] Results are as good, the patient's compliance is more easily gained, and cost and side effects are less. If, in the future, you get another bladder infection that requires treatment with antibiotics, ask your doctor about the new single-dose therapy.

Here are some antibiotics that are used in the single-dose therapy.

SINGLE-DOSE ANTIBACTERIAL AGENTS FOR UNCOMPLICATED BLADDER INFECTIONS

ANTIBIOTIC	SINGLE DOSAGE
amoxocillin (Amoxil and others)	3 grams
sulfisoxazole (Gantrasin and others)	2 grams
trimethoprim/sulfamethoxazole (Septra DS, Bactrim DS)	160/800 milligrams

A single urinary tract infection in a man can be a sign of a more serious disease than is likely to be found in women. Such an infection in a man should be subjected to a thorough medical evaluation.

What is glomerulonephritis? Can you tell me how I got this disease?

Glomerulonephritis is a disease of the kidneys that is marked by inflammation of groupings of capillaries called *glomeruli*. This condition is one of several that are considered to be antigen-antibody complex diseases. In this case, complexes—that is, combinations of two or more substances found in the person's body—eventually lodge in the glomeruli, causing inflammation and destruction of surrounding kidney tissues. The disease affects primarily the membranes between the capillaries and the tubules of the kidney. Both known and unknown sources of the antigens that form these complexes have been found. The best known are streptococcal bacteria, parasites, viruses, foreign proteins that happen to be injected into the body during immunizations, and certain foods.[4] When the injury from the complexes lasts for only a short time, then a case of acute glomerulonephritis occurs, and the kidneys usually recover fully. But if the injury persists for a long time, then the chronic form of glomerulonephritis develops, and the damage to kidney tissues is great and continuing. Eventually, the kidney tissues that are lost to injury are replaced by nonfunctioning scar tissues.

I don't have any kidney infections that I know of, and I haven't had any immunizations in years. If something I have eaten is the cause of this, could changing the things I eat possibly help?

Foods certainly should be considered in searching for the cause of any chronic disease when no other obvious reason can be found. Protein molecules and other components derived from foods can pass through the intestinal wall into the bloodstream, even in normal healthy children and adults.[5-12] These proteins and food derivatives can act as antigens to form antigen-antibody complexes that are distributed in the circulating blood.

According to investigations, several kinds of active diseases of the glomeruli can be caused by antigen-antibody complexes that include proteins from food. A minor kidney ailment called *orthostatic albuminuria*—which means that protein called albumin appears in a patient's urine when standing and sitting but is not released when lying down—occurs in some children after they have eaten milk products and eggs.[13] Antibodies against proteins from these foods were detected in the children's blood. When these foods were excluded from their diet, the condition disappeared or improved remarkably.[13]

People suffering with a much more serious kidney disease called *nephrotic syndrome* lose large amounts of proteins through their kidneys all the time and eventually develop edema, the swelling of their body tissues. Many different factors have been blamed for this disease. Allergic reactions and immune complexes are suspected in some cases. Older children with severe kidney disease and nephrotic syndrome have shown pronounced improvement, often in a single week, when certain food proteins were eliminated from their diet.[14] Challenging these convalescent young patients with as little as one ounce of milk provoked a worsening of their condition.

More severe injury to the glomeruli by antigen-antibody complexes is believed to result in many cases of glomerulonephritis. An estimated 70 to 80 percent of the cases of glomerulonephritis from immunologic causes result from antibodies complexed with circulating antigens that deposit in vessels and filtering structures of the kidney.[15] Antigen-antibody complexes derived from food antigens have been found in the circulating blood of patients with chronic glomerulonephritis of unknown cause.[11,12]

The foods most likely to form antigen-antibody complexes are dairy products and other animal-derived proteins. Elevated levels of antibodies to cow's proteins and antigen-antibody complexes containing cow's proteins have been found in the blood of patients suffering from a variety of immune complex diseases, including rheumatoid arthritis, lupus erythematosus, and glomerulonephritis.[11,12,16,17] The antigen-antibody complexes that persist in the bloodstream are trapped in the tiny blood vessels of the kidney glomeruli and also in the joints and the skin. Wherever they are caught, they cause inflammation, and therefore, trouble.

Your diet may be detrimental to the health of your kidneys in other ways also. Progressive kidney failure from a variety of causes may be aggravated by the fats and cholesterol you eat. After inflicting an initial injury upon the kidneys, such as the one caused by antigen-antibody complexes, fats and cholesterol infiltrate the kidneys' blood vessels and other tissues, further impairing their health and function.[18,19] An increase of 75 percent in the fat content of the kidney membranes over normal is found in cases of glomerulonephritis.[18] There is evidence that fats and cholesterol may actually be toxic to the kidney tissues and cause progressive destruction and loss of those essential cells.[18]

My other doctor never paid much attention to diet. He just gave me some pills to take.

Food proteins are usually overlooked as sources of the antigens in this potentially fatal disease. Most physicians treat the symptoms of glomerulonephritis and pay little attention to searching for the cause. Medicines are prescribed, such as corticosteroids that impair the immune system, with the hope that these drugs will reduce the inflammation and subsequent loss of kidney tissues.

Unfortunately, for most cases of long-standing kidney disease little effective drug treatment is available. Once chronic kidney failure has begun, the course of events is all but decreed: a steady decline in function, at a constant rate, allowing an accurate prediction of the date when end-stage kidney failure will be reached and the patient will need the help of a kidney machine in order to survive.[20,21]

Because the disease is progressive and, at present, is untreatable by surgery or drugs, the opportunity should not be overlooked to help the patient by recommending a change in diet. Studies have not yet been done to establish the exact role of foods in the cause and possible treatment of chronic glomerulonephritis. However, it is important that the investigations be performed soon, since confirmation of the role of food in glomerulonephritis holds the potential for a safe and effective method of prevention and treatment for this often fatal disease. Since this therapy is entirely safe and cost-free, a change in diet should be tried under their doctor's supervision by anyone with chronic glomerulonephritis of unknown cause. The elimination of all dairy products will likely give the greatest results for people with antigen-antibody complex diseases. But there are many other foods that are involved in allergic diseases that can affect the kidneys such as eggs, meats, wheat, and corn. *The Elimination Diet* should be used to search out trouble-making foods. (See appendix for details of the Elimination Diet).

Even though the potential benefits from eliminating food sources of antigen-antibody complexes and lowering the cholesterol and fat in the diet have received too little scientific study, the role of another dietary nutrient has been convincingly established in helping people with glomerulonephritis and other forms of chronic kidney disease. The greatest help from a dietary change is gained when the total protein content of meals is reduced. Not only are the waste products from proteins, such as urea, reduced in amount, but in most cases the progression of the underlying disease can be halted or slowed, especially when the change is begun early in the course of the disease.[22-48]

My other doctor half-heartedly suggested a low-protein diet. But don't I need more protein now that I'm sick and losing protein in my urine?

People with kidney disease usually lose protein as a result of leakage through their damaged kidneys into the urine.[23] Because of this loss, some doctors and dietitians mistakenly recommend a high-protein diet, assuming that the extra protein will compensate for the amounts lost. But this added protein is not needed. All natural diets, whether based on vegetables or on animal products, provide more than enough proteins to meet our needs in times of health or disease. Proteins we eat are converted in the liver and other tissue cells into the substances we need for all our metabolic functions of growth and maintenance. Adding more proteins in the diet won't make the metabolic systems work any better. Replacement of lost proteins is not accomplished by this effort. In fact, the excessive amounts of proteins actually will worsen the kidney disease. The way to stop the loss of proteins into the urine is to stop the injury to the glomeruli.

How could a little extra protein hurt me? I figure that my body can store the extra amount for those days when I might not eat much.

Among the most subtle and important toxins you can force upon your kidneys are the excessive amounts of proteins that are eaten daily by the average American.[22-26] Excess proteins are not stored in the body in the way that excess calories are stored as body fat; excess proteins have to be eliminated quickly. The by-products of proteins that are not used for body repair and growth spill over into the bloodstream and remain there until they are removed by the liver and kidneys. The parts of the kidneys that filter them out of the blood stream are called *nephrons*. Destruction of the nephrons is believed to be caused directly by the remnants of the excess protein. These by-products raise fluid pressures in the nephrons and affect the flow of both blood and waste materials in, through, and out of the kidneys. The increase in glomerular pressures and flows is believed to accelerate the destruction of kidney tissues, leading to more rapid loss of kidney function.[24]

This damage is not limited just to individuals who already have diseased kidneys, but is believed to be the cause of the progressive loss of kidney tissues and functions that affects people as they age.[24-26] The damage can be so serious that, in an otherwise healthy person, half the functional capacity of the kidneys can be destroyed after spending seven or eight decades living on the high-protein American diet.[24] Even so, fortunately for us, the remaining half of our kidneys can dispose of the waste products of body metabolism, and they do not accumulate to the level that leads to symptoms of kidney failure. The kidneys are designed in such a way that they have a tremendous reserve capacity. Even when three-quarters of the kidney function has been lost, an individual may show little systemic evidence of disease.[27] The remaining quarter of the kidneys is quite able to eliminate all the body's wastes and unneeded water without being overwhelmed. Despite our abuse of them, our bodies are very forgiving. Not until the very end-stages of kidney failure, when the kidney function falls below 5 percent of normal, will a life-threatening buildup of potassium occur.[28] When that happens, the person with kidney failure will either die or be dependent upon a kidney machine for the rest of their life.

I guess a high-protein diet would be especially harmful in someone like me who already has kidney damage.

More than thirty-five years ago a famous kidney specialist recommended that the protein intake be restricted in a patient with kidney failure, in order to minimize further loss of kidney function.[29] This kidney-damaging effect of a high-protein diet, actually the level of protein consumed daily by a typical American, becomes a life and death matter in someone who has lost kidney tissues from another cause, such as glomerulonephritis, diabetes, high blood pressure, atherosclerosis, chemical poisoning, injury, or surgical loss through donation or disease.[29-45] Some evidence indicates that certain kinds of kidney disease are benefited more than others by restricting intake of proteins. For example, disease of the kidney tubules and surrounding tissues, called *tubulointerstitial nephritis,* seems very responsive to this therapy.[30] Other investigators report significant benefit for chronic glomerulonephritis, which is your condition.[31,32] The earlier these dietary restrictions are started, the more effective the therapy is likely to be.[33]

The timely introduction of a low-protein diet can keep someone with progressive kidney disease like yourself off the kidney machine for a longer time, if not forever. Many reports have appeared in the medical literature indicating the remarkable benefits that restricting protein intake achieves in slowing or even halting the progress of kidney failure.[30-45] A recent study of 228 kidney patients who were placed on only a moderate restriction of protein intake showed three to five times slower progress of kidney disease compared with patients who were not given this dietary advantage.[31] Many of the patients in this study had the same disease as you do, chronic glomerulonephritis. Furthermore, other kinds of kidney diseases also benefited from the moderate protein diet. These conditions included polycystic kidney disease, interstitial nephritis, nephrosclerosis, loss of kidney tissues after surgery or disease, and others.

Many of the beneficial effects of a low-protein diet have been observed in animals as well. For example, a low-protein diet protects the kidneys of experimental animals with glomerulonephritis.[23,46,47] During the last forty years, improvements in patients with chronic glomerulonephritis who were placed on a low-protein diet suggest a protective effect from the basic disease processes for people also.[29-45]

Instruction about the usefulness and application of a low-protein diet is a critical aspect of medical education for the care of patients who have lost any part of their kidney function. Too few of us in the medical and nutritional fields have emphasized enough the importance of proper or improper diets for our patients with kidney diseases. Many patients are never given this information at all. As a direct result, their conditions steadily worsen and their future prospects are bleak to say the least.

I've noticed that I have lost my desire for meat and fish since I've become ill. Is there anything else besides the danger of too much protein that I should know about my diet?

Many patients with kidney failure have similar naturally acquired aversions to meats and fish.[48] But remember that other dietary factors are also important for people with kidney failure. Phosphates, which are found in highest concentrations in meats, dairy products, food additives, and certain soft drinks, are thought to worsen kidney failure. Restriction of phosphates has slowed and stopped progress of kidney failure in animals and possibly in people.[48,49] High levels of blood calcium, along with the high levels of phosphates, are believed to worsen kidney failure, possibly by forming calcium deposits in the kidney tissues.[48] You may notice the similarity between high-phosphate and high-protein foods as being animal products and expect that you would gain benefit from restricting the intake of both kinds of ingredients. However, of all the components of the foods we eat that are found to be harmful to the kidneys, available evidence indicates that the *primary* benefits from a dietary change come from lowering the protein content.[22]

Restricting the animal products in your diet has other important benefits for the rest of your body's health. Your cholesterol level should be kept as low as possible by eliminating all animal products from your diet, not only because doing so may slow the progress of the kidney disease but also because the rest of your body is harmed by cholesterol. Atherosclerosis and associated complications of heart attacks and strokes are more common in patients with kidney failure, especially in those who have reached the terminal stage and are on a kidney machine.[50-53]

Once a person has deteriorated from kidney failure, the body is weakened to the point where many systems fail, particularly those dealing with repair and defense. Infections are common, especially after a patient needs the help of a kidney machine. Bone loss is also more severe in kidney patients. A diet that best supports health in every way possible should be greatly appreciated by a patient with failed kidneys and fast-failing health.

Is there anything that can be done for my swollen feet? My blood pressure has recently gone up. Could a low-salt diet help both these problems?

Yes, you should cut down on your salt intake. Salt is eliminated by the kidneys. If the capacity of the kidneys is decreased to the point where more salt is taken in than can be eliminated, then this mineral compound will accumulate in the body. Water is retained in proportion to the amount of salt accumulated, and the body tissues swell. The parts that are affected more by gravity, such as the feet and legs, are the first to swell, but soon swelling is noticed around the eyes, especially after the patient has been sleeping while lying down. Lowering salt intake to a level the kidneys can accommodate will reduce the swelling in a few days. Sometimes, a low level of protein in the blood that occurs with protein-losing kidney disease will also cause swelling. Some rare forms of kidney disease are known in which large amounts of salt are lost from the body. In these cases, salt restriction is unwise.

The kidneys are important regulators of blood pressure, and when they are damaged the blood pressure frequently rises, sometimes to very high levels. The restriction of salt, animal fats, and proteins can be very beneficial in lowering the blood pressure through a variety of mechanisms.[43-45] These strategies can reduce or eliminate the need for medications used to treat high blood pressure. Without medications, of course, side effects are avoided. A change in diet, which benefits the entire body as well as the kidneys, will relieve much of the suffering endured by people with kidney failure.

If a low-protein, low-fat diet can keep me off a kidney machine, it would be worth doing. How does a kidney machine work, anyway?

Kidney machines perform a filtering process of the blood that is called *dialysis*. This process removes toxic waste products that are accumulating in the body. Products of the breakdown of proteins, a large part being blood urea nitrogen or BUN, potassium, and salt, are removed during the three- to six-hour filtering that must take place several times a week. A life tied to a kidney machine is miserable for most patients and expensive for our overburdened health-care system.

People who are on dialysis often take the attitude that they can eat anything they want because the machine will compensate for their over-indulgence. However, the machine can undo only a part of the damage that dietary abuse will provoke.

Many benefits of a low-protein, low-fat, no-cholesterol, low-salt diet are gained for patients who are tied to a kidney machine. People on dialysis can decrease the levels of waste products such as blood urea nitrogen (BUN) through sensible eating and thereby decrease the frequency and the length of dialysis treatments they are obliged to have.[54] Valuable time can be spent away from the kidney machine, doing more interesting things, more comfortably.

Potassium is a problem for dialysis patients as well as for those with very severe kidney failure. Fruits and most vegetables are high in potassium content. Grains are lower in potassium, and they should be the main starchy foods for these patients. Naturally, a close watch is kept on the blood potassium level of a patient near end-stage kidney disease or on dialysis.

Dialysis patients often have high blood pressure that is treated by a variety of drugs which have some pretty serious side effects. Sensible eating can reduce or eliminate the need for many medications. Diabetes is a common disease of kidney patients, and this condition can be improved and sometimes eliminated altogether with a high-carbohydrate, high-fiber, low-fat diet. However, much of the damage done by many years of diabetes is not reversible. Dialysis patients have worse atherosclerosis, leading to premature death and disability from strokes and heart attacks.[50-53] A low-fat, no-cholesterol diet will give these people a better chance for a longer, and more nearly normal, functional life.

I have seen many people with skin sores, undiagnosed aches and pains, and other indeterminate feelings of illness who are relieved when attention is paid to feeding them a diet that supports health and healing processes, instead of one that burdens all the body's systems. Kidney patients are often surprised by what they gain from such a simple maneuver as a change in foods.

The kidney machine sounds like an expensive method of treatment that brings many new problems for a patient. Is there much chance of someone who is put on a kidney machine ever getting off it? Maybe by a kidney transplant?

At present, about 50,000 people each year are on kidney dialysis machines in the United States. In Great Britain, however, the cost of such care is too heavy a burden on the government-supported medical care system. Many people are denied access to kidney machines for reasons that Britain's health-care officials consider to be practical and justifiable.[55]

One hope for many of those people who have reached end-stage kidney failure is a kidney transplant. Thousands of people have had this operation. When the new kidney is donated by a close relative, then the success rate is 75 to 90 percent one year after surgery. Kidneys obtained from nonrelatives function only 50 to 60 percent of the time at the end of one year. Transplant patients have to be maintained on powerful drugs that suppress the immune system and prevent the body from rejecting the donated kidney. Cancer and microbial infections are more common in kidney transplant patients because of those suppressive drugs. These people certainly don't need the added burden of the American diet, overfilled with kidney-damaging proteins and atherosclerosis-producing cholesterol and fats.[51]

I have always wondered what happens to the donor of a kidney.

Usually no short-term adverse effects are felt by the person who donates a kidney. However, remember that the donor's kidney function is suddenly lessened by half after the surgery. Fortunately, half of the normal kidney activity is adequate for maintaining a normal life under normal conditions. However, the donor must take care to preserve intact that precious remaining kidney in all its parts and functions. Real threats await this person in the guise of microbial infections, injuries, and toxic substances that can change a generous donor into the recipient of a transplanted kidney. One important kidney toxin that is easy to avoid and yet is too often overlooked in most transplant recipients and donors is excess dietary protein.[24] Both donors and recipients must be given instruction about the foods they eat that will help them to sustain their bodies in the best possible health. Today, however, most patients are not given this absolutely essential information.

I have also suffered with kidney stones. Can I do anything to prevent another painful attack?

To know how to prevent them from coming again, you have to know what type of stones they are and something about the conditions in your body that caused them to form. When they do form, they are likely to be accompanied by severe pains in the abdomen and the back and at least microscopic blood in the urine. Most often they occur in men over thirty years of age, but women can have them too. Statistics indicate that stones will form in about 12 percent of our population.[56] Stones grow in the upper portion of the collecting system of a ureter, which is located within the related kidney. When these kidney stones break loose from that upper drainage system and get lodged in the narrow stretches of the ureter, they can cause indescribable pain. The two most common types of stones seen in the United States, called calcium stones and uric acid stones, are named for the dominant mineral ingredient in each kind. Calcium oxalate and calcium phosphate stones comprise 75 to 85 percent of the total and uric acid stones account for 5 to 8 percent. Other types of stones are rare and can be the result of metabolic defects or infections.

I had the calcium type. What causes those stones?

Calcium stones are found mostly in developed countries, where people can afford to eat like royalty twenty-one or more times a week.[57] Throughout the world, the incidence of kidney stones can be correlated with the wealth of a country, especially as it is defined by expenditures for foods. The dietary factor that is most strongly related to the formation of kidney stones is animal proteins.[58] After World War I and II, when food became more abundant again, near epidemics of stones occurred in many countries in Europe.[59] In Japan, since the change toward a Western-type diet began after World War II, the incidence of kidney stone formation has been rising.[60] Formation of stones in the kidneys and the upper ureters is almost unknown in underdeveloped societies whose people follow a starch-based diet that is low in animal products.[61,62] In the United States, modern-day vegetarians have about half the incidence of stones as the general population.[63]

The effect of proteins on the body, especially animal proteins, increases the excretion of calcium through the kidneys into the urine.[64] The calcium comes from the foods eaten and from the stores of its depository found in the bones. The urine carries calcium in high concentration. As the urine becomes saturated with calcium and other minerals, microscopic crystals form, and around these core crystals stones will grow to a visible and very troublesome size.[65]

Eating meats also increases the amount of oxalate in the urine. Oxalate is the second mineral component in the most common form of kidney stone in this country. The increase in oxalate may result from an increase in absorption from the intestine or from an increased production of it in the body by way of the metabolic breakdown of certain amino acids present in great amounts in meat proteins.[66]

Even though plant foods, especially green leafy vegetables, are high in oxalates, in a normal person the oxalates are poorly absorbed, because in the intestine almost all of this substance is in the insoluble form of calcium oxalate.[67] Fats from meat or any other source will assist the absorption of oxalates by forming so-called soap complexes with the calcium found in the calcium oxalate present in foods. When the calcium is combined with fats, the oxalate is freed for absorption.[67]

High concentrations of oxalate in the urine and frequent formation of kidney stones occur in people who have diseases of the small intestine such as Crohn's disease. This is because of the large amounts of fat present in their intestinal contents caused by malabsorption of dietary fats resulting from their illness. When these patients are placed on a low-fat diet, the amount of oxalate in their urine decreases, and so does the likelihood of their forming kidney stones.[68]

There are other components of the rich American diet that have been incriminated in the formation of stones. All of these fit the worldwide observation that stone disease is common in people who consume a rich diet. Refined grains lacking in fiber and phytates, uric acid found in high concentrations in meats, and a high salt intake have each been considered as possible factors that increase stone formation in people living in affluent Western nations.[69-72]

Once I was told that I had "idiopathic hypercalcuria." What does that mean?

The word *idiopathic* refers to a disease of unknown cause, peculiar to an individual. The origin of *hypercalcuria* is certainly not known by very many physicians practicing today. Hypercalcuria means high levels of calcium in the urine. Idiopathic is an incorrect term for this problem, because in most cases the cause is known.[57,64,65,70,73-75] However, since nutrition is usually a neglected part of a physician's education, we seldom give much thought to the probability that the high level of proteins in a patient's diet has caused the elevated levels of calcium in the urine. Until physicians and dietitians stop thinking about causes of common diseases under the mistaken notion that the well-balanced American diet offers correct nutrition, we will be handicapped both in our attempts at diagnosis and in our ability to provide effective treatments for our patients.

The presence of calcium in high levels in the urine is resolved in almost every case by lowering the protein content of the patient's diet.[57,64,65,73-75] The effects of this approach on the concentration of urine calcium are detected in only a few hours. Reducing the intake of proteins from animal sources is especially important. Meat proteins consist of large amounts of sulfur-containing amino acids, which have a very powerful calcium-losing effect on the kidneys.[74] Reducing the intake of meats will also reduce other components in the urine, such as uric acid, that favor stone formation and the probability of recurrent calcium stones.[66]

Keeping the natural bran on the grains by avoiding refining processes will preserve the fibers and phytates in the foods. Phytates, especially, decrease the absorption of calcium by the intestine, which in turn decreases the amount of calcium that eventually ends up in the urine.[69,70]. It has been observed that adding rice bran to the diet of patients with a history of kidney stones is an effective way to lower urine calcium levels and dramatically decrease stone formation.[70].

Can uric acid stones also be prevented with a proper diet?

A low-protein, low-purine diet is an accepted therapy prescribed by some physicians and dietitians for the prevention of uric acid stones. Uric acid is a breakdown product of purines, which are the basic building blocks of DNA and RNA. However, the dietary programs now used most often could be more effective if they were changed to eliminate animal products altogether. Red meats, poultry, fish, and other seafoods are all rich in purines, but most practicing medical doctors and dietitians still permit meat in the diet of a patient who forms kidney stones. In part this is because many so-called experts in the health professions can't imagine that anyone else can eat foods that are different from the ones they themselves gorge upon. And they can't imagine going without all those mouth-watering delicacies, like steak and lobster, baked potatoes loaded with sour cream or butter, topped off with marvelous rich chocolate mousse bedecked with whipped cream, washed down with espresso coffee and a fine imported brandy. The works! All preceded, of course, by a couple of hours of boozing and stuffing themselves with the latest and richest kinds of canapés. Patients are trapped by this indulgence into receiving less than the best attention from their physicians.

Can kidney stones be dissolved with a good diet?

Doctors are just starting to investigate treatment of actual stones by means of proper foods. Uric acid stones can be dissolved by making the urine more alkaline. This is accomplished by decreasing the intake of animal protein, increasing the amount of potassium contributed by vegetable foods, and drinking more water.[76] A medication called allopurinol is recommended in addition to potassium salts. In one small study this approach was 100 percent effective.[76] Future studies will determine how effective dietary control will be in dissolving all types of stones.

For now, however, in most patients painful kidney stones are removed by surgical procedures. A new ultrasonic technique has been tried recently, which pulverizes a stone to a size that easily passes through the ureter. With this merciful kind of intervention, the need for surgery is eliminated.

If I have to limit my intake of proteins, cholesterol, and salt—and later potassium—what is left for me to eat?

Your diet for now should be centered around a variety of starchy foods such as potatoes, sweet potatoes, corn, rice, and other whole grains. To this central starch staple, you should add fruits and vegetables low in proteins. Foods from the legume family, such as beans, peas, and lentils, are high in proteins and should be limited or eliminated altogether.

When kidney disease has progressed to the point where less than 5 percent of the kidney function remains, then the kidneys cannot eliminate all the potassium that is taken in from the diet. Occasionally, a dangerous buildup of potassium can occur even earlier than at the point where only 5 percent function remains. This may happen when a patient follows a diet high in potassium or takes potassium supplements. Therefore, people with less than 25 percent function, who are on a diet high in fruits and vegetables, should have their blood potassium level checked regularly. Salt substitutes, which replace sodium with potassium, should be avoided. People requiring further restriction of potassium intake should arrange their meals around grains instead of starchy vegetables. Certain fruits and vegetables are lower in potassium than others. Natural sugar can be used liberally by most patients to supply required calories without need for proteins, cholesterol, table salt, potassium, or phosphates.

The trouble with Americans today is that they want to eat every day all those rich and harmful foods that their grandparents never even had the chance to eat, that their parents worked hard to buy for only very special occasions, but that they themselves can order up at the flash of a credit card and swallow without a thought for tomorrow. No wonder the body's systems break down under the load!

I hope that information about this new and painless way of treating people with kidney disease and kidney stones spreads quickly among both doctors and patients so that more people can be helped. I'll have no trouble following a low-protein diet now that I realize its importance.

Most of the information I've shared with you was reported forty years ago to physicians in meetings and medical journals. On January 13, 1946, Walter Kempner, M.D., of Duke University read before the New York Academy of Medicine the results of his treatment of patients afflicted by a variety of diseases using a simple dietary approach. He reported that 203 of 322 patients with kidney disease, other diseases of the urinary tract, and hypertension, most of whom had previously tried other kinds of therapies, showed measurable improvement with his dietary therapy. Of the 100 patients with primary kidney disease, 65 showed objective improvement. Of the 222 patients with blood vessel disease caused by hypertension, 62 percent improved. Of the 31 patients with inverted T-waves on their EKGs, a sign of heart disease, the T-waves of 11 became upright, in other words, normal. In 77 of the 87 with blood vessel disease because of severe hypertension, the enlarged hearts became smaller. Dr. Kempner pointed out to his colleagues that the relationship between high blood cholesterol levels and high blood pressure had been stressed repeatedly by others, especially with regard to vascular eye disease, coronary artery disease, and atherosclerosis. In 53 of his patients with blood vessel disease and cholesterol levels above 220 milligram percent, 52 showed a drop after a change in diet, the average decrease being 74 milligram percent in blood cholesterol.

Dr. Kempner treated with a rice-based diet many patients with acute and chronic glomerulonephritis, other kinds of kidney disease, heart disease, hypertension, obesity, and diabetes. Fruits and fruit juices supplemented the rice. His diet provided approximately 2000 calories from rice and table sugar, fruits, and fruit juices supplemented with vitamins and iron. The addition of the "empty-calorie" sugar and fruit juice effectively reduced the 40 grams of proteins that would have been present in 2000 calories of rice alone to the required 20 grams. By limiting the proteins in the diet, little is left to yield waste products that damage and otherwise overburden the capacity of the remaining kidney tissues.

These days much research is being reported that confirms and expands upon the benefits that Dr. Kempner saw in his patients during more than forty-seven years of research and clinical care. The success of this pioneer, researcher, and thinker has never been surpassed. And yet few patients today are offered the advantages of a simple, safe, and inexpensive therapy.

Is a change in diet simply too much for a doctor to suggest to a patient? Perhaps more of us in the health professions should give our patients a chance to answer this question and to choose this highly effective therapy.

℞

•A low-protein, low-purine, low-fat, low-sodium, no-cholesterol, high-fiber diet is the basic method for preventing and treating most kidney diseases and most kinds of kidney stones.

•Your basic meal plan is to be centered around starches, with the addition of fresh fruits and vegetables. Legumes (beans, peas, and lentils) are restricted.

•The Elimination Diet should be tried by people who have a kidney disease that may be caused by an allergic or antigen-antibody reaction. (See the appendix for detailed explanation of the Elimination Diet). Often a change as simple as elimination of all foods that contain animal products will eliminate the disease.

•A low-protein, low-fat, low-phosphate, no-cholesterol diet is essential for slowing or stopping the progress of most kinds of kidney failure.

•Patients near the end-stages of kidney disease, or on dialysis should base their diet upon grains and fruits low in potassium to avoid buildup of fatal levels of potassium in the blood. A doctor's supervision and frequent blood tests are necessary for someone who is this sick.

•Surgery or pulverization is necessary for removing kidney stones that cause pain. In some less insistent cases, the doctor and patient may try to dissolve stones with a change in diet.

•People with kidney disease frequently are on medications that require adjustment of dosages. These adjustments should always be made under a doctor's supervision.

•Uncomplicated bladder infections can be treated with copious amounts of cranberry juice taken orally. If an antibiotic is required, it should be given in a single dose whenever possible.

•Women with recurrent bladder infections should stop using soaps for washing the genital area.

REFERENCES

[1]Ravnskov U. Soap is the major cause of dysuria. *Lancet* 1:1027, 1984.

[2]Bodel P. Cranberry juice and the antibacterial action of hippuric acid. *J Lab Clin Med* 54:881, 1959.

[3]Treatment of urinary tract infections. *Med Lett Drugs Ther* 23:69, 1981.

[4]Theofilopoulos A. Evaluation and clinical significance of circulating immune complexes. *Ann Prog Clin Immunol* 4:63, 1980.

[5]Walker W. Uptake and transport of macromolecules by the intestine. Possible role in clinical disorders. *Gastroenterology* 67:531, 1974.

[6]Hemmings W. Transport of large breakdown products of dietary protein through the gut wall. *Gut* 19:715, 1978.

[7]Delire M. Circulating immune complexes in infants fed on cow's milk. *Nature* 272:632, 1978.

[8]Paganelli R. Immune complexes containing food proteins in normal and atopic subjects after oral challenge and effect of sodium cromoglycate on antigen absorption. *Lancet* 1:1270, 1979.

[9]Paganelli R. Detection of specific antigen within circulating immune complexes: validation of the assay and its application to food antigen-antibody complexes formed in healthy and food-allergic subjects. *Clin Exp Immunol* 46:44, 1981.

[10]Brostoff J. Production of IgE complexes by allergen challenge in atopic patients and the effect of sodium cromoglycate. *Lancet* 1:1268, 1979.

[11]Cairns S. Circulating Immune complexes following food: delayed clearance in idiopathic glomerulonephritis. *J Clin Lab Immunol* 6:121, 1981.

[12]Sancho J. Immune complexes in IgA nephropathy: presence of antibodies against diet antigens and delayed clearance of specific polymeric IgA immune complexes. *Clin Exp Immunol* 54:194, 1983.

[13]Matsumura T. Significance of food allergy in the etiology of orthostatic albuminuria. *J Asthma Res* 3:325, 1966.

[14]Sandberg D. Severe steroid-responsive nephrosis associated with hypersensitivity. *Lancet* 1:388, 1977.

[15]Wilson C. The renal response to immunological injury. In: Brenner BM, Rector FC (eds): *The Kidney,* vol 2. Philadelphia, WB Saunders, 1976, p 838

[16]Parke A. Rheumatoid arthritis and food: a case study. *Br Med J* 282:2027, 1981

[17]Carr R. Antibodies to bovine gamma globulin (BGG) and the occurrence of a BGG-like substance in systemic lupus erythematosus sera. *J Allergy Clin Immunol* 50:18, 1972.

[18]Kelley V. Enriched lipid diet accelerates lupus nephritis in NZBxW mice. Synergistic action of immune complexes and lipid in glomerular injury. *Am J Pathol* 111:288, 1983.

[19]Moorhead J. Lipid nephrotoxicity in chronic progressive glomerular and tubulo-interstitial disease. *Lancet* 2:1309, 1982.

[20]Mitch W. A simple method of estimating progression of chronic renal failure. *Lancet* 2:1326, 1976.

[21]Oska H. Progression of chronic renal failure. *Nephron* 35:31, 1983.

[22]Laouari D. Adverse effect of proteins on remnant kidney: Dissociation from that of other nutrients. *Kidney Int* 24 (suppl 16) S-248, 1983.

[23]Neugarten J. Amelioration of experimental glomerulonephritis by dietary protein restriction. *Kidney Int* 24:595, 1983.

[24]Brenner B. Dietary protein intake and the progressive nature of kidney disease: The role of hemodynamically mediated glomerular injury in the pathogenesis of progressive glomerular sclerosis in aging, renal ablation and intrinsic renal disease. *N Engl J Med* 307:652, 1982.

[25]Kennedy G. Effects of old age and over-nutrition on the kidney. *Br Med Bull* 13:67, 1957.

[26]Baldwin D. Chronic glomerulonephritis: nonimmunologic mechanisms of progressive glomerular damage. *Kidney Int* 21:109, 1982.

[27]Epstein F. The treatment of reversible uremia. *Yale J Biol Med* 27:53, 1954.

[28]Papper S. *Clinical Nephrology*, 2nd ed. Little, Brown & Co. Boston, 1978. p 106.

[29]Addis T. *Glomerular nephritis: diagnosis and treatment*. New York: Macmillan, 1948.

[30]Nahas A. Selective effect of low protein diets in chronic renal diseases. *Br Med J* 289:1337, 1984.

[31]Rosman J. Prospective randomised trial of early dietary protein restriction in chronic renal failure. *Lancet* 2:1291, 1984.

[32]Williams A. Protein restriction in chronic renal failure. *Lancet* 1:102, 1985.

[33]Maschio G. Effects of dietary protein and phosphorus restriction on the progression of early renal failure. *Kidney Int* 22:371, 1982.

[34]Levin D. Metabolic effects of dietary protein in chronic renal failure. *Ann Intern Med* 63:642, 1965.

[35]Mitch W. The effect of nutritional therapy on progression of chronic renal failure: quantitative assessment. *Clin Res* 24:407A, 1976.

[36]Barsotti G. Effects on renal function of a low-nitrogen diet supplemented with essential amino acids and ketoanalogues and of hemodialysis and free protein supply in patients with chronic renal failure. *Nephron* 27:113, 1981.

[37]Gretz N. Low-protein diet supplemented by keto acids in chronic renal failure.: a prospective controlled study. *Kidney Int* 24 (suppl 16):S-263, 1983.

[38]Alvestrand A. Retardation of the progression of renal insufficiency in patients treated with low-protein diets. *Kidney Int* 24 (suppl 16):S-268, 1983.

[39]Maschio G. Early dietary protein and phosphorus restriction is effective in delaying progression of chronic renal failure. *Kidney Int* 24 (suppl 16): S-273, 1983.

[40]Barsotti G. Restricted phosphorus and nitrogen intake to slow the progression of chronic renal failure: a controlled trial. *Kidney Int* 24 (suppl 16):S-278, 1983.

[41]Walser M. Supplements containing amino acids and keto acids in the treatment of chronic uremia. *Kidney Int* 24: (suppl 16):S-285, 1983.

[42]Mitch W. The effect of a keto acid-amino acid supplement to a restricted diet on the progression of chronic renal failure. *N Engl J Med* 311:623, 1984.

[43]Kempner W. Treatment of kidney disease and hypertensive vascular disease with rice diet. *N Carolina Med J* 5:125, 1944.

[44]Kempner W. Compensation of renal metabolic dysfunction. Treatment of kidney disease and hypertensive vascular disease with rice diet, III. *N Carolina Med J* 6:61, 1945.

[45]Kempner W. Compensation of renal metabolic dysfunction. Treatment of kidney disease and hypertensive vascular disease with rice diet, III. Part 2. *N Carolina Med J* 6:117, 1945.

[46]Farr L. The effect of dietary protein on the course of nephrotoxic nephritis in rats. *J Exp Med* 70:615, 1939.

[47]Friend P. Dietary restrictions early and late: effects on the nephropathy of the NZBxNZW mouse. *Lab Invest* 38:629, 1978.

[48]Walser M. Does dietary therapy have a role in the predialysis patient? *Am J Clin Nutr* 33:1629, 1980.

[49]Ibels L. Preservation of function in experimental renal disease by dietary restriction of phosphate. *N Engl J Med* 298:122, 1978.

[50]Spencer E. Atherosclerosis in dialysis and renal-transplant patients. *Lancet* 1:591, 1980.

[51]Chan M. Atherosclerosis in dialysis and renal-transplant patients. *Lancet* 1:591, 1980.

[52]Kishore B. High density lipoproteins, premature atherosclerosis, and renal failure. *Lancet* 1:1252, 1980.

[53]Editorial: Uraemia, lipoproteins, and atherosclerosis. *Lancet* 2:1151, 1981.

[54]Gombos E. Dietary programs and chronically uremic patients on and off dialysis. *Am J Clin Nutr* 21:574, 1968.

[55]Douglas J. Renal failure and the law. *Lancet* 1:1319, 1985.

[56]Sierakowski R. The frequency of urolithiasis in hospital discharge diagnoses in the United States. *Invest Urol* 15:438, 1978.

[57]Robertson W. Should recurrent calcium oxalate stone formers become vegetarians? *Br J Urol* 51:427, 1979.

[58]Robertson W. The role of affluence and diet in the genesis of calcium-containing stones. *Fortschritte der Urologie and Nephrologie* 11:5, 1979.

[59]Prien E. The riddle of urinary stone disease. *JAMA* 216:503, 1971.

[60]Andersen D. Historical and geographical differences in the pattern of incidence of urinary stones considered in relation to possible aetiological factors. In: Hodgkinson A, Nordin BEC, eds. *Renal stone research Symposium*. London: Churchill, 1969, p-7.

[61]Wise R. Urinary calculi and serum calcium levels in Africans and Indians. *S Afr Med J* 35:47, 1961.

[62]Coetzee T. Urinary calculus in the Indian and African in Natal. *S Afr Med J* 37:1092, 1963.

[63]Robertson W. Prevalence of urinary stone disease in vegetarians. *Eur Urol* 8:334, 1982.

[64]Licata A. Effects of dietary protein on urinary calcium in normal subjects and in patients with nephrolithiasis. *Metabolism* 28:895, 1979.

[65]Diet and urinary calculi. *Nutr Rev* 38:74, 1980.

[66]Robertson W. The effect of high animal protein intake on the risk of calcium stone-formation in the urinary tract. *Clin Sci* 57:285, 1979.

[67]Williams H. Oxalic acid and hyperoxaluric syndromes. *Kidney Int* 13:410, 1978.

[68]Andersson H. Fat-reduced diet in the treatment of hyperoxaluria in patients with ileopathy. *Gut* 15:360, 1974.

[69]Modlin M. Urinary phosphorylated inositols and renal stone. *Lancet* 2:1113,1980.

[70]Ohkawa T. Rice bran treatment for patients with hypercalciuric stones: experimental and clinical studies. *J Urol* 132:1140, 1984.

[71]Coe F. Hyperuricosuric calcium oxalate nephrolithiasis. *Kidney Int* 13:418, 1978.

[72]Modlin M. The aetiology of renal stone: a new concept arising from studies on a stone-free population. *Ann Roy Coll Surg Engl* 40:155, 1967.

[73]Urinary calcium and dietary protein. *Nutr Rev* 38:9, 1980.

[74]Brockis J. The effects of vegetable and animal protein diets on calcium, urate and oxalate excretion. *Br J Urol* 54:590, 1982.

[75]Linkswiler H. Protein-induced hypercalciuria. *Fed Proc* 40:2429, 1981.

[76]Rodman J. Dissolution of uric acid calculi. *J Urol* 131:1039, 1984.

[77]Kempner W. Some effects of the rice diet. Treatment of kidney disease and hypertension. *The Bulletin* 22:358, 1946.

EPILOG

Susan, in control of the decisions to be made for her breast cancer:

I thought it all over very thoroughly and even went to several other doctors and asked their opinion. Each doctor I saw I asked, "Do you have evidence that cutting off my breast will keep me alive longer than if I had a simple lumpectomy?" All but one admitted they had none. One doctor mumbled something like, "There hasn't been enough time yet to prove that lumpectomy, or even lumpectomy with radiation, will be as good as the time-honored mastectomy." Well, I was ready for that answer. I'm all too familiar with the horrible record for that form of mutilation.

The radiotherapist I saw told me that if I had a recurrence in my breast after the lumpectomy he would have no trouble treating it at that time.

The biggest problem I had was with the chemotherapy specialists. One told me that if I didn't take chemotherapy I would be three times as likely to die of breast cancer and that he rarely saw serious side effects from the year-long treatments he gave many patients. From what I saw going on in his office I can easily guess why he saw so few side effects from the chemotherapies he was giving. Only the nurses gave the injections and talked to the patients, not the doctor. If I were seriously considering that kind of therapy I would have asked the patients or some of the nurses about the side effects of the therapy. The other chemotherapy specialist doctor I saw freely admitted that the use of chemotherapy after breast cancer surgery was experimental, and that the benefits were far from convincing.

I sure learned a lot from the time I spent talking to those doctors. I'm glad I took the trouble, because now I'm confident that I've made the right choices. I do have a serious problem, cancer, but why rub salt into a wound? I see no reason to live the remainder of my life deformed by a therapy that, as far as I am concerned, is proved to be a failure after ninety years of experimentation on several million women. Nor am I going to spend the next year taking pills and shots that would make me violently ill. This sounds more like a trial by fire and water, than a humanitarian treatment of another person.

Not a single doctor asked about my diet or mentioned that it would be advisable to cut down on the fats I ate. In fact, I had a home visit by a breast cancer patient from a program to help women with breast cancer make adjustments to life easier. This person was very insistent that diet had nothing to do with breast cancer and that I was foolish to give up all those tasty foods. I know better and I'm angry that the way I've eaten in the past has caused a disease that now threatens my life in my most productive years. Simply out of rebellion I would change my diet, even if I didn't have the hope a better diet would help me live longer. I have no doubt I will live healthier. My daughters deserve better also. After they saw what I went through and I explained to them the importance of foods on their health they had no trouble making the changeover to a low-fat, starch-based meal plan.

I'm still a little frightened, but in time I'm sure I will worry less. I feel like every step I'm taking is a positive one towards better health. I'm already picking up the pieces and every day looks more hopeful.

Martha, willing and able to avoid osteoporosis:

Changing to a low-protein diet and getting more exercise was very little adjustment for me. My friends had more difficulty with my change in eating than I did. Some of them actually acted defensive, like I was doing something that threatened them. A few closer friends told me I was just on another one of my "kicks," this time health food. At first, I would eat a little chicken or fish when we went out to lunch together, mostly to be sociable. However, now I find the flesh just gets caught in between my teeth and I don't like the taste anymore. If it weren't for all the grease in the sauces, I would just as soon they would put the sauce they used on the chicken or fish over a potato or some rice. The sauce is where all the spice and flavor in the meal is found anyway.

I had one interesting experience. My doctor sent me to the hospital dietitian for an analysis of my new diet. This nice young man told me I wasn't getting enough protein to stay healthy from only rice and potatoes. I challenged him to calculate out how much protein I was actually getting and he was surprised. He then told me I wasn't getting a proper balance of amino acids. Well I didn't know exactly how to answer him. He was such a nice person and seemed so interested in my health that the next day I went out and bought him a copy of *The McDougall Plan*. I asked him to read the chapter on protein and this would explain to him about the fact that nature designed the foods complete with all the necessary amino acids and proteins long before they reached the dinner table. I pointed out the challenge in the protein chapter, that it was virtually impossible to design a diet based around any single unprocessed starch that failed to give all the protein and amino acids that any child or adult would possibly need. I told him to call if there were any problems. Well, I haven't heard from him yet.

In addition to less concern I now have over breaking my bones, I have gained many side benefits from better eating and exercise. No more constipation or morning headaches and I've lost an unwelcome ten pounds. I think I will have my bones checked at the hospital every six months for awhile with their little photon machine. They have a program where I can get a reading for about $50 dollars. The results of the test will give me confidence that I am doing well and don't need any other therapy. I wouldn't change my diet and lifestyle now anyway and I don't plan on taking any pills either, unless absolutely necessary. Maintaining good health should be this simple.

Henry, never too late to stop the destruction of his arteries:

Giving up the chicken and fish wasn't easy at first, I'll admit. I really couldn't visualize what I was supposed to eat. It all seemed the same to me, just a bunch of vegetables. Every time I tried a recipe that first week I felt like something was missing from my meal. I didn't feel full and I was in the refrigerator all the time looking for more food to nibble on. After three weeks those cravings went and I now feel very satisfied. Part of the problem was I started out just trying to eat plain potatoes, plain rice, and boiled vegetables. That was hard to enjoy. However, once I started to make some of Mary McDougall's recipes I really discovered how good things tasted. She has a section in the back of each book entitled "Quick and Easy." I can make some of these in less than 15 minutes. I don't have any blood pressure trouble so I add a little salt over the food at the table and that helps a lot with the taste. I also wasn't eating enough food when

I first started. I thought I should stick to the same size portions or I'd gain weight. I couldn't have been more wrong. I now eat two to three times as much food as before and stay trim.

My blood test improved in one way and got worse in another. My cholesterol fell over 100 points, but my triglycerides went up. However, as soon as I stopped eating seven fruits a day, the fruit juice and the honey on my cereal and got a little more exercise, they came right down to normal.

I'm confident the atherosclerosis will reverse, though all I really care about is that it doesn't get any worse. After all, the blood vessels I have now are adequate, since all my parts are getting enough blood to keep me functioning pretty normal. In just this few short weeks I have noticed I can walk longer without leg pains. Amazing how forgiving the old body is. I'll see my doctor once in a while to check on the size of that aneurysm, but no other tests, except for the blood, unless I get some new trouble.

George, finally found motivation to get his life in order—bypass surgery:

I left that doctor's office so enthused about changing my diet and getting out of that bypass surgery, but somehow things just didn't work as easy as I had planned. It was close to Christmas season and there were all those office parties. I couldn't be unsociable, could I? My wife didn't have any real health problems and she couldn't really see the need for the whole family to change their diet. At first every night she would cook two separate meals, but soon I got back into eating whatever was on the table. It wasn't that I didn't like the new foods. It was just too much trouble.

It wasn't that the diet didn't work either. All my chest pains went away after the first week and I was walking five miles a day. I lost twenty pounds the first month. I can really recommend the program to anyone with a little more will power than I had.

A couple of months after I got off the diet I had a real bad chest pain at work an hour after lunch. The ambulance took me to the hospital and I found myself in the coronary care unit. Before I knew it, I had an angiogram done and the doctors told me that I had better have the bypass surgery. I was told I had had my chance with my vegetarian diet, and I failed. I resented that, but I was scared and figured that I could have the best of both treatments. After the surgery I was going to restart my diet.

The bypass surgery was no picnic. They had to take me back to the operating room twice after the initial surgery because of bleeding problems in my chest. I was in the hospital a total of ten days. Otherwise, everything else seems to have gone well. I have no more chest pain, even when I walk. There is only one thing different that concerns me. I'm an accountant and I work with figures all day long. Since the surgery I find I just can't seem to remember as many numbers as I used to. Maybe some of this will come back in time?

One thing the operation did do for me is to make me realize that my health is worth the effort. I have started the diet again and this time my wife is with me. She realizes that she doesn't want to lose this nice warm body that keeps her secure at night, and helps her pay the bills and raise the kids. We're going to make it a family project this time. Only the right foods will be served in our home. If anyone feels they have to satisfy a craving there are plenty of restaurants just down the block they can go to for an occasional "pig out." With all the problems I have to face with getting my health back, the family can see I need all the support I can get. Besides, the children want to have better health than their parents when they grow up. I have one primary goal and that's to deprive those bypass surgeons of any more of my blood and money. I'm not planning to support any undertakers soon either.

John, fully functional without pills or high blood pressure:

There was little decision to be made when it came to my manliness or a better diet. My sexual interests and functions came back as soon as I got off those pills. The contrast in how I feel is quite dramatic, and now I realize what those drugs were doing to me. I went to the doctor who put me on the pills and told her what I wanted to do and to my surprise she was all for it. Her only hesitation was she had never taken patients off of drugs before and wasn't sure where to begin. I gave her the book to read and she could find no reason not to give it a try.

I had no problems at all. My blood pressure went down and stayed down just days after I changed my diet. I could have decreased the pills on my own, but it sure was nice to have the help and support of my doctor. She was so excited by my success that she is going to try a diet and exercise approach on some of her other patients. She even ordered *The McDougall Plan, The McDougall Health-Supporting Cookbooks,* and *McDougall's Medicine* from the publisher and she's going to sell or give them away to her patients who are interested.

I think the one who is most pleased with my renewed vigor is my wife. She's due with our first baby in four months. She says if beans and rice keeps me performing sexually this well, she'll only let me eat junk when she goes to visit her parents during the summer. I hope she doesn't ask me to take those pills while she's gone too.

Kim, needing a better future than diabetes offers and willing to work for it:

I started having low blood sugar reactions three days after I started eating starches, vegetables, and fruits even though I had cut my insulin in half the first day. But I guess that wasn't enough. After a few of those hypoglycemic reactions my doctor stopped my insulin altogether. I've done just fine. My urine checks mostly negative. I've had several blood tests. While my sugar's still not perfect, the levels are no worse than when I was taking insulin or diabetes pills. I'm real excited about my cholesterol, triglycerides, and weight; they're all down after only a month. I've lost ten pounds and I've stuffed myself.

The biggest problem I had was what to eat when I was away from home, which is a lot of the time. Now I know where most of the salad bars are in town. I found a vegetarian restaurant just one block from where I work. I was really surprised to see how much cheese, eggs, and oil these so called health-food people put in their food. They do make a vegetable bean soup that is free of oil and fat that I enjoy when I go there. They always have brown rice and I order a whole wheat bread sandwich with sliced tomato, onion, cucumber, lettuce and shredded carrots. Lately I've been walking to the other side of town, about a mile away, on my noon lunch break for some Chinese food. The cook will make me a delicious vegetable chow mein without the oil. They only have white rice, but I'm working on them to start serving brown also. I solved my snacking problem by carrying baked potatoes wrapped in aluminum foil or a piece of fruit in my purse. I've really learned to like this way of eating and my change in taste happened faster than I had imagined it would. The few times I have had oily foods have been real eye openers. The grease gets on my face and hands and I can hardly wait to get to the restroom and wash. I can imagine now how tough fats and oils must be on my insides. Usually the way I feel afterwards leaves me little doubt that I did myself some harm.

I've spent many years getting myself into this trouble. I'm amazed at how quickly I've felt better. I still have a few pounds to lose, but I'm confident that the weight will continue to shed as effortlessly as it has so far. By the time I'm trim I should also have my blood sugar and cholesterol down to healthy levels. It feels good just to know that for a change I'm getting healthier every day instead of digging my grave with my knife and fork.

Adele, leaving her arthritis behind and getting more from life everyday:

My joints already feel better. Maybe it's all in my head, but I don't think so. I don't have to wake up in the middle of the night and take aspirin so I will be able to move in the morning. As a matter of fact, I only take an occasional aspirin anymore. I've told my two friends who have rheumatoid arthritis about the diet and both of them had doctors who insisted that diet has nothing to do with arthritis. One has changed her diet, the other had no interest. So far my one friend reports the change has been very helpful for her.

There isn't much incentive for me to cook most of the time, because I live alone. I've found that cooking a large pot of soup or sauce once or twice a week makes it easy. I keep very busy outside my house and when I get home in the evening I don't have to look forward to preparing dinner since I already have something in the refrigerator or freezer that I can warm up in the microwave. Baked potatoes are fast to cook this way too.

Even if my arthritis wasn't better I still wouldn't change back to eating all that meat, cheese and white bread. Do you know how many times the subject of "occasional irregularity," in other words, constipation, is the topic of our social gatherings? I'm relieved that I no longer have anything to contribute to that conversation.

Karen, important dietary changes are keeping her a long way from the kidney machine:

The change I made in my diet was really drastic from what I had been eating, but the change in my health was just as great. Now if I cheat even a little, I can tell in how I feel. I wasn't convinced that I needed to eat simply and sensibly until I visted the hospital's dialysis unit and saw first hand just how these unfortunate people look and imagined how life must be for them. Anybody who isn't convinced of the importance of taking good care of their kidneys should have a similar eye-opening experience.

I've read *The McDougall Plan* and Mary's recipes and I wish I could have all those delicious foods most other people get to enjoy. I'm pretty much limited to grains, vegetables, and fruits with no salt and no legumes. I can use all my favorite spices, and quite honestly I am getting to really enjoy the food, as simple as it is.

My blood tests are better; the BUN has fallen almost to normal and this is probably why I feel so good. A urine check showed much less protein and fewer red blood cells for the first time since I got kidney trouble. My family and friends think I look better too. I'm happy for the chance to recover any health I can, because I will never get used to living with that kidney machine.

Dr. McDougall, still full of hopes and dreams, but less disappointments:

Individual patient care over the past thirteen years has brought me many rewards. The past seven years of practice with principles of diet and lifestyle have been particularly satisfying. I have learned much about the behavior of people in relation to their health. There are a certain number of people, let's guess 20%, who enjoy their life and appreciate their health, and will expend any effort to preserve both. All these people need is the information on how to heal and stay healthy, and then they can't be stopped. These are usually people who have demonstrated success in other areas of their life, such as business, education, family, arts, recreation, and personal relationships. They see every reason to succeed in their health also. These people don't smoke, drink minimally, and always wear their car safety belts. Once they understand the foods that support health, appropriate changes are made and the feast again becomes a special occasion.

There is a large group of people who haven't found a reason to change their lifestyle significantly, yet. Let's say 40 percent of the American population. Many will make some changes and in time a few will gradually find that taking care of themselves is easier than the inconvenience of being sick and/or fat. However, the vast majority need motivation to help them to appreciate their health. They have to lose it and often be confronted with a threat of dying before deciding that change is necessary and worth their while. Unfortunately, until they find the reason, all the talking in the world by you or me will not cause them to make significant changes. (Even though you will find most do agree with us about the importance and the validity of a better diet and lifestyle.)

The last 40 percent are hopeless. No amount of education and convincing argument will start people in this group on a healthier path. Many of these people are involved in other self-destructive behaviors, not only with their health, but in their social, family and business relationships.

Early on in my career I came to the realization that I couldn't have everyone see things as I do. I now realize that this unified view of the problems of health and health-care would not even be desirable. However, I do believe that people should have the opportunity to know and understand that they do have an option to being ill and to many of the treatments offered today. Then whatever they choose is their business. For example, thirty years ago many smokers didn't realize the dangers of tobacco as they watched sports figures and sexy models advertise cigarettes. Today only a rare smoker is unaware of the health consequence of this habit. People who choose to smoke arouse little concern from me, because they are informed and making a choice based on widely available facts. This freedom of choice is not available to people in many areas of health care, particularly when it comes to diseases related to our foods and the treatments prescribed by health professionals. I have provided what I believe is the information you need in these two areas in the books *The McDougall Plan* and *McDougall's Medicine*. For those of you who have read and understand the information in these two books, I feel I have fulfilled my obligation to you as a doctor and a health educator. And I see a healthy future for you and your family.

I see my most valuable role in education. My efforts over as many years as I am fortunate to have left will be spent in this field through writing, radio and television appearances, and, hopefully, working with other people, possibly you, with similar interests in the health field. As a practicing physician I would like to work with all my colleagues to improve health care and honestly hope I find very little of my time spent in contesting with opponents. Much more change will occur much more rapidly if we can all work together to improve health and health-care for everyone.

UNDERLYING AND REPEATING THEMES

There are several underlying themes that are repeated throughout this book that focus on the problems of health and the health-care system. These problems are so basic and prevalent that they can be identified in almost every area of the practice of medicine today. With these in mind you may wish to reread part or all of this book. People who grasp the principles discussed throughout the book will understand more about the cause, cure, and treatment of the epidemic of degenerative disease than I did as a young doctor, even after three years of general practice and caring for a population of over 5000 patients.

CAUSE AND PREVENTION OF DISEASE

● People are intended to be healthy and fully functional throughout their normal lifespan, an average of about eighty-five years.

● Diet and lifestyle are the causes of most of the deaths and disabilities that people suffer in the United States today. In particular, they are the causes of most of the degenerative diseases, which include most cancers, osteoporosis, atherosclerosis and its complications such as heart disease and strokes, hypertension, diabetes, arthritis, and kidney disease. Knowing the cause is the first step toward prevention and treatment.

● Diet and lifestyle practices that support the health of people are known by the scientific community. Research done over the last eighty years clearly identifies what are good health habits and what causes disease. You are not a helpless victim waiting for illness to strike without provocation or reason.

• A health-supporting diet is based upon starches, with the addition of fresh or fresh-frozen fruits and vegetables. These foods provide calories primarily as carbohydrates.

• Health-supporting lifestyle practices include moderate exercise, adequate rest, comfortable psychological relationships, and an environment providing clean air and clean water.

• The components of the food that cause injury can be separated out somewhat artificially, into several categories. The categories are fats, proteins, cholesterol, salt, simple sugars, additives, and processed-refined foods. Antigen-antibody complexes from certain foods, especially animal products, are distributed by the blood and, wherever they lodge, they damage large and small blood vessels and surrounding tissues.

• Arguments exist over which of the basic components of the American diet is causing disease. These differences are of little concern to us as consumers. The foods that support health because they provide no cholesterol, little fat, moderate protein, and require little processing are the starches, vegetables and fruits. These are easy to distinguish from the feast foods that are laden with cholesterol, fat, protein, and contamination, and are deficient in fiber. Red meats, poultry, fish, and refined and processed foods loaded with additives, including salt, are easy to recognize and avoid.

• Feast foods have become the only meal items known to the American consumer. They are tasty, primarily because we have learned to like them. However, we have the capacity to relearn to enjoy foods that support our health instead of destroying it. The components of food that people enjoy most are saltiness and sweetness, innate physiological desires expressed on the tastebuds of our tongue. Our noses enjoy the aroma of (plant-derived) spices. Unsalted and unseasoned meat, cheese, butter and other fats are unappealing. All three components that do bring us pleasure in our foods can be a part of a healthy diet. Some adjustment will be required at first.

• The love for and exclusive indulgence in feast foods keeps most of us, including health professionals and policy makers, from seeing the actual culprits that prevent good health. Real change will come only after people in charge of dispensing information on health and dictating health-policies see the wisdom of changing their personal diet.

● The health problems that plague people in affluent societies are not isolated diseases of specific name and cause. The same people that have diabetes are also the ones with hypertension and atherosclerosis. It is no coincidence that obesity is linked to all these chronic diseases, including cancer. Instead of identifying the diseases as hypertension, atherosclerosis, adult-onset diabetes and so on, a more descriptive term may be to call all of them *diseases of rich eating and unhealthy living.* Then have subcategories to identify where the body failed first.

● Genetics does play a role in disease, but only to determine the susceptibility one person has for the damaging effects of the American diet and other detrimental lifestyle practices. Almost everyone was given at birth a body that will resist chronic degenerative diseases if it is not subjected to unnatural stresses like daily hamburgers, milk shakes, cigarettes and cocktails.

● We inherit more from what we learn than from what is passed along in genetic material from our parents. Parents teach their children what foods to like and how to cook them.

● Each and every one of us has control over what we eat and whether or not we smoke or drink excessively. None of us can control our genetic makeup. Emphasis should be placed on the things we can control. Uncontrollable factors should be largely ignored. Even the efforts spent looking for viruses as the cause of disease will yield little actual gain for the patients, because there is no cure yet for any viral illness. Only good food and a good lifestyle are the ''magic pills'' available to us today.

● Prevention is the key to lowering the incidence of illness, not early detection. Most often early detection only increases the time a person is aware of the illness, but fails to actually prolong life. (This is largely because the treatments are ineffective.) Besides, the incidence of disease is not reduced by treatment (with extremely few exceptions). The only ways in which disease has been reduced in prevalence has been by protecting the individual through immunizations and improved nutrition, and by eliminating causative factors in the environment. It has been estimated that less than one-third of 1 percent of the health budget in the United States is devoted to prevention of disease (reference-Burkitt D. ''Headed in the wrong direction.'' *Lancet* 2:1475, 1984).

ILLNESS-ORIENTED TREATMENTS

• The present modes of treatment fail to result in a cure or even significant improvement in most cases because they fail to deal with the cause. The harmful components of diet and lifestyle that cause disease also promote disease and thus the disease progresses unchecked.

• Present modes of therapy are intended to cover up symptoms and signs rather than relieve the cause of disease.

• Present forms of therapy are very powerful and as a result many changes take place in the patient. The more powerful and extensive the therapy, the more the changes. Unfortunately, along with any positive effects come negative ones.

• Therapies of unproven worth in saving lives, including most uses of bypass surgery, mastectomies, chemotherapy, diabetes pills, and antihypertension medications, are unleashed upon the American public and prescribed almost by reflex by many doctors. Patients unwittingly believe that these therapies have been thoroughly tested and are of proven value. Because of the controversies that rage among medical authorities, many therapies prescribed widely today should still be at a stage of laboratory animal experimentation or clinical trial with selected, properly-informed and consenting patients.

• The burden of proof of the value of a therapy lies with those who recommend treatments that mutilate and debilitate the patient. The evidence that supports such therapies must show the benefits are greater than the side effects, including financial costs for the patient. In reality, therapies of unproven worth are now being prescribed and the burden of proof has been placed on those who question their worth.

• The present practice of medicine is expensive and as long as there is a profit to illness, the business will flourish. Removing the profit from sickness and placing it on health will rapidly and dramatically change the health-care system and the care you and your family receive. This change in payment for services is being accomplished by health maintenance organizations (HMOs) and through government and private health insurances.

• The most rewarding accomplishment for most doctors is to see their patients regain health and find relief from their suffering. Unfortunately, we have been deprived of the tools to gain these ends through our early and ongoing medical education.

HEALTH-SUPPORTING TREATMENTS

• The normal state of the body is health not illness. The body has an innate ability to heal and maintain health once the factors causing the disease are removed. Since dietary and lifestyle factors cause most chronic diseases, the key to regaining health is to correct these factors. Without a strong body, with the capacity to mend itself, no amount of medication will regain health.

• You are only a helpless victim of your poor health because of the information you lack and, possibly, the lack of will to bring about the necessary changes.

• Most people have the capacity to recover from chronic degenerative diseases to the point where they can function fully and look and feel healthy. However, there is a point at which disease processes have gone past a point of reversal. Even for these people there is still reason to eat a proper diet and maintain a supportive lifestyle in order to attain and maintain the highest level of health that is possible under the circumstances.

• In most cases the least that can be done to accomplish the immediate purpose is the best. This applies to surgery for cancer, for example. The smallest surgery that removes all of the obvious tumor is all that needs to be performed in most cases of solid tumors. Also, a change in diet to relieve chest pains is a lot less therapy than bypass surgery which provides pain relief only after an awful lot of pain.

• The understanding of disease processes and the humane treatments recommended in this book are supported by many voices in the medical community. Unfortunately, they are the quieter voices because they don't have a message that brings profits to big business. When an investigator shows benefit from a product of the drug or food industry, the advertising and public relation departments make sure every doctor and potential customer knows about it. Many times the research itself is funded by the industry involved.

• This knowledge concerning the basic treatment of disease by correcting the causes of disease and using simple dietary and lifestyle changes is not new. These principles have been written in the modern medical literature and discussed by doctors for thirty to sixty years and they resurface at regular intervals. The treatments are uncontested for the most part.

• The reason these simpler, more humane, treatments fail to become popular is not because they lack scientific and clinical validity. They fail to reach your attention because few people, except those afflicted with the condition, can see any real gain. Industry sees no profit in the message; why should it waste valuable time and dollars telling people about this non-profit approach? Giving responsibility and control of health back to the patient relieves the doctor of many rewards. Many doctors find personal, and monetary, gratification from controlling the health of their patients. Furthermore, doctors and scientists who eat the American diet can't imagine why anyone would want to, or how anyone could possibly, eat differently than themselves. Why burden the patient with the information is too often the attitude these professionals take.

● Powerful medicine is at the hands of the physician who realizes that one of his or her greatest therapies is in educating patients how to care for themselves.

HOW TO CHOOSE AND USE A DOCTOR

The physician you choose for you and your family may be more important than any other person influencing your lives. Therefore, take your time to choose and never hesitate to choose again, when necessary. There is no way to guarantee that your choice will be the right one, but there are some things to know that will increase the likelihood of your finding someone who will provide you with good care.

Doctors right out of school rarely have matured enough through experience to exercise judgment that will give you the best results. It takes two to five years of practice before most doctors become seasoned enough to really understand the consequences of their decisions. It's not that they gain any more book knowledge, but the practical knowledge is only acquired with time. Doctors with years of practical experience tend to be more conservative, and not rush into extensive testing, surgery, and multiple drug therapy. Let young doctors learn on someone else other than you and your family.

On the other hand, don't choose a doctor who is too old and may be incompetent because of mental deterioration or education that is too far out of date. Someone between these extremes in age would be the safest choice.

Education is important. A ''prestige'' medical school or postgraduate medical internship and residency programs have little to do with the quality of the professional you are choosing. However, the medical school and postgraduate programs he or she received training from should be fully accredited. There are qualifying tests called board examinations that test for a minimal level of knowledge that a physician has acquired during schooling. These are referred to as a "Board Certification" in a particular field. Pick a doctor who is board certified. Also, many specialties have recertification exams. Doctors may be required to take these, but usually these exams are voluntary. You might inquire about ongoing education and any recertification of the person you're considering to be your doctor. The American Medical Association publishes *The Directory of Medical Specialists* and there are other directories that tell how doctors are trained. These books are found in most libraries or at your local chapter of the American Medical Association.

When you visit a prospective doctor, look around for the type of journals he or she subscribes to. *The New England Journal of Medicine, JAMA, The Lancet* and *Annals of Internal Medicine* should be your doctor's favorites, not Medical Economics, Diversions, or other recreation or drug company supported publications.

The specialty of the doctor you choose will have a lot to do with the kind of treatment that will be prescribed. For example, if you see a surgeon first for a problem, you are more likely to hear a surgical solution. Why would you expect otherwise? Generally, a family practitioner or an internist would be the best person to have as an initial contact for everyday health problems. Some women may consider their gynecologist as their general doctor.

What you're looking for is a competent doctor, who generally has successful results for his or her patients. You also want someone you can reach in time of need. To find this person you may ask your friends about who they think is a good doctor, but this is not always a reliable source of information because their opinions are likely based on a few personal experiences. The people who work with doctors know best how doctors perform. The best source of reliable information is the nurses working in a hospital. They have first hand experience with the many successes and failures of all the doctors in their hospital and little goes on that they don't hear all about. If you don't know a nurse working in a hospital, then anyone else employed in the medical field may have a fair idea about who delivers quality care. Several positive recommendations would be much more valuable than a single one.

Other doctors can be a good source of information for a competent specialist for a particular problem. Unfortunately, a lot of politics goes on with referring patients that may not always result in finding the best doctor for you. Some doctors refer to others based on whether or not they return the favor. Medical groups are notorious for their patterns of referral to members only within their group. This may not be all bad, because a medical group has a reputation to build and keep, and therefore may strive to have only top quality doctors on its staff. Sometimes sticking with a group with an excellent reputation is the safest way to assure uniformly good care. However, the opposite can also hold true for a group of poor doctors.

Another source of information on the quality of a doctor can also be gleaned from the honors bestowed upon one by fellow physicians. For example, the chief of the staff of a hospital or the chief of a particular department such as medicine, pediatrics, or surgery will likely be a quality physician as far as his or her colleagues are concerned. However, part of this honor may be a personality contest also. When you call a hospital for this information, ask for the names of chiefs of staff and chiefs of departments you're interested in for the past several years. Doctors involved in medical education, who teach in a nearby hospital or medical school, would also likely have an extra measure of competence.

There may be other qualities of a doctor that are important for you. For example, many women say they can feel comfortable only with a female doctor. Many people feel that the doctor's religious faith is important. When you are dealing with personal matters and serious events, like life and death, a person who views the world similar to the way you do can be a real comfort. Don't feel that any issue is too trivial when you are making this decision. If it is important to you, then pursue it.

You will probably have difficulty finding a doctor who is nutritionally-oriented because of the lack of this training in medical schools and post-graduate training programs. Don't let this stand in your way. You need someone who can treat your immediate health care problems competently. You don't need someone to tell you what to eat, that you need daily exercise, that you should cut down on your drinking of alcohol and coffee, and quit smoking. You already know these things and they are your personal responsibility, not your doctor's. You might get a good idea about how your doctor feels about these issues just by observing his or her personal appearance. This may stop you from ever asking how he or she feels about these health issues.

After you have narrowed your choice down to a few prospective candidates based on education, experience, reputation, and personal traits, then it's time to talk to the doctors personally. Call and leave a message to return your call. Explain that you are looking for a new physician for you and your family and would like to talk to the doctor. Don't expect the doctor to interrupt his patient visits at that moment. However, any doctor worth having is one you can reach. Not returning your introductory call is a poor beginning.

Have some questions ready that you would like answers to. Ask how he or she treats your particular problem. In general, you might ask if the doctor encourages people to eat well and to exercise to maintain health. Then ask what he or she considers "eating well." Many doctors will tell you flat out they think food has little or nothing to do with health. Don't expect the doctor to be a nutrition expert, but do expect a little understanding for your beliefs and preference. If your questions anger the doctor or cause an unpleasant defensive reaction, don't expect the relationship to improve with time. The doctor business has become a consumer's market. You have the right and opportunity to pick and choose the doctor you will trust and feel confident with.

You may want to have an initial in-person interview before choosing a doctor. However, this may be too much to ask of a busy professional. Don't turn down the doctor if he or she politely declines a free get-to-know-you visit, but instead, next time you need a health professional, give the new prospect a try.

Doctors are professionals who perform a service and provide an opinion for which you pay dearly. Keep the relationship at this level, until trust has been built up by your experience with the doctor. This trust should not be automatically attached to the M.D. title. You need a doctor who will take the time to explain things to you. You need to be involved in all the decisions and not told that this is the way things will be done. If you feel rushed, you usually have been. Health care is not that precise and the treatments are not at all perfect in most cases. You really shouldn't have to ask to be brought into the discussion, but because of years of tradition in the doctor-patient relationship that needs to change, you will likely have to insist on a discussion, and make clear that you are the one to make the final decisions. It's your life and your body. But you don't want to be foolish and reckless, so you need the best professional advice. Consider also that your doctor wants a good relationship with you for many reasons.

If you are having something elective done by the doctor, get all your questions and concerns discussed before the time of the procedure. This may be particularly important with surgery or the delivery of a baby. If you have special requests, make them clear so that there are no misunderstandings and hard feelings later. Always feel you have had time to talk to your doctor and that you were understood. If this has not been the case, tell your doctor how you feel. After all, he or she may be completely unaware that you feel slighted. Doctors are not mind readers. Be fair: communication must be in both directions.

Health-care is a unique business in that the failures and the mistakes made are not just a few lost dollars or an appliance that doesn't work. Human lives are on the line and both joy and suffering result from events that are beyond anyone's control and from the decisions made. Have someone working with you that you feel always has your interest in mind and does their best for you at all times. With this kind of relationship both patients and doctors always gain the most.

THE ELIMINATION DIET

If you suspect that you suffer from a food allergy, the most accurate and least expensive way to discover the cause is to follow an elimination diet. The Elimination Diet, which is also all-around health-supporting, consists of the foods that are least likely to cause an allergic reaction and are also low-fat, no-cholesterol, high-fiber, and high-carbohydrate. About one week is needed to completely clear the bowel of foods which were eaten before beginning the diet. By this time most people will either be relieved, or begin to see signs of relief, from the problems caused by their food allergies. The Elimination Diet should be centered around brown rice, sweet potatoes, winter squash, taro (or poi) and/or tapioca, which are the starches least likely to cause a reaction in most people. Rice flour and puffed rice are also allowed. Cooked peaches, cranberries, apricots, papaya, plums, prunes, and cherries can be used freely. However, no citrus fruits are allowed. Cooked fruits are used because cooking alters the proteins in the fruit, making them less likely to act as allergens. Cooked beets, beet greens, chard, summer squash, carrots, artichokes, celery, string beans, asparagus, spinach, and lettuce are allowed. Salt, if not contraindicated for other reasons, may be used for flavoring. All other spices and condiments are excluded. Water is the only acceptable beverage. Some sensitive individuals may be allergic to one or more of the foods listed for the elimination diet. For the week of the elimination these persons should keep their diet very simple, such as a single starch and vegetable least suspected of causing trouble.

After a week, most problems due to food allergies should have ended. Then you begin adding other foods to the diet already found "safe", one at a time, on an empty stomach, to determine which of them cause your allergic reactions. Each "new" food should be eaten in large amounts three times a day for two days. If the food does not cause a reaction, it is considered to be non-allergic and can be kept in the diet. Most reactions occur within a few hours, but some do not show up for several days. Each food must be tested individually: *do not introduce two new foods at once*. When you do have an allergic reaction to a specific food, you must wait 4 to 7 days before testing the next item. This interval gives you the time you need to clear your system of that allergy-causing food.

Assuming that you are not interested in testing animal products, begin the introduction of new foods with either wheat or corn, which are the vegetable foods most commonly causing allergy. Next, try fresh citrus fruits, such as oranges or grapefruits. Then add oats, beans, peas, or lentils. Cooked vegetables, such as white potatoes, onions, or green peppers can be tested last. They are the least likely to be a cause of an allergy problem.

If the elimination diet seems too drastic for you right now, you can first try a simpler procedure. Just avoid entirely the foods that were mentioned above (in the second paragraph of this chapter) as the leading causes of allergy. Doing so will relieve most people of their allergy symptoms. For many people just the elimination of dairy products and eggs will result in a dramatic improvement.

INDEX

osteoporosis and, 61, 63, 64
Menstruation, age at beginning of, 22-23
Metastases, 32
Methionine, 76
Methyldopa, 192
Metoprolol, 192
Micronesia, diabetes and, 211-212
Milk, 8
   calcium balance and, 78-79
   hypertension and, 188-190
   rheumatoid arthritis and, 244
Miller's bran, diabetes and, 215-216
Mineral balance, negative, 73
Minoxidil, 192
Modified radical mastectomy, definition of, 29
Mueller, C. Barber, 31

N

Nadolol, 192
National Academy of Sciences, 45
National Cancer Institutes, 45, 47
National Dairy Council, 8, 66, 78, 189
National Heart, Lung, and Blood Institute, 116
National Institutes of Health, 66, 75
National Livestock and Meat Board, 78
Nauru, diabetes and, 211-212
Nephritis, tubulointerstitial, 261
Nephrons, 260
Nephrotic syndrome, 257-258
New Guinea, hypertension and, 172
New York Academy of Medicine, 269-270
New York Heart Association, 186
Niacin, cholesterol and, 115-116
Noninsulin-dependent diabetes mellitus,
   204-205, 209
Nonsteroidal antiinflammatory drugs, 248
Norway, 120, 121

O

Obesity
   breast cancer and, 22, 45-46
   diabetes and, 215
   estrogens and, 21, 87
   osteoporosis and, 87
Oil
   corn, 114
   fish, 111-112, 117-118, 243
   safflower, 114
Opposite breast, cancer and, 33-34
Oral hypoglycemic drugs, 210
Orthostatic albuminuria, 257
Osteoarthritis, 232, 237-239
Osteoporosis, 8, 60-94, 239
   androgens and, 64, 87
   bone density and, 62-63
   calcitonin and, 86

   calcium and, 65, 66-94
   calcium balance and, 8
   calcium supplement pills and, 66, 69-70
   dairy products and, 67-70
   diet and, 64-65
   effect of
      age on, 62
      cultural differences on, 64-65
      nutrients on, 65
   estrogen pills and, 11-12
   estrogens and, 63
   exercise and, 85-86, 87
   fluorides and, 65-66
   heredity and, 64
   hip fractures and, 62
   loss of function of ovaries and, 63
   in men, 61, 64
   menopause and, 63, 64
   obesity and, 87
   occurrence of, 61-62
   phosphorus and, 65-66
   proteins and, 8, 65, 72-73, 74, 75, 76-77, 87
   vegetables and, 70
   vitamin D and, 65
   weakening of bones in, 63
   in women, 60-94
   wrist fractures and, 62
   X-rays in diagnosis of, 62-63
Ovary
   cancer of, 47
   estrogen production and, 42-43
   loss of function of, osteoporosis and, 63
   removal of, estrogens and, 42-43, 82-83
Oxylates, calcium and, 70

P

Pain, chest; *see* Chest pain
Pancreas, 217
   cancer of, 47
Partial mastectomy, definition of, 29
D-Penicillamine, 248
Pericarditis, 136
Persantine, 117
Phosphates, 211
   kidney disease and, 262
Phosphorus
   calcium loss and, 77-78
   osteoporosis and, 65-66
Photon absorptiometry bone scanner, 62-63, 87
Photons, 62-63
Physical examination in detection of cancer, 26
Phsyicians, advertising by, 9
Physicians Desk Reference, 185
Phytates, 267-268
   calcium and, 70
Pituitary gland, estrogen production and, 42-43
Plankton, 242

A BRIEF SUMMARY OF THE McDOUGALL PLAN

The *McDougall Plan* encourages you to adopt the diet and lifestyle which best supports your natural tendencies to heal and stay healthy. This supportive environment is based around proper foods, moderate exercise, adequate sunshine, pure air and water, and surroundings comfortable to your psychological wellbeing.

The primary component, the diet, is centered around a variety of starchy plant foods such as rice, potatoes, and pastas with the addition of fresh or frozen fruits and vegetables. Animal-derived foods and plant products that are refined or otherwise processed are not health-supporting and are placed in the category called delicacies. Other plant foods that are also considered delicacies are those high in fat such as nuts, seeds, and avocados; and foods high in unprotected simple sugars; for example, honey, molasses, and maple syrup. These delicacy foods are to be reserved for special occasions and consumed only by healthy individuals. There are relative degrees of harmfulness among delicacies. No portions are recommended for the meal plan except that a starch should provide most of the calories. The quantity consumed each day is variable among individuals and governed by our highly efficient hunger drive. Foods that support your health easily make the most interesting and delicious meals you can imagine.

Additions and modifications of the basic meal plan include:

1. Supplementation of a nonanimal source of vitamin B-12 after three years on the plan or if you are pregnant or nursing.

2. Addition of foods concentrated in calories (dried fruits, nuts, seeds) to the basic diet of healthy individuals with unusually high caloric needs.

3. Elimination of foods that cause adverse reactions such as an allergy or an irritation.

4. Limitation of foods high in protein (legumes) to one cup a day for most people and further restriction in persons with certain illnesses (osteoporosis, gout, kidney stones, liver or kidney failure).

5. Fruits may have to be limited in those very sensitive to simple sugars (elevated triglycerides and hypoglycemia). In general three fruits a day is reasonable for most people.

6. One teaspoon of added salt over the surface of the foods is permitted in the daily diet of those who do not suffer from salt sensitive conditions (high blood pressure, heart or kidney disease, and edema).

7. Children are solely breastfed until the age of six months, solid foods are then supplemented, but breast milk still constitutes 50-25% of the childs diet until age two. After this age, starches, vegetables, and fruits provide for the basic nutritional needs.

PERSONS WHO ARE ILL OR ON MEDICATION WHO WISH TO CHANGE THEIR DIET SHOULD DO SO ONLY UNDER THE DIRECTION OF A PHYSICIAN FAMILIAR WITH THE EFFECTS OF DIET ON HEALTH. Otherwise you are encouraged to start today this meal plan and lifestyle that have provided excellent support for the health of most of our ancestors from the beginning of time and will do the same for you.

Companion books:

The McDougall Plan, New Century, 1983

The McDougall Health Supporting Cookbook—Vol I, New Century, 1984

The McDougall Health Supporting Cookbook—Vol II, New Century, to be released early 1986.

These books are found in better book stores throughout the country. However, further information and assistance in obtaining books can be obtained by writing:

John McDougall M.D.

P.O. Box 1761

Kailua, Hawaii 93734